A *sociology of*

mental health and illness

Second edition

Mary Forrett
28 Clement Court
Auchtermuchty
KY14 7LB.

Praise for the first edition of *A Sociology of Mental Health and Illness*

'I would recommend this book highly as an essential text for Mental Health Branch nursing students and others seeking to understand the complex and contradictory issues behind the identification of mental health problems and the responses of society to these problems. It is clearly written, and supported by comprehensive references.'

Philip Lister, Nurse Tutor, The Hereford & Worcestershire College of Nursing and Midwifery

'Pilgrim and Rogers' text offers an excellent starting point for those wanting an overall introduction to the sociological issues, covering a wide range of perspectives. Written with undergraduates and mental health professionals in mind, it fills a huge void in the literature, as most introductory textbooks in health and health care still focus primarily on somatic health, and most critical analyses of psychiatry do not sufficiently connect up to broader sociological discourses. The strength of their approach lies in the fact that they raise the key issues from the outset . . . *A Sociology of Mental Health and Illness* provides not just students, but also grateful "old hands" like myself an indispensable vantage point from which to explore mental health issues from a sociological perspective.'

Mick Carpenter, Department of Applied Social Studies, University of Warwick

'This is a welcome addition to the growing literature on social aspects of mental illness and mental health. It is aimed at social science undergraduates and trainee mental health workers. As such, the text covers a wide range of issues and a diversity of perspectives that can offer a broad foundation of understanding . . . Given the introductory intention of the authors, this book will provide a more than useful starting point for the target audience. People already working or intending to work in the area of mental health and mental illness should read it.'

Lawrence Whyte, *Health Matters*

A *sociology of*
mental health and illness

Second edition

David Pilgrim
and
Anne Rogers

Open University Press

Open University Press
McGraw-Hill Education
McGraw-Hill House
Shoppenhangers Road
Maidenhead
Berkshire
SL6 2QL
United Kingdom

email: enquiries@openup.co.uk
world wide web: www.openup.co.uk

and
Two Penn Plaza
New York, NY 10121-2289, USA

First Published 1993
Reprinted 1994 (twice), 1996, 1997

First published in this second edition 1999
Reprinted 2000, 2001, 2002, 2004

A catalogue record for this book is available from the British Library.

ISBN 0 335 20347 7 (pb)   0 335 20348 5 (hb)

Library of Congress Cataloging-in-Publication Data
Pilgrim, David, 1950–
    A sociology of mental health and illness / David Pilgrim and Anne Rogers.
    – 2nd ed.
        p.   cm.
    Includes bibliographical references and index.
    ISBN 0–335–20348–5 (hbk.). – ISBN 0–335–2347–7 (pbk.)
        1. Social psychiatry. 2. Mental illness–Social aspects.
    3. Psychiatric epidemiology. I. Rogers, Anne. II. Title.
    RC455.P49   1999   98–44939
    616.89–dc21   CIP

Typeset by Graphicraft Limited, Hong Kong
Printed and bound in Great Britain by Biddles Ltd, King's Lynn, Norfolk

For Steven and Jack (again!)

Contents

5 Age   84

6 The mental health professions   100

9   Psychiatry and legal control   165

Preface to the Second Edition

The demand for this book since 1993 has provided us with the gratifying opportunity to update our earlier thoughts and report new work in the field, including some of our own research subsequent to the first edition. The first edition reflected our working academic context at the end of the 1980s. Sociological debates about mental health and psychiatry were not as salient as they had been during the 1960s and 1970s. During those decades, mental illness had been subject to considerable scrutiny and was used as an exemplar in mainstream sociological theorizing on deviance and social control. The popularity of sociological work about psychiatry during those 'counter-cultural' decades was also fuelled by radical critiques from some mental health professionals, who questioned their own traditional theory and practice.

The 1980s witnessed sociological interest in health and illness turning more and more to mainstream topics of physical and chronic illness. Sociology's reputation for being an intellectual fellow traveller of, or contributor to, 'anti-psychiatry' had diminished. Even in the mid-1970s, with the zenith of 'anti-psychiatry', the eclipse was occurring. The decline was signalled first in 1976 by the appearance of Clare's *Psychiatry in Dissent*, which defused the libertarian and Marxian resonances of psychiatry's critics by incorporating them into a new eclectic orthodoxy of a 'biopsychosocial' portmanteau model. By 1978 there was a more explicit return to psychiatric tradition in *Reasoning about Madness* by Wing, an eminent social psychiatrist. It contained a contemptuous dismissal of the ideas of Foucault (an emerging doyen within medical sociology). Wing's defence of his profession helped to deflate sociological confidence about the study of mental health and illness.

Now, in the late 1990s, we live at a time when several contradictions co-exist: in mental health service practices; in civil society's interest in mental health; and in the analyses sociologists deploy in understanding these social relationships. During the mid-1990s issues around mental health and illness re-emerged for sociologists. Consumerism and user participation within the NHS and wider society has found a particularly strong voice within mental health campaigns. Sociological work on the problematic history of institution-alization and deinstitutionalization and women's mental health have been reinvigorated by a series of government social policy considerations, as well as by the rise of feminist ideas within community care debates. At the same time, recently within psychiatry, biological ideas have found a fresh vigour with a renewed interest and enthusiasm for psychopharmacology, hi-tech brain photography, behavioural genetics and post-mortem brain slicing. After its professional dismissal as a therapeutic abomination, psychosurgery, which involves the destruction of healthy brain tissue, has returned to near respectability within NHS medical practice.

Despite this return to traditional biological psychiatry, other parts of the mental health professions have been influenced by philosophical and socio-logical ideas and have eschewed the trend towards bio-determinism. Some academic psychiatrists have argued that we now live in a post-psychiatric society and that their own profession 'can no longer claim any privileged understanding of madness, alienation or distress' (Bracken and Thomas, 1998). We now have 'post-psychiatry', rather than 'anti-psychiatry', in tension with maintream bio-medical views. Additionally, a further trend to note is the increasing integration of sociological ideas about mental health and illness with ideas and practices from other disciplines concerned with mental health. Feminist psychologists have, for example, drawn on social history and social constructionism to analyse gender and mental health. In mental health nurs-ing there is evidence too of the integration of key concepts associated with the sociological analysis of mental health.

The increasing salience of the 'psy complex' and the popularity of socio-logical analyses, which focus on the ontological status of emotions and intimacy in everyday life, sit alongside evidence of the increasing social exclusion and stereotyping of the emotional lives and status of people with severe and enduring mental health problems. The rise in popularity of coun-selling, psychological therapies and psychoanalytical ideas and the view that 'regulatory systems' in contemporary society promote rather than crush sub-jectivity are evident. But so too are the old anti-psychiatric themes about control and surveillance, such as 'assertive outreach' and the 'care programme approach'. Similarly, a concern with risk and risk assessment, which pervades sociological and cultural analysis generally has found a peculiar expression in the mental health field.

Social research has consistently shown the importance of social support networks and employment in the community and the risk to mental health when these are absent. Yet approaches to treatment inside and outside of hospital are still dominated by a narrow preoccupation with medication. Additionally, as work undertaken by Philo and colleagues (1996) in the Glas-gow University Media Group demonstrates, public, media and policy con-cerns have been limited in the main to the risk that mental patients pose to others. In contrast there has been less concern with the evidence we have that people with mental health problems are at risk of victimization in their childhood, in the patient role during service contact, and when living in open community settings. Sociologists of health inequalities such as Wilkinson (1996) who have highlighted the relationship between agency and structure in understanding health inequalities provide a rich conceptual basis from which to progress thinking about the interplay between self-identity, per-sonal experience and people's material and social circumstances in inequal-ities in mental health.

We emphasized in the first edition that this was *A*, not *The*, *Sociology of Mental Health and Illness*. This remains the case. Moreover, as the sources we draw upon are often outside sociology, the book's roots and its relevant audience are inter-disciplinary. Any book which only used sociological literature to examine our topic would be relatively short. However, from the outset we interpret all material used sociologically, emphasizing social theory and concepts. Also, we explore each chapter in ways which are probably more familiar to sociologists than, say, psychiatrists or psychologists. As a consequence, this book is more than just a digest of our chosen topic for students, be they sociology undergraduates or postgraduate mental health workers. It does provide this function but it also reflects our own sociological analysis of a complex body of inter-disciplinary knowledge about a contested topic.

The chapter structure has been more or less maintained from the first edition, with two exceptions. First, we provide overviews for the reader at the start of each chapter. Second, further reading is offered at the end of each chapter as a focus for essay work. Each list has been constructed to reflect a mixture of general texts which extend the discussion of some aspect of the chapter and specialist references which explore some aspect in more depth. The further reading lists also contain a mixture of recent works for students to access and older durable articles or books which have retained contemporary relevance.

Here we will briefly outline the revisions made to the original text. This is done sequentially for readers (especially for course tutors rather than students) who may wish to compare and contrast the editions chapter by chapter. We were rightly taken to task by reviewers for underplaying social class in the first edition. We have upgraded the status of this topic from being a section in the first chapter to a whole chapter (now Chapter 2). This chapter deals with social class and mental health in the context of wider debates and theorizing about health inequalities which have expanded recently in the sociology of health and illness. As a consequence, the new edition has ten, rather than nine, chapters. We have also expanded the discussion of perspectives in the first chapter to include material on critical theory, social realism and an enlarged account of social constructivism. The recent burgeoning literature on the sociology of the emotions is also noted.

The chapters on gender, race, age and the mental health professions have been updated. New material on treatment has been included to reflect shifts in psychiatric knowledge and to examine the question of equality of access to treatment. The chapter on the organization of psychiatry includes a new discussion about the crisis of acute psychiatric units. The chapter on psychiatry and legal control provides a new focus about coercion in the light of an expanding Anglo-American interest in this field. Finally, the chapter on service users provides fresh material on relatives of psychiatric patients, an emerging role of users as providers of mental health care, and the role of the mass media in sustaining negative images of mental illness.

Although we have had to be selective about a wide and complex topic, we hope that all the changes in the new edition have done justice to most of the appropriate literature appearing in the last five years.

David Pilgrim
Anne Rogers

List of figures and tables

Chapter **1**

Perspectives on mental health and illness

Chapter overview

This chapter will make some necessary conceptual clarifications about the vexed question of terminology. Our assumption at the outset is that terminology remains such a controversial issue for the sociology of mental health and illness because there are markedly differing ways of speaking about mental normality and abnormality in contemporary society. Rather than assuming that there are competing claims about the same issue, or set of issues, we need to take a step back and check on different frameworks of understanding. In other words, what perspectives or discourses do we need to understand at the outset about normal and abnormal mental life?

This question will be answered by addressing a variety of perspectives. The chapter will cover the following perspectives outwith sociology:

- The lay view
- Psychiatry
- Psychoanalysis
- Psychology
- The legal framework

The chapter will then cover the following perspectives within sociology:

- Social causation
- Social reaction (labelling theory)
- Critical theory
- Social constructivism
- Social realism

The perspectives outwith sociology

The lay view

In every culture there is some notion of emotional or psychological difference. Not all cultures identify these differences in exactly the same way, nor
do they use identical terms. Equally, however, no culture is indifferent to
those who are sad, frightened or unintelligible in their conduct (Horwitz
1983). It is a well-rehearsed argument that in Europe, from the seventeenth
to the twentieth century, such differences were accounted for less and less by
demonic possession and more and more by medical notions. This is sometimes known as the period when madness became 'medicalized' (Scull 1979)
or when psychiatry became possible (Foucault, 1965).

With or without an expertise in the field of mental abnormality, most
people know madness when they see it. Equally, most of us can identify for
ourselves when we are sad or anxious. Any of us might be directly involved
in invoking a medical diagnosis for a friend, a relative or even a stranger in
the street acting in a way we find perplexing or distressing. Any of us might
reach a point where we decide our own distress warrants a visit to the doctor
or other expert for help. Everyday notions of 'nervousness' suggest that a
concept does prefigure a psychiatric label of phobic anxiety or some other
version of neurosis. Likewise, if people act in a way others cannot readily
understand they run the risk of being dismissed as a 'nutter', a 'loony',
'crazy', 'mad' or even 'mental'. Again, these prefigure notions of psychosis
within a professional discourse.

The term 'mental distress' has found favour in Britain in the past few years
with service users (see Chapter 10). A problem with this term is that it
alludes only to the pain of the patient and it gives no notion that they can
be distressing, frustrating or frightening to others at times. Indeed, from the
lay but non-patient perspective, the latter is often the preoccupying concern.

There is considerable overlap between lay and psychiatric notions of
mental health and illness. For example, in psychiatric disease categories, such
as anorexia nervosa, where there is uncertainty about the cause and a large
cultural component to the diagnosis, lay and psychiatric epistemologies have
been found to be similar (Lees 1997). However, there are also differences
between lay perspectives and disciplinary and formal knowledge. Notions
about antisocial behaviour sometimes appear to be less readily accommodated within the lay discourse of distress and oddity. Two examples of this
appeared in Britain in the early 1980s when juries were asked to consider the
states of mind of two mass murderers and rejected expert psychiatric views
that the men were mentally disordered. Peter Sutcliffe (the so-called York-
shire Ripper) murdered several women on the pretext of being on a mission
from God. Jurors were not prepared to allow him the excuse of mental ill-
health and found him guilty of malice aforethought. What confirmed the
difference in this case between lay and expert views of mental abnormality
was that the expert witnesses for both the defence and the prosecution were
of the view that he was schizophrenic. A similar discrepancy between lay
and psychiatric discourses about antisocial behaviour emerged in the trial of
Denis Nilsen, who killed, dismembered and stored the remains of 15 young

men in his home in London. The jury found him guilty of murder. Forensic psychiatrists acting as defence witnesses failed to persuade ordinary people that Nilsen was a psychopathic personality.

The lay discourse contains a contradiction about mental abnormality and antisocial conduct. As Rosen (1968) points out, in Ancient Rome and Athens madness was defined in pre-psychiatric times by two characteristics: aimless wandering and violence. In Laos, 'crazy' people are called 'baa'. Westermeyer and Kroll (1978) studied villagers' perceptions of the 'baa' people at a time when the country had no mental hospital or mental health professionals. They found that non-'baa' people adjudged their deviant fellows to be violent in 11 per cent of the cases, before their change of character, but, this attribution went up to 54 per cent after 'baa' was identified.

In France, a 'family colony' has existed at Ainay-le-Chateau since 1900. These psychiatric patients are fostered by families in the community instead of being inside an institution. Jodelet (1991) studied the ways in which citizens construed the patients in their midst. She found that the patients were segregated not by walls but by personal constructions – mainly based on fear of contamination by the illness and fear of unpredictable danger. This fear is so great that a taboo has emerged in the colony about patients marrying non-patients. (When sexual relationships of this type have developed over the years, which is rare, this has led to the couple being banished from the locality.)

As we will see in Chapter 9 the relationship between 'mental illness' and dangerous acts is minimal. However, public views tend to exaggerate the extent and link between violence and schizophrenia. This is a cross-cultural phenomenon. In the US, which has been called a 'psychiatric society' by Castel *et al.* (1979), the public has mixed views about the association of mental disorder and violence. For instance, 61 per cent of a sample of 1500 people agreed with the following statement: 'A person who is diagnosed as schizophrenic is more likely to commit a violent crime than a normal person' (Field Institute 1984). However, the violent image was less pronounced in another survey (DYG Corporation 1990), which found that only 24 per cent of 1000 respondents thought that mentally ill people were more dangerous than others. Forty-five per cent of the sample thought that mentally ill people were less violent than others. In Britain, studies have also suggested a strong link between violence and mental disorder which are predicated on a complex relationship between a combination of personal experience, beliefs and media messages (Philo *et al.* 1996).

Psychiatry

Psychiatry is a specialty within medicine. Its practitioners, as in other specialties, are trained to see their role as identifying sick individuals (diagnosis), predicting the future course of their illness (prognosis), speculating about its cause (aetiology) and prescribing a response to the condition, to cure it or ameliorate its symptoms (treatment). Consequently, it would be surprising if psychiatrists did not think in terms of illness when they encounter variations in conduct which are troublesome to people (be they the identified patient or those upset by them). Those psychiatrists who have rejected this illness framework, in whole or in part, tend to have been exposed to, and have accepted, an alternative view derived from another discourse (psychology, philosophy or sociology).

As with other branches of medicine, psychiatrists vary in their assumptions about diagnosis, prognosis, aetiology and treatment. This does not imply, though, that views are evenly spread throughout the profession, and as we will see later in the book, modern Western psychiatry is an eclectic enterprise. It does, however, have dominant features. In particular, diagnosis is considered to be a worthy ritual for the bulk of the profession and biological causes are favoured along with biological treatments.

This biological emphasis has a particular social history, which is summarized in Chapter 7. However, this should not deflect our attention from the capacity of an illness framework to accommodate multiple aetiological factors. For instance, a psychiatrist treating a patient with antidepressant drugs may recognize fully that living in a high rise flat and being unemployed have been the main causes of the depressive illness, and may assume that the stress this induces has triggered biochemical changes in the brain, which can be corrected by using medication.

The illness framework is the dominant framework in mental health services because psychiatry is the dominant profession within those services (see Chapter 6). However, its dominance should not be confused with its conceptual superiority. The illness framework has its strengths in terms of its logical and empirical status, but it also has many weaknesses. Its strengths lie in the neurological evidence about madness: bacteria and viruses have been demonstrably associated with madness (syphilis and encephalitis). Such a neurological theory might be supported further by the experience and behaviour of people with temporal lobe epilepsy, who may present with anxiety and sometimes florid psychotic states. The induction of abnormal mental states by brain lesions, drugs, toxins, low blood sugar and fever might all point to the sense in regarding mental illness as a predominantly biological condition.

The question begged is what is medicine to do with that wide range of mental problems that elude a biological explanation? Indeed, the great bulk of what psychiatrists call 'mental illness' has no proven bodily cause, despite substantial research efforts to solve the riddle of a purported or assumed biological aetiology. These illnesses include the anxiety neuroses, reactive depression and the functional psychoses (the schizophrenias and the affective conditions of mania and severe or endogenous depression). Whilst there is some evidence that we may inherit a vague predisposition to nervousness or madness, there are no clear-cut laws evident to biological researchers as yet. Both broad dispositions run in families, but not in such a way as to satisfy us that they are biologically caused. Upbringing in such families might equally point to learned behaviour and the genetic evidence from twin studies remains contested (Marshall 1990).

It may be argued that biological treatments that bring about symptom relief themselves point to biological aetiology (such as the lifting of depression by ECT or the diminution of auditory hallucination by major tranquillizers). However, this may not follow: thieving can be prevented quite effectively by chopping off the hands of perpetrators, but hands do not cause theft. Likewise, a person shocked following a car crash may feel better by taking a minor tranquillizer, but their state is clearly environmentally induced. The thief's hands and the car crash victim's brain are merely biological mediators in a wider set of personal, economic and social relationships. Thus, effective biological treatments cannot be invoked as necessary proof of biological causation.

A fundamental problem with the illness framework in psychiatry is that it deals, in the main, with symptoms not signs. That is, the judgements made about whether or not a person is mentally ill or healthy focus mainly (and often singularly) on the person's communications. This is certainly the case in the diagnosis of neurosis and the functional psychoses. Even in organic conditions, such as dementia, brain damage is not always detectable post-mortem (see Chapter 5). In the diagnosis of physical illness the diagnosis can often be confirmed using physical signs of changes in the body (e.g. the visible inflammation of tissue as well as the patient reporting pain).

However, it is possible to over-draw these distinctions between physical and mental illness. For example, an internal critic of psychiatry, Thomas Szasz, has argued that mental illness is a myth (Szasz 1961). He says that only bodies can be ill in a literal sense and that minds can only be sick metaphorically (like economies). And yet, as we noted earlier, physical disturbances can sometimes produce profound psychological disturbances. Given that emotional distress has a well-established causative role in a variety of psychosomatic illnesses, like gastric ulcers and cardiovascular disease, the mutual interplay of mind and body seems to be indicated on reasonable grounds.

It is true (following Szasz 1961) that the validity of mental diagnosis is undermined more by its over-reliance on symptoms (see Chapter 4) and by the absence of detectable bodily signs, but this can apply at times even in physical medicine. For instance, a person may feel very ill with a headache but it may be impossible to appeal to signs to check whether or not this is because of a toxic reaction, for instance a 'hangover', or a brain tumour. Also, people with chronic physical problems have much in common, in terms of their social role, with psychiatric patients – both are disabled and usually not valued by their non-disabled fellows. Finally, the absence of a firm biological aetiology is true of a number of physical illnesses, such as diabetes and multiple sclerosis. Thus, the conceptual and empirical uncertainties that Szasz draws our attention to, legitimately, about mental illnesses, can apply also to what he considers to be 'true illnesses'.

Psychoanalysis

Psychoanalysis was the invention of Sigmund Freud. It has modern adherents who are loyal to his original theories but there are other trained analysts who adopt the views of Melanie Klein (see Chapter 4); others take a mixed position, borrowing from each theory. Thus, psychoanalysis is an eclectic or fragmented discipline. Its emphasis on personal history places it in the domain of biographical psychology. Indeed, Freud's work is sometimes called depth or psychodynamic psychology, along with the legacies of his dissenting early group such as Jung, Adler and Reich. Depth psychology proposes that the mind is divided between conscious and unconscious parts and that the dynamic relationship between these gives rise to psychopathology. (This will be considered further in Chapter 4.)

Like other forms of psychology, psychoanalysis works on a continuum principle – abnormality and normality are connected, not disconnected and separate. To the psychoanalyst we are all ill to some degree. However, the medical roots of psychoanalysis and the continued dominance of medical analysts within its culture have, arguably, left it within a psychiatric, not psychological, discourse. It still uses the terminology of pathology ('psycho-pathology' and its 'symptoms'); assessments are 'diagnostic' and its clients 'patients'; people do not merely have ways of avoiding human contact, they have 'schizoid defences' and they do not simply get into the habit of angrily blaming others all of the time, instead they are 'fixated in the paranoid position'. The language of psychoanalysis is saturated with psychiatric terms. Thus, the discipline of psychoanalysis stands somewhere between psychiatry and psychology.

Psychoanalysis, arguably, has two strengths. First, it offers a comprehensive conceptual framework about mental abnormality. Once a devotee accepts its strictures, it offers the comfort of explaining, or potentially explaining, every aspect of human conduct. Second, there is a symmetry between its causal theory and its corrective programme. That which has been rendered unconscious by past relationships can be rendered conscious by a current relationship with a therapist.

Its first weakness is the obverse of biological psychiatry. The latter tends to reduce psychological phenomena to biology, whereas psychoanalysis tends to psychologize everything (i.e. the biological and the social as well as the personal). A person with temporal lobe epilepsy or a brain tumour would be helped little by a psychoanalyst. The brain-damaged patient would certainly give the analyst plenty to interpret, but the analyst would be wrong to attribute a psychological, rather than a neurological, cause. Likewise, socially determined deviance (like prostitution emerging in poor or drug-using cultures) may be explained away psychoanalytically purely in terms of individual history (Pilgrim 1992 and 1998). A second weakness of psychoanalysis as a frame of reference is that it can do no more than be wise after the event. It has never reached the status of a predictive science.

Psychology

Psychoanalysis has competed with other psychological accounts of mental abnormality. Moreover, because psychology, as a broad and eclectic discipline, focuses, in the main, on 'normal' conduct and experience it has offered concepts of normality as well as abnormality. Buss (1966) suggests that psychologists have put forward four conceptions of normality/abnormality:

- the statistical notion
- the ideal notion
- the presence of specific behaviours
- distorted cognitions

The statistical notion

The statistical notion simply says that frequently occurring behaviours in a population are normal – so infrequent behaviours are not normal. This is akin to the notion of norms in sociology. Take as an example the tempo at which people speak. Up to a certain speed, speech would be called normal. If someone speaks above a certain speed they might be considered to be 'high' in ordinary parlance or 'hypomanic' or suffering from 'pressure of thought' in psychiatric language. If someone speaks below a certain speed they might be described as depressed. Most people would speak at a pace between these upper and lower points of frequency.

A question begged, of course, is who decides on the cut-offs at each end of the frequency distribution of speech speed and how are those decisions made? In other words, the notion of frequency in itself tells us nothing about when a behaviour is to be adjudged normal or abnormal. Value judgements are required on the part of lay people or professionals when punctuating the difference between normality and abnormality. Also, a statistical notion may not hold good across cultures, even within the same country: for example, slow speech might be the norm in one culture, say in rural areas, but not in another, such as the inner city.

The statistical notion of normality tells us nothing in itself about why some deviations are noted when they are unidirectional rather than bidirectional. The example of speech speed referred to bidirectional judgements. Take, in contrast, the notion of intelligence. Brightness is valued at one end of the distribution but not at the other. Being bright will not lead, in itself, to a person entering the patient role, but being dim may well do so.

In spite of these conceptual weaknesses, the statistical approach within abnormal psychology remains strong. Clinical psychologists are trained to accept that characteristics in any population follow a normal distribution and so the statistical notion has a strong legitimacy for them. This acceptance of the normal distribution of a characteristic in a population means that in psychological models there is usually assumed to be an unbroken relationship between the normal and abnormal. However, this notion of continuity of, say, everybody being more or less neurotic, may also assume a discontinuity from other variables. For instance, in Eysenck's personality theory (Eysenck 1955) neurosis and psychosis are considered to be personality characteristics that are both normally distributed but separate from one another.

The ideal notion

There are two versions of this notion: one from psychoanalysis and the other from humanistic psychology. In the former case, normality is defined by a predominance of conscious over unconscious characteristics in the person (Kubie 1954). In the latter case, the ideal person is one who fulfils their human potential (or 'self-actualizes'). Jahoda (1958) drew together six criteria for positive mental health to elaborate and aggregate these two psychological traditions:

1 Balance of psychic forces
2 Self-actualization
3 Resistance to stress
4 Autonomy
5 Competence
6 Perception of reality

The problem is that each of these notions is problematic as a definition of normality (and, by implication, abnormality). The first and second are only meaningful to those in a culture who subscribe to their theoretical premises (such as psychoanalytical or humanistic psychotherapists).

The resistance-to-stress notion is superficially appealing but what of people who fail to be affected by stress at all? We can all think of situations in which anxiety is quite normal and we would wonder in such circumstances why a person fails to react in an anxious manner. Indeed, the absence of anxiety under high stress conditions has been one defining characteristic of 'primary psychopathy' by psychiatrists. Likewise, those who are excessively autonomous (i.e. avoid human contact) might be deemed to be 'schizoid' or be suffering from 'simple schizophrenia'.

As for competence, this cannot be judged as an invariant quality. As we will see when discussing young adults and mental health in Chapter 5, norms of competence vary over time and place. Likewise with perceptions of reality. In some cultures, seeing visions or hearing voices is highly valued, and yet it would be out of sync with the reality perceived by most in that culture. In other cultures the hallucinators may be deemed to be suffering from alcoholic psychosis or schizophrenia.

The presence of specific behaviours

The emergence of psychology as a scientific academic discipline was closely linked to its attention to specifiable aspects of conduct. It emerged and separated from speculative philosophy on the basis of these objectivist credentials. Behaviourism, the theory that tried to limit the purview of psychology to behaviour and eliminate subjective experience as data, no longer dominates psychology but it has left a lasting impression. Within clinical psychology, behaviour therapy and its modified versions are still common practices. Consequently, many psychologists are concerned to operationalize in behavioural terms what they mean by abnormality.

The term 'maladaptive behaviour' is part of this psychological discourse, as is 'unwanted' or 'unacceptable' behaviour. The strength of this position is that it makes explicit its criteria for what constitutes abnormality. The weakness is that it leaves values and norms implicit. The terminology of specific behaviours still begs questions about what constitutes 'maladaptive'. Who decides what is 'unwanted' or 'unacceptable'? One party may want a behaviour to occur or find it acceptable but another may not. In these circumstances, those who have more power will tend to be the definers of reality. Thus, what constitutes unwanted behaviour is not self-evident but socially negotiated. Consequently, it reflects both the power relationships and the value system operating in a culture at a point in time.

Distorted cognitions

The final approach suggested by Buss emerged at a time when behaviourism was becoming the dominant force within the academic discipline. However, during the 1970s this behavioural emphasis declined and was eventually displaced by cognitivism. As a result, psychologists began to treat inner events as if they were behaviours (forming the apparently incongruous hybrid of a 'cognitive-behavioural' approach to mental health problems) or they increasingly incorporated constructivist, systemic and even psychoanalytical views (e.g. Bannister and Fransella 1970; Guidano 1987; Ryle 1990). It is not clear even now whether the ascendency of 'cognitive therapy' within clinical psychology during the 1980s was driven by cognitivism or was merely legitimized by it. So much of the seminal writing on cognitive therapy came not from academic psychology but from clinicians, some of whom were psychiatrists, not psychologists, offering a pragmatic and a-theoretical approach to symptom reduction (e.g. Beck 1970; Ellis 1970).

The legal framework

Mental disorder represents the main point of contact between psychiatry and the law. The early days of psychiatry in the nineteenth century were heavily influenced by eugenic considerations – it was assumed that a variety of deviant conducts could be explained by a tainted gene pool in the lower social classes. This degeneracy theory, which characterized early biological psychiatry, linked together the mad, the bad and the dim. However, during the First World War and its aftermath such an underlying assumption began to falter. In the forensic field, there emerged a resistance to the old eugenic ideas of degeneracy, which accounted for criminality in terms of an inherited disposition to bad conduct (Forsythe 1990). This was replaced by an increasing interest in environmental or psychological explanations for lawbreaking. Since that time, psychiatric experts have played a major role in identifying and explaining criminal conduct.

In Britain the law has a definition of mental disorder, which includes four separate conditions: mental illness, mental impairment, severe mental impairment, and psychopathic disorder. The first of these is not defined; the second and third are references to people with learning difficulties who are additionally deemed to be dangerous; the fourth refers to antisocial individuals who are 'abnormally aggressive' or who manifest 'seriously irresponsible conduct'.

The legal framework is thus parasitical on psychiatric opinion in two senses. First, the absence of a definition of mental illness accepts tautologically that its presence in law accords with, or is identical to, what psychiatry calls mental illness. (Although at times of doubt the lay view of madness may be incorporated – see below.) Second, in particular cases being tried in court, psychiatric opinion is offered as the expert view on the presence or absence of any of the four legal categories. Unlike Sutcliffe's jurors, discussed earlier, the legal framework does accept that certain forms of badness can be a medical condition. This condition permits offenders the defence of mental disorder and hence absolves them from personal responsibility (although it gives no guarantee that the person will be treated benignly).

Because mental illness is not legally defined, judges have sometimes resorted to the lay discourse. In 1974, Judge Lawton said that the words 'mental illness' are 'ordinary words of the English language. They have no particular medical significance. They have no particular legal significance'. Lawton refers to the dictum of Lord Reid in a case where the defendant's mental state was being considered: 'I ask myself what would the ordinary sensible person have said about the patient's condition in this case if he had been informed of his behaviour? In my judgment such a person would have said "Well the fellow is obviously mentally ill"' (cited in Jones 1991: 15). This lay conception of legal insanity has been called 'the-man-must-be mad' test (Hoggett 1990).

In one sense, therefore, the legal framework accepts a psychiatric framework, but when the latter is found lacking then ordinary language definitions are invoked. It also raises the question about whether madness is simply, for legal and lay purposes, incomprehensible conduct. 'Normal' criminal acts are clearly goal directed. 'Mentally disordered' criminal acts are not directed towards mere material gain.

However, in practice, two ambiguities emerge about such a simple legal distinction. First, sex offenders may end up either in prison or in secure psychiatric units, showing that sexual gratification as a criminal motive confuses those prescribing a judicial response. Second, some murderers are adjudged commonsensically to be sane, despite the contrary view of expert witnesses. The cases already discussed (Sutcliffe and Nilsen) highlight this uncertainty. If the legal framework looks to lay people through a jury system to clarify the presence or absence of mental abnormality, then this ambivalence is likely to be reflected in their judgements. Lay people may argue that, on the one hand, a person must be 'sick' to perpetrate heinous acts but, on the other, that the acts warrant severe punishment or even death.

Notwithstanding the failure of the legal framework to adopt a definition of mental illness, its strength is that it literally spells out in black and white what is being discussed under the rubric of 'mental disorder'. However, these explicit categories are then still open to dispute in terms of their being the basis for diagnosis in particular cases. Also, the legal framework delegates powers of identification of mental abnormality to psychiatrists in these cases. By implication it internalizes psychiatry and its conceptual strengths and weaknesses. However, this dominant medical presence at the outset of legal considerations does diminish thereafter. When an abnormal offender is considered for release or 'discharge', non-medical people are party to the judgement (lawyers and lay people attending Mental Health Review Tribunals).

The legal framework is also relevant in a more general sense in psychiatry. It defines the conditions under which mental health professionals can and cannot detain patients and compulsorily treat them. These conditions will be dealt with in more detail in Chapter 8.

A final point to note in this section is that the 1983 Mental Health Act is soon to be revised. This may have a bearing on some of the points of our discussion above. In particular, definitions of both mental illness and psychopathic disorder are being reviewed by the British government which may be incorporated into new legislation.

Conclusion about the perspectives outwith sociology

The expert perspectives on mental health and illness all have a certain persuasiveness. Equally, we have noted some credibility problems that each encounters. The illness and legal frameworks emphasize discontinuity (people are ill/disordered or they are not) whereas the other perspectives tend to emphasize continuity. It is a matter of opinion whether a continuous or discontinuous model of normality and abnormality fits our knowledge of people's conduct and whether one or other is morally preferable. Traditional psychiatrists might argue that, unlike psychoanalysts, they do not see abnormality everywhere. Psychoanalysts might argue that the pervasive condition of mental pain connects us all in a common humanity.

Our concern here is not to resolve these questions but to record them in order to demonstrate that the topic of mental health and illness is highly contested. There are no bench marks that experts from different camps can agree on and discuss. Thus 'mental disorder' or 'mental illness' or 'maladaptive behaviour' or simply being 'loony' do not necessarily have a single referent. It is not *only* a matter of terminology, although it is in part. It is not simply like the difference between speaking of motor cars and automobiles. In our discussion, each perspective may be warranting certain types of reality but not others. What we have is a fragmented set of perspectives, divided internally and from one another, which occasionally enter the same world of discourse. Given this, the first perspective we considered, that of lay people, should not necessarily be construed to be inferior to so-called expert views.

A final comment on the five perspectives is that all of them have difficulty in sustaining notions of mental health and illness which are stable, certain or invariant. In each case, the caveat of social relativism has to be registered. Judgements about health and illness (physical as well as mental) are value-laden and reflect specific norms in time and place.

The perspectives within sociology

Having discussed perspectives about mental health and illness from outside of sociology, we now turn to contributions within the latter academic discipline. Five major sociological perspectives will be outlined: social causation, societal reaction (labelling theory), critical theory, social constructivism and social realism. These five perspectives bear the respective imprints of major contributions from Durkheim, Weber, Freud, Foucault and Marx. These influences are not linear but cross-cut and are mediated by the work of later contributors such as Sartre and Mead. Different theoretical perspectives have been popular and influential at different times. However, it is important to acknowledge that there is no set of boundaries to neatly periodise disciplinary trends. Rather, there are sedimented layers of knowledge which overlap unevenly in time and across disciplinary boundaries and professional preoccupations. The social causation thesis arguably peaked in the 1950s when a number of large-scale community surveys of the social causes of mental health problems and of the large psychiatric institutions were undertaken

(Pilgrim and Rogers 1994). However, one of its most quoted exemplars appeared in the late 1970s and early 1980s (Brown and Harris 1978) and studies in the social causation tradition were set to proliferate in the late 1990s with an explicit government policy agenda which is designed to tackle the social, economic and environmental causes of mental health problems (*Our Healthier Nation*, DoH, 1998). Similarly, there is no absolute distinction between sociological knowledge and other forms of knowledge. In relation to lay knowledge/perspective some sociological perspectives (such as symbolic interactionism) in large part draw on the meaning and understandings of lay people. More recently, and in line with a re-found enthusiasm for psychoanalytical approaches applied to sociology, the sociological perspective of 'social constructionism' within sociology has been treated 'as if it were a client presenting itself for psychoanalysis' (Craib 1997). According to Craib social contructionism (discussed in more detail below):

> . . . can be seen as a manic psychosis – a defense against entering the depressive position . . . Sociologists find it difficult to recognise the limitations of their discipline – the depressive position – one reason being that we do not actually exercise power over anybody; social constructionism enables us to convince ourselves that the opposite is true, that we know everything about how people become what they are, that we do not have to take account of other disciplines or sciences, but we can explain everything . . . a non-psychotic theory is one which knows its own limitations.
>
> (Craib 1997: 1)

The five sociological perspectives will now be considered.

Social causation

This response from sociologists essentially accepts schizophrenia or depression as legitimate diagnoses. They are given the status of facts in themselves. Once these diagnoses are accepted, questions are then asked about the role of socially derived stress in their aetiology.

The emphasis within a social causation approach is upon tracing the relationship between social disadvantage and mental illness. Given that many sociologists have considered the main indicator of disadvantage, to be low social class and/or poverty, it is not surprising that studies investigating this relationship have been a strong current within social studies of psychiatric populations. The next chapter will outline this in more detail. Social class has not been the only variable investigated within this social causation perspective. Disadvantage of other sorts, related to race, gender and age have also been of interest. These studies will be picked up in Chapters 3, 4 and 5.

The advantage of this psychiatric epidemiological perspective is that it provides the sort of scientific confidence associated with objectivism and empiricism (methodological assurances of representativeness and pointers towards causal relationships). Four main disadvantage of the approach can be identified. First, pre-empirical conceptual problems associated with psychiatric knowledge are either not acknowledged or are evaded (see for example Brown and Harris 1978). Second, psychiatric epidemiology investigates correlations between mental illness and antecedent variables. However, correlations are not necessarily indicative of causal relationships. Third, the investigation of large subpopulations cannot illuminate the lived experience of mental health problems or the variety of meanings attributed to them by patients and significant others. Fourth, medical epidemiology proper attempts to map the distributions of *causes* of diseases not merely the *cases* of disease. Because most of psychiatric illness is described as 'functional' (i.e. it has no known biological marker and its cause or causes are either not known or contested), then psychiatric epidemiology cannot fulfil the general expectation of mapping causes.

Societal reaction (labelling theory)

Labelling theory was highly influential during the 1960s but has now fallen out of fashion. Essentially, this theory was concerned with documenting the ways in which the patient role was negotiated and maintained. The emphasis was on how others reacted to and categorized deviance. The wider theoretical context of this was the version of sociology called 'symbolic interactionism', which is concerned with mapping out ways in which social reality is negotiated by people. Thus, an emphasis is placed on the roles people take up and the meanings that are exchanged with others when occupying these roles. A failure to act appropriately in a role then becomes a critical point of understanding for those involved.

According to labelling theorists, when people deviate from conduct expected of them, a common reaction in others is to deny the deviation in order to keep the person in their existing role. For instance, Yarrow *et al.* (1955) found that the wives of men eventually labelled as schizophrenic ignored and rationalized their husbands' symptoms for varying periods of time before seeking help. Similar denials can be found in the relatives of people with drink problems (Lemert 1967). If this is true, it would be predicted that the incidence of symptoms would be much higher than the incidence of formal diagnoses. Evidence certainly exists for this position from community surveys leading to the assumption of the 'clinical iceberg' (Wadsworth *et al.* 1971; Hannay 1979) in both physical and mental illness. That is, doctors only diagnose as ill a small proportion of people in a population who manifest symptoms. Up to this point, labelling theorists are talking about primary deviance or variations in conduct which involve rule-breaking.

The next consideration for labelling theorists is how symptoms become diagnosed as mental illnesses so that the person takes on a deviant role (secondary deviance). The answer given is in terms of contingencies. That is, the same behaviour, under some circumstances, will be ignored whilst in different circumstances it will provoke concern and the need for expert help. The transition between these two sets of circumstances can be linked to either a one-off crisis or a series of gradual shifts. The latter is a bit like water reaching boiling point after being heated for a long time.

For instance, the wives in the Yarrow *et al.* (1955) study tolerated deviance but gradually began to re-construe their husbands. Eventually, a point was reached when their spouses' strange or stressful conduct could be tolerated no more. In other circumstances, though, a single event might lead to the ascription of deviance. Rosenhan (1973) showed that 'pseudo-patients' were hospitalized for simply reporting hearing the words 'empty', 'hollow' and 'thud', when presenting themselves voluntarily to psychiatric facilities. This was the only odd behaviour they presented to psychiatric professionals. In all other respects they behaved sanely. Likewise, where deviance is visible and threatening, a single event like smashing a window may cause a member of the public to call the police, who will then refer the offending person to a psychiatrist. According to Lemert (1951) the more visible the symptoms, the greater the chance of labelling, but the latter is also contingent upon varying tolerance levels of deviance in a particular culture. For instance, the more conformist a society (i.e. intolerant of breakdown in public decorum) the higher the levels of mental hospital admission.

As well as visibility being part of the contingent picture of labelling, so too is the relative importance of the labelled person. For instance, Hammer (1968) found, in taking retrospective accounts of patients' roles in their family prior to hospital admission, that a young mother with children would be admitted at an earlier point than an older woman with fewer family responsibilities. In the latter case, symptoms may go unnoticed for longer. Thus, the amount of dependency expressed towards a person by others may mean that they are adjudged to fail or be deviant at an earlier point in time than less needed people. To indicate how contingencies vary from context to context, Brown and Harris (1978) found that tiredness might be normalized by GPs who fail to refer depressed women with children.

Those emphasizing labelling do not concur as to who are the significant labellers. For Scheff (1966) it is psychiatrists; for Goffman (1961) it is the family plus professionals plus the total institution. However, there is an agreement that, once labelled, this significantly alters the person's identity and social status. Once a person is seen to have lost their reason, then they will never be quite the same again in the eyes of others (Garfinkel 1956). They are stripped of their old identity and a new one takes its place in what Goffman calls a 'status degradation ceremony'. Part of such a process then leads to the labelled person internalizing the new identity ascribed to them.

Thus, according to the societal reaction position, the psychiatric patient's role is then maintained by a new set of role expectations. The person in the patient role plays at being a patient and those looking on construe all of the person's conduct in terms of the patient role. The pseudo-patients in Rosenhan's study logged their ward experiences, and the clinical notes on them recorded that they indulged in 'excessive writing behaviour': a mutually reinforcing process then keeps the person locked into their deviant role. However, this can be disrupted by new contingencies emerging – hence the findings alluded to in Chapter 2 when discussing social causation about the improvements of patients who can gain employment.

Despite the demise of the asylum, the institutional context for Goffman's notion of the 'betrayal funnel', which entailed significant others propelling an individual towards a patient career and identity, the impact of labelling in community settings is still evident. A quote from a patient diagnosed as schizophrenic, who took part in a recent qualitative study (Rogers *et al.* 1998) examining the use and views of medication by patients, illustrates the link between violence and mental illness that is commonly linked in the public eye (see earlier discussion of the lay view), as well as the internalization of a labelled identity:

... the word (schizophrenia) frightened me to death because books I've read and programmes on telly like when I heard the word 'schizophrenic' at that time it meant to me 'not bloody safe, I'm a dangerous person' and that sort of thing and I'm likely to be talking nice and calm to someone and the next minute I'm going to be getting a knife or something like that to them you know. . . . That word does frighten people, if you were to tell somebody that I was a schizophrenic, oh my God, you know the first thing they'd say is, 'I think you better keep away from him'.

What then are the weaknesses of labelling theory that might account for it losing its popularity within sociology? The following may be relevant:

1 Critics of labelling theory point out that it understates the underlying power of the causes of primary deviation (Gove 1970, 1975). For instance, Rosenhan's pseudo-patients, whose primary deviance was invented, not authentic, did not become trapped in their role once the experiment was over. This may suggest that the 'push from behind' of the underlying reasons for primary deviance may sometimes outweigh the impact of labelling, which is 'pulling from the front'. Having said this, it is also acknowledged by most parties involved in psychiatric services that hospital life does induce odd behaviour ('institutional neurosis' (Barton 1959)).

2 If lay people play such an important role in identifying and creating mental illness by their reactions to primary deviance, we would expect everyday stereotypes of mental illness to be consistent with the range of behaviours displayed by psychiatric patients. However, studies of stereo-typing of mental illness by ordinary people only partially confirm this assumption. For instance, Jones and Cochrane (1981) found that stereo-types conform only loosely to what psychiatrists diagnose as schizophrenia. The common diagnosis of depression was not included in everyday stereo-typing. Likewise, Bean (1979) found that psychiatrists do not always concur with the ascription of deviance already identified by the family of a patient. When this is the case, Goffman's notion of a 'betrayal funnel' of professional and lay labellers conspiring against the incipient patient would seem to be unfounded.

3 Labelling theory does not really provide us with a clear picture of what the salient contingencies are that make the difference between deviance being ignored or being ascribed. On the other hand, this may simply reflect the inherently fluid nature of contingencies. They cannot be laid out accur-ately because they emerge and wane in complex social systems which are in flux and which have rules or norms that fluctuate over time. Having said this, there do appear to be some circumstances that more regularly predict the ascription of mental illness taking place. One of these is the gender of those labelled. Horwitz (1977) found that women are more likely to be labelled than men in lay networks (though not by husbands). Horwitz (1983) also points out that the greater the personal gap in terms of class, race, culture and gender between labellers and the potentially labelled, the greater the chances of ascription taking place and the more devaluing the label.

This question of contingencies and labelling connects the social reaction position to social constructivism (see below). Labelling theorists are basically arguing that secondary deviance is socially negotiated or constructed. They accept, though, that primary deviance may have *causes* which may be social, psychological or biological. Social constructivism also examines the categories of primary deviance in terms of their social construction. The epistemological proximity of labelling theory to social constructivism has led Bowers (1998) to take us to task for hair splitting. He argues that labelling theory is a variant of social constructivism and that the latter actually was elaborated from the former in social science. We would argue that the distinction should still be maintained for academic clarity.

Critical theory

During the twentieth century, a number of writers have attempted to account for the relationship between socio-economic structures and the inner lives of individuals. One example was the work of Sartre when he developed his 'progressive-regressive method' (Sartre 1963). This method was an attempt to understand biography in relation to its social context and understand social context via the accounts of people's lives. This existential development of humanistic Marxism competed with another and more elaborate set of discussions about the relationship between unconscious mental life and societal determinants and constraints. Within Freud's early circle, a number of analysts took an interest in using their psychological insights in order to illuminate societal processes. This set a trend for later analysts, some of whom tended to reduce social phenomena to the aggregate impact of psychopathology (e.g. Bion 1959). The dangers of psychological reductionism were inevitable in a tradition (psychoanalysis) which had a starting focus of methodological individualism. Moreover, the individuals studied by psychoanalysis were from a peculiar social group (white, middle-class, European neurotics).

Out of this tradition emerged a group of Freudo-Marxists who came to be known as 'critical theorists', most of whom were associated with the Frankfurt Institute of Social Research which was founded in 1923 and led after 1930 by Horkheimer (Slater 1977). This group accordingly came to be known as the 'Frankfurt School'. The difference between the work of the Frankfurt School and most of clinical psychoanalysis was the focus on the interrelationship between psyche and society. In an early address to the Institute, Horkheimer set out its mission as follows:

> What connections can be established, in a specific social group, in a specific period in time, in specific countries, between the group, the changes in the psychic structures of its individual members and the thoughts and institutions that are a product of that society, and that have, as a whole, a formative effect upon the group under consideration?
> (Horkheimer 1931: 14)

These interrelationships between the material environment of individuals and their cultural life and inner lives were subsequently explored by a number of writers in the Institute, including Marcuse, Adorno and Fromm. In addition, there were contributions from Benjamin (who was a marginal and ambivalent Institute member) and Reich, a Marxist psychoanalyst and outsider. These explorations had an explicit emancipatory intent and were characterised by anti-Stalinist as well as anti-fascist themes. Within the Frankfurt School, Freudianism was accepted as the only legitimate form of psychology which was, potentially at least, philosophically compatible with Marxism. (Both Freud and Marx were atheists and materialists, although Freud's materialism was barely historical.) The compatibility was explored and affirmed though by one member in particular who was a psychoanalyst – Fromm. The integration of Freudianism was selective and critical, filtering out or querying elements such as the death instinct (a revision of classical psychoanalytical theory by Freud himself (Freud 1920)) and questioning the mechanistic aspect of instinctual drive-theory.

The role of this group of critical theorists in social science has been important and seemingly paradoxical. For a theory which drew heavily, if selectively, upon clinical psychoanalysis, the raft of work associated with the Frankfurt School (which was largely relocated in the USA with the rise of Nazism) focused not on mental illness but instead upon what Fromm called the 'pathology of normalcy'. It was only seemingly paradoxical because psychoanalysis was (and still is) concerned with the notion that we are all ill – psychopathology for Freud and his followers was ubiquitous, varying between individuals only in degree and type. Accordingly, the concerns of this group of Freudo-Marxists were about life-negating cultural norms associated with authoritarianism and the capitalist economy and the ambiguous role of the super-ego as a source of conformity and mutuality. These norms were said to be mediated by the intra-psychic mechanism (especially the repression) highlighted in Freud's theory of a dynamic unconscious.

Critical theory is exemplified in studies of the authoritarian personality (Adorno *et al.* 1950), the mass psychology of fascism (Reich 1933; Fromm 1942) and the psychological blocks attending the transitions from capitalist to socialist democracy (Fromm, 1955). When Habermas came to review the project of the early Frankfurt School (Habermas 1989), he suggested a six-part programme of topic focus: forms of integration in post-liberal societies; family socialisation and ego development; mass media and culture; the social psychology behind the cessation of protest; the theory of art; and the critique of positivism and science.

The work of the Frankfurt School eventually fragmented, with Horkheimer recanting his younger Marxism, and Fromm and Marcuse in post-war USA taking divergent and mutually critical paths about the programme summarized in Horkheimer's mission statement cited above (Marcuse 1964; Fromm 1970). The continuation of a project to examine a 'critical theory of society' was maintained by Habermas and Offe in the 1970s and 1980s (Habermas 1972, 1975, 1987; Offe, 1984). Moreover, resonances of critical theory can be found in a variety of leftist Freudian projects which continued to explore the relationship between economics, culture and the psychopathology of the individual (Sennett and Cobb 1973; Jacoby 1975; Holland 1978; Lasch 1978; Richards 1984; Kovel 1988), as well as 'anti-psychiatry' (Cooper 1968; Laing 1967). There is a continuing body of work which examines the way in which contemporary western society is developing in a pathological direction – through the culture of narcissism or the fragmented self represented in the metaphor of schizophrenia (Harvey 1989). Thus, critical theory is included here as an important sociological current of relevance to this book because it has been an influential framework for connecting the psyche and society.

The problems of critical theory have been twofold. First, as was indicated earlier, the theoretical centre of gravity of this project (the Frankfurt School) fragmented. Second, the meaningfulness of any hybrid of dialectical materialism and psychoanalysis requires social scientists to accept the legitimacy of *both* of its component parts *and* their conceptual and practical integration. This requires a triple act of faith or theoretical commitment which leaves many unconvinced, dubious or even hostile to the expectation.

The German version of Freudo-Marxism (the Frankfurt School) emerged in the first half of the twentieth century and its traces in social science, with the exception of Habermas and Offe, tend recently to be faint and influenced by other theoretical positions. For example, the long list of post-war American and British writers cited above have been part of a theoretical tradition which is still psychoanalytically orientated but reflects changes such as the impact of Klein and later object-relations theorists. Another Freudo-Marxian hybrid can be found more recently in French intellectual life, especially following the work of Althusser and Lacan (Elliot 1992). This current moved in a different direction from the Frankfurt School and contributed to the emergence in the 1970s of post-structuralism – a variant of the next perspective we summarize.

Social constructivism

One of the most influential theoretical positions evident in the sociology of health and illness over the past 20 years has been social constructivism – as mentioned above, it sometimes appears as 'social constructionism', especially, though not only, in psychological literature. A central assumption within this broad approach is that reality is not self-evident, stable and waiting to be discovered, but instead it is a product of human activity. In this broad sense all versions of social constructivism can be identified as a reaction against positivism and naïve realism.

Brown (1995) suggests three main currents within social constructivism:

1 The first approach is not concerned with demonstrating the reality or otherwise of a social phenomenon but with the social forces which *define* it. The approach is mainly traceable to sociological work on social problems (Spector and Kitsuse 1977). To investigate a social problem, such as drug misuse or mental illness, is to select a particular aspect of reality and thus implicitly concede the factual status of reality in general (Woolgar and Pawluch 1985). In particular, the lived experience of social actors, those inside deviant communities or those working with and labelling them, are the focus of sociological investigation. The social problems' emphasis, which gave rise to this version of social constructivism, has been associated, like societal reaction theory, with methodologies linked to symbolic interactionism and ethnomethodology.

2 The second approach is tied more closely to the post-structuralism of Foucault and is concerned with *deconstruction* – the critical examination of

language and symbols in order to illuminate the creation of knowledge, its relationship to power and the unstable varieties of reality which attend human activity ('discursive practices'). Foucault's early work on madness, however, was not about such discursive concerns (Foucault 1965). The latter have been the focus of interest of later post-structuralists (see below).

3 The third approach is associated neither with the micro-sociology of social problem definition nor with deconstruction but with understanding the production of scientific knowledge and the pursuit of individual and collective professional interests (Latour 1987). This science-in-action version of sociology is concerned with the illumination of *interest work*. This version of social constructivism examines the ways in which scientists and other interested parties develop, debate and use facts. It is thus interested in the networks of people involved in these activities. Unlike the post-structuralist version of social constructivism noted above, it places less emphasis upon *ideas* and more upon action and negotiation (e.g. Bartley *et al.* 1997). This approach is thus compatible with both symbolic interactionism and social realism (see next section).

These three versions of constructivism are not neatly divided within many studies within medical sociology. Bury (1986) notes that the notion of social constructivism subsumes many elements, some of which are contradictory. However, certain core themes can be detected across the three main types described by Brown. The first is that if reality is not rejected as an epiphenomenon of human activity (as in very strict constructivism) it is none the less problematized to some degree – hence the break with positivism. The second relates to the importance of reality being viewed, in whole or part, as a product of human activity. What constructivists vary in is whether this activity is narrowly about the cognitive aspects of human life (thought and talk), or it is conceived in a broader sense in relation to the actions of individuals and collectivities. The third is that power relationships are inextricably bound up with reality definition. Whether it is the power to define or the power to influence or the power to advance some interests at the expense of others, this political dimension to constructivism is consistent.

When we come to examine sociological work on mental health and illness these three core elements are evident. Constructivists problematize the factual status of mental illness (e.g. Szasz 1961). They analyse the ways in which mental health work has been linked to the production of psychiatric knowledge and the production of mental health problems (e.g. Parker *et al.* 1995). Also, they establish the links which exist in modern society with the coercive control of social deviance by psychiatry on the one hand and the production of selfhood by mental health expertise on the other (e.g. Miller and Rose 1988).

The final point to be made about social constructivism is that it does not *necessarily* have to be set in opposition to social realism (the view that there is an independent existing reality) or social causationism (the view that social forces cause measurable phenomena to really exist). It is certainly true that strong social constructivism challenges both of these positions (see e.g. Gergen 1985). However, a number of writers who accept some constructivist arguments point out that strictly it is not *reality* which is socially constructed but *theories of reality* (Greenwood 1994; Brown 1995). So much of the

apparent opposition between constructivist and realist or causationist arguments in social science results from a failure to make this distinction. This
brings us to our next perspective.

Social realism

The final perspective to be discussed in this chapter is that of social realism
– a perspective held by the authors (Pilgrim and Rogers 1994) as well as
others working in the field of mental health and the social psychology of
emotions (Greenwood 1994). Bhaskar (1978, 1989) outlines the philosophical basis of realism and we will draw out, briefly, the implications of his work
for a sociology of mental health and illness. His version is called 'critical
realism'.

As the name implies, critical realism accepts that reality really does exist
(*contra* strict constructivism). However, the 'critical' prefix suggests that it
diverges from social causationism. The latter follows the Durkheimian view
that external social reality impinges on human action and shapes human
consciousness. The Weberian view emphasizes the opposite process – that
human action inter-subjectively constructs reality. Critical theory, following
Freud, emphasizes the role of unconscious processes, especially repression,
and is rooted in methodological individualism (clinical psychoanalysis). By
contrast to all of these, critical realism attends to conscious action or agency
and is critical of methodological individualism. Bhaskar argues, following
Marx, that human action is neither mechanically determined by social reality nor does intentionality (voluntary human action) simply construct social
reality. Instead, society exists prior to the lives of agents but they become
agents who reproduce or transform that society. Material reality (the biological
substrate of actors and the material conditions of their social context) constrains action but does not simply determine it. Social science and natural
science warrant different methodologies and social phenomena cannot be
reduced to natural phenomena, even though the latter may exert an influence
on the former and are a precondition of their existence.

Bhaskar highlights the difference between natural and social science in the
light of this basic starting point. Here we quote three major differences
between natural and social structures and then draw out the implications for
the topic of this book:

1 social structures, unlike natural structures, do not exist independently of
   the activity they govern;
2 social structures, unlike natural structures, do not exist independently of
   the agents' conceptions of what they are doing in their activity;
3 social structures, unlike natural structures, may be only relatively enduring
   so that the tendencies they ground may not be universal in the sense of a
   space-time invariant (Bhaskar 1989: 79).

The implication of point 1 is that mental health work is part of a social
structural set-up so that objective or disinterested descriptions and action
within that work are untenable. Point 2 follows closely in its implication –

the professional knowledge perspectives we rehearsed earlier in the chapter contribute to the constitution of mental health work and the health and welfare structures they inhabit. Point 3 implies that mental health work must be understood within its specific context of time and place – it is historically and geographically situated. As a consequence of points 2 and 3 social psychiatric investigations should be accepted tentatively. They may supply useful information about the relationship between social variables such as gender or class (see later chapters) but they cannot be credited with the same scientific status as, for example, knowledge claims from biochemistry or physiology.

Because critical realism is a materialist, rather than idealist, basis for social science (cf. the Kantian idealism underlying the work of Weber and Foucault and their followers) it can accommodate material causation (e.g. temporal lobe epilepsy) alongside a critical analysis of the interests being served by the way mental health problems are described and conceptualized in a society at a point in time (e.g. a critique of the interests served by psychiatric knowledge). Such a critical reading comes near to the deconstruction emphasis of post-structuralism and the critiques of interest work found in critical studies of the production of scientific knowledge, but differs in its position during the exercise about the factual status of reality. As will become clear, we consider that evidence of social structural influences on mental health can be furnished by methodologies rooted in Durkheimian sociology. Equally, the concerns of social constructivists can furnish critical readings which give insights into the interests being served by discourses (what Bhaskar calls the 'agents' conceptions'). In other words, all sorts of methodologies used by sociologists to study mental health and illness can furnish illuminative information and, potentially, can be subjected to a critical reading (Pilgrim and Rogers 1999).

The relevance and applicability of sociological theory are themselves influenced by the particular time and social context in which they are used. More and more sociologists are employed in applied research contexts which lie outside their core disciplines. Sociology has also influenced generations of health workers including medical practitioners, nurses, psychologists and social workers. In comparison, 'pure' sociologists are a small minority of those who have had access to sociological knowledge through their socialization and education as health and social welfare professionals. Additionally, working in the field of mental health and health services research is a largely interdisciplinary endeavour. Thus, social realism allows co-existing explanations to exist about mental health.

Discussion

In this chapter we have rehearsed different perspectives, both outside and inside sociology, about the topic of mental health and illness. More will be said in the following chapters about how sociology has addressed a variety of questions about the identification and treatment of mental ill-health. Before we move to this, a final clarification is worth making about the relationship between sociology and the other perspectives discussed above. It may seem, at first reading, that sociology is somehow a separate and recent commentator on mental health and illness. This is only partially true. Over the past 40 years newly trained sociologists have contributed to knowledge about psychiatry and the mental patient, but this may give the false impression that sociology is merely responding to the dominant discourse on health and illness, coming from medical and paramedical professionals.

Social science existed at the beginnings of medicine. Before the latter settled down to become preoccupied with individual bodies and their parts, social medicine emerged in the eighteenth century as a programme of political intervention to prevent ill-health (Rosen 1979). Indeed, Foucault (1980) argues that medical surveys of society in the early nineteenth century were the true roots of modern sociology, not its reputed fathers like Comte, Marx, Durkheim and Weber. For a wider discussion of this topic see Kleinman (1986) and Turner (1990).

In the particular case of mental health, so much research of the epidemiological variety was intertwined with medical research. The discipline of social psychiatry demonstrates this overlap (Goldberg and Morrison 1963; Warner 1985). Also, some of the seminal epidemiological work of the 1950s and 1960s involved the collaboration of sociologists (e.g. Hollingshead and Brown) with psychiatrists (e.g. Redlich and Wing). However, it is also true that the more recent response of sociologists has been seen as oppositional by those inside clinical psychiatry. During the late 1960s, sociologists became part of 'antipsychiatry' or 'critics of psychiatry', according to leaders of the offended profession, such as Roth (1973). Thus, sociologists are in an ambivalent relationship to psychiatry. On the one hand, they have contributed to an expanded theory of aetiology, in tracing the social causes of mental illness; on the other, they have set up competing ways of conceptualizing mental abnormality.

The bulk of the work we have reviewed in this chapter reflects a dominant sociological interest in mental abnormality and in psychiatry. By comparison, over the past hundred years, there has been much less sociological (and for that matter general social scientific) interest in ordinary emotional life, non-deviant conduct and professional knowledge outside of the governance of psychiatric experts. However, this is changing. One major shift about this became evident in the work of post-structuralists (e.g. Rose 1986, 1990). Although this had mental health experts as a central focus (the 'psy complex'), it did demonstrate, under the prompt of Foucault, the diffuse and widespread influence of 'the confessional' and other personalizing discourses in everyday life.

Outside of post-structuralist frameworks we find a more pluralistic sociological interest in ordinary emotions (Elias 1978; Hochschild 1983; Freund 1988; James 1989; Giddens 1992; Beck and Beck-Gersheim 1995; Bendelow and Williams 1998). This range itself may reflect an aspect of postmodernity – diverse commentaries on personal life are becoming increasingly legitimate and demanded. For example, not only was it widely acknowledged that the mass emotional response to the death of Diana, Princess of Wales in 1997 was an extraordinary event in an undemonstrative British cultural context, but this reaction became a focus of extensive professional commentary. A whole edition of *The Psychologist* (the in-house journal of the British

Psychological Society) was devoted to a range of academic and clinical accounts of the phenomenon. We also find commentaries with resonances of psycho-analytical ideas about ordinary emotional life (Craib 1998) and those which bridge psychoanalysis and social constructionism (Lupton 1998).

Within this shift in social science, there has developed a sociological inter-est in the ways in which society has followed the trend of the fast food chain McDonald's in a whole range of cultural process (including sexual activity, health care 'delivery', and dying). This 'McDonaldization thesis' (Ritzer 1995 and 1997) reflects a shift in society towards consumerism. Within this thesis, it is suggested that the emotions, like food, have become subject to both commercial pre-packaging and increasing everyday interest to ordinary people.

Our brief concluding point here is not to analyse the contents of these commentaries and the events they respond to and construct, but that their increasing *existence* reflects a social scientific departure from a tradition which tended, by and large, to ignore the normal in favour of the abnormal. At the beginning of the next chapter we pick up this point about mass psychology and mental health.

To conclude

This chapter has rehearsed and summarized a set of perspectives about mental health and illness both inside and outside of sociology. The very existence of such a wide range of viewpoints highlights that the field of mental health and illness is highly contested. As a result, any discussion of the topic cannot take anything for granted – one's own assumptions, and those of others, need to be checked at the outset and at each stage of a dialogue or analysis thereafter.

Questions

1 Why are lay views about mental health and illness important?

2 What are the strengths and weaknesses of the legal perspective on mental illness?

3 Compare and contrast two approaches to mental health and illness within sociology.

4 Discuss the relevance of the Frankfurt School to contempory discus-sions about mental health.

5 Compare and contrast social constructivism with social realism when conducting sociological studies of mental health and illness.

6 Discuss recent developments in the sociology of the emotions.

For discussion

Consider your own views about mental health and illness. How do they relate to the range of perspectives offered in this chapter?

Further reading

Giddens, A. (1992) *The Transformation of Intimacy*. Cambridge: Polity Press.
Kleinman, A. (1988) *Rethinking Psychiatry*. London; New York: Free Press.
MacLachlan, M. (1997) *Culture and Health*. London; New York: Free Press.

Chapter **2**

Social class, inequalities, and mental health

Chapter overview

This chapter focuses on the key variables and concepts associated with socio-logical work on health inequalities and mental health. It will cover:

- The general relationship between social class and health status
- The relationship between social class and diagnosed mental illness
- The relationship between poverty and mental health status
- Social class and mental health professionalism
- Lay views about mental health and social class
- Conceptual problems of psychiatric epidemiology

The general relationship between social class and health status

Establishing the relationship between social class, social and economic conditions and poor mental health has been a dominant trend in both social psychiatry and sociology. A close association between sociology and medicine is evident within this tradition traceable to nineteenth-century social medicine (Kleinman 1986). One of the earliest studies in psychiatric epidemiology, which sought to establish a link between schizophrenia and social class (Faris and Dunham 1939) was carried out in the context of the development of 'human ecology' as a theoretical trend within the Chicago School of Sociology (Park 1936) and since then sociologists have continued actively to cooperate with psychiatrists. There are other ways in which a link between social conditions and milieu have been made. Some theorists have made a link between social conditions and the collective psychological well-being of a society. This was a feature of the work of Fromm, a member of the Frankfurt School (discussed in Chapter 1). More recently this has been expressed in analyses of the 'feel bad factor' which was associated with the social, economic and political context of the mid-1990s. This is succinctly put by Lashmar (1995):

> ... there has been an irrevocable shift in the national psyche. 'The Feel Bad Factor' is not only caused by job insecurity, but also by long term and widespread fears about finance – mortgages, negative equity, crime, social security, pensions and the cost of ill health in old age. A few prosper, the majority worry. This has created a new *zeitgeist,* reflected most poignantly by a dramatic increase in mental health problems, which I call the 'Feel Psychotic Factor'.
>
> (Lashmar 1995: 57)

This focus also appears in the developing area of the 'sociology of emotions' and the analytical links being made between the unconscious dimensions of human experience and identity in postmodern societies (discussed at the end of the last chapter). Mental health is part of a wider topic (health). Before we examine mental health this wider relationship between social class and ill-health will be summarized.

In the previous chapter we noted the social causation position in medical sociology. The empirical case for this position is at its strongest in relation to the correlations which have been established between social class and ill-health. Link and Phelan (1995) summarized 40 years of work in medical sociology which has supported the social causation of disease by noting that:

> Lower SES [socio-economic status] is associated with lower life expectancy, higher overall mortality rates and higher rates of infant and perinatal mortality ... Moreover, low SES is associated with each of the 14 major cause-of-death categories in the International Classification of Diseases as well as many other health outcomes including major mental disorders.
>
> (Link and Phelan 1995: 81)

However, the authors go on to note that the social causation case is not limited to considerations of class. Other social variables are implicated such as gender. Men have higher mortality rates at all ages, higher rates of coronary heart disease, respiratory disease and ulcers. Women have higher rates of diagnosed mental illness (see Chapter 3) and hypertension (the raised prevalence reflecting greater longevity in women). In relation to race, African Americans have higher rates of mortality at all ages, renal failure and stroke but lower rates than whites of coronary heart disease. In Britain, people who emigrated from the Caribbean and their British-born offspring have significantly higher rates of diagnosed major mental illness (see Chapter 4).

A recent British study comparing community samples of 15, 35 and 55-year-olds found a class gradient on a number of health indicators throughout the life span. However, class differences were not found in the youngest group in relation to chronic physical illness and mental health (Ford *et al.* 1994). Another study focusing on lower-class adolescents – 1000 young, unemployed people (15–21yrs) in Scotland – found that a third of the males and two-fifths of the females were exhibiting evidence of 'psychological morbidity' by 18 years of age (Sweeting and West 1995).

The importance of the life course perspective in understanding the determinants of inequalities in mental and physical health is succinctly put by Bartley and her colleagues (1998):

> The more data we have which show . . . how early circumstances contribute to health in later life, the clearer it becomes that 'social class' at any given point is but a very partial indicator of a whole sequence, a 'probabilistic cascade' of events which need to be seen in combination if the effects of social environment on health are to be understood. Different individuals have arrived at any particular level of income, occupational advantage or prestige which have different life histories behind them. Variables such as height, education and ownership of additional consumer goods act as indicators of these past histories.
>
> (Bartley *et al.* 1998: 573)

Traditionally, both inequalities in physical and mental health have been explained with reference to four main factors which were originally identified in the Black Report (DHSS 1980).

- *Artefact explanations* suggest that inequalities are an artefact of the way in which official statistics have been collated (Illsley 1986). By implication the artefact explanation attacks the assumption that health inequalities exist at all and that there is a causal relationship between social conditions and health. However, new methods available for validating the existence of class inequalities, using longitudinal Census data on health inequalities and linking these to death certification and cancer registration, have confirmed that health inequalities are not likely to be due to statistical bias (Bartley *et al.* 1998).
- *Selection explanations* suggest that long-term illness or 'health capital' in early life constrains social mobility and continued inequalities in illness in adulthood (Power *et al.* 1996). In other words health status determines

socio-economic position (Illsley 1986) (as in the 'social drift' hypothesis discussed in more detail below).
* *Cultural/behavioural explanations* suggest that lifestyle and health related behaviours (such as cigarette smoking, diet and lack of exercise amongst manual groups) lead to health inequalities.
* *Materialist explanations* emphasize the differential exposure to health threats inherent in society over which people have little control. Thus, this explanation suggests that a person's socio-economic position, and material deprivation in particular, leads to poorer health amongst people in lower social classes.

Over the last two decades there have been extensions elaborating on this four-fold typology. The debates about the causes of inequalities in health and illness have moved beyond simplistic unitary explanations and have incorporated more complex theories and concepts from mainstream sociology and the sub-discipline of the sociology of health and illness. The use of other indicators and proxies for social class (e.g. use of housing tenure and car ownership), which have produced similar socio-economic gradients in health, has lessened the strength of the artefact explanation (Davey Smith *et al.* 1990). The importance of time, biography and longitudinal life course research (Blaxter forthcoming, Shaw *et al.* 1998; Mheen *et al.* 1998) and of 'place' (e.g. the types of spatial effects which may impact on health status (Macintyre *et al.* 1993; Curtis and Jones 1998)) may act to reinforce inequalities in health status and health care operating within a locality. There is a greater emphasis too on the relationship between social structure and human agency in gaining insights into the nature of health inequalities. Recent sociological analyses have made use of the notions of social capital, personal identity and the situated actions and decisions made by individuals, when exploring health inequalities. The lack of 'social capital', which refers to 'features of social life-networks, norms and trust that enable participants to act together more effectively to pursue shared objectives' (Putnam cited in Wilkinson 1996: 221), implies that the quality of social relationships and, most importantly, our perceptions of where we are relative to others in the social structure, are likely to be important psycho-social mediators in the cause of inequalities in health (Wilkinson 1996). Informed by this approach, Nettleton and Burrows (1998) have recently theorized how the experience of mortgage debt and insecure home ownership results in higher rates of primary care consultations for mental health problems. They point to the way in which people's notion of home and home ownership are part of their sense of identity and aspirations, which provide a basis for what Laing (1959) called 'ontological security'. A threat to the latter may occur when, for example, mortgage arrears impact negatively on an individual's mental health.

As part of this transition in theorizing about health inequalities more generally, greater importance has been attributed to social-psychological factors and the role of emotions as mediators in health inequalities (Williams 1998). Emotions have come to be seen as central to the relationship between social structure and health.

> . . . the fact that socio-economic factors now primarily affect health through psychosocial rather than material pathways, places emotions

centre-stage in the social patterning of disease and disorder in advanced Western societies. In this sense, emotions, as existentially embodied modes of being in the world and the *sine qua non* of causal reciprocity and exchange, provide the 'missing link' between 'personal troubles' and broader 'public issues' of social structure.

(Williams 1998: 133)

One final point with regard to the broader research agenda about health inequalities and ill-health is the politicized context within which social and medical research has recently been undertaken. During the 1980s, ideological pressure, intended perhaps to gloss over the persistent and growing relative inequalities between rich and poor, found expression in a change of official terminology. There was also a seeming imbalance between work, which prioritized cultural individual and artefact explanations, compared to work which focused on material deprivation (Davey Smith *et al.* 1990). During this period, the term 'inequalities' was replaced by the preferred official (Conservative) government term 'variations' in health. With an incoming Labour health administration in 1997, not only was there a reversal to the previous terminology, but there was the appointment of a public health minister and Green Paper with the aim of tackling inequalities and unmet need (DoH 1998).

The relationship between social class and diagnosed mental illness

Class remains a predictable correlate of mental ill-health. A class gradient is evident in mental health status across all the diagnostic groups but it is not a neat inverse relationship. For example, affective disorders are diagnosed fairly evenly in all social classes, whereas a very strong correlation exists between low social class and the diagnosis of schizophrenia.

Faris and Dunham (1939) studied the intake of patients to hospital from different parts of Chicago. They found higher rates of illness for schizophrenia, alcoholism and organic psychosis in those groups from poor areas. The greatest difference was in the diagnosis of schizophrenia. There was seven times the rate of schizophrenic diagnosis for people from poor inner city districts compared with middle-class suburban areas. The investigators concluded that the combination of poverty plus a lack of social cohesion in a locality precipitated schizophrenic breakdown. They argued that those vulnerable to breakdown are those who, for developmental reasons, became socially isolated during childhood. The stress of poverty and social disorganization then pushes these vulnerable individuals into psychosis. Faris (1944) then elaborated this 'social isolation' theory of schizophrenia.

After the Second World War, Dunham (1957) drew attention to several studies that confirmed the role of social isolation in the aetiology of schizophrenia; there were exceptions though. Clausen and Kohn (1959) did not find the relationship between isolation and psychosis in the small city of Hagerstown, Maryland. Also, Weinberg (1960) studying the histories of schizophrenic patients did not find a pattern of social isolation. Gerard and Houston (1953)

found that divorced and single people who already had a diagnosis of schizophrenia moved to inner city areas. At this stage the controversy over 'social
drift' emerged. Its proponents argued that mentally ill people drift into poverty.
Its opponents argued that poverty precipitates illness.

Lapouse *et al.* (1956) and Hollingshead and Redlich (1958) did not find
in their surveys that people diagnosed as schizophrenic drifted into poor
areas, but they confirmed the class gradient in the diagnosis of schizophrenia. Overall, the epidemiological evidence does strongly point to an over-
representation of patients considered to have schizophrenia in lower-class
samples (e.g. Tietze *et al.* 1941; Stein 1957; Goldberg and Morrison 1963).
These patients are particularly over-represented at the bottom of the social
scale (Dunham 1964). The question is, why does this class gradient exist?

Broadly, there have been two competing hypotheses about why mental
illness is diagnosed more in poorer populations. The first is the 'drift' hypothesis and the other is the 'opportunity and stress' hypothesis. The 'drift'
hypothesis, which suggests that illness incapacitates social competence, itself
has two aspects. One has already been mentioned – that psychotic patients
perhaps drift into poorer urban areas. The other is that patients drift down
the social scale. Here the assumption is that patients from all classes above
that of the lowest stratum (the unskilled and the unemployed) who become
mentally ill cannot maintain their class position and they sink to the bottom
of society, in class terms.

Empirical work suggests that the different causal explanations vary according to the type of mental health problem under investigation. A large-scale
epidemiological study in Israel (Dohrenwend *et al.* 1992) concluded that
social causation was stronger than social selection in producing the inverse
association of socio-economic status to severe depression in women, substance abuse and antisocial personality in men. However, in relation to those
who carried a diagnosis of schizophrenia the epidemiological evidence was
more supportive of the social selection explanation.

Investigations to date have not resolved the drift versus stress debate.
Given the mixed evidence for both, there have been some attempts to integrate elements of each of them. For example, the mixed model of Kohn is
assessed by Cochrane (1983).

The hypothesis relating to stress and opportunities suggests that these
differentially affect lower-class people compared with those from the middle
and upper classes. Srole *et al.* (1962) and Langer and Michael (1963) in their
large-scale community surveys of mental health in the US found that lower-
class people were more likely to have psychotic symptoms and middle-class
people were more likely to have neurotic symptoms. They accounted for this
difference in part by suggesting that middle-class children are over-inhibited
compared with their lower-class equivalents. Their sexual and aggressive
impulses were considered to be more controlled. This was thought to lead to
problems of anxiety and guilt appearing more often in non-lower-class groups.
Also, the emphasis on self and identity was found to be a stronger preoccupation during upbringing in non-lower-class families. This may mean that a
sense of identity is stronger in these groups. By contrast, identity strength
may be lower, on average, in lower-class groups. Lower-class people may be
more readily vulnerable to the loss and fragmentation of their sense of self
and thus may become psychotic.

These speculations about psychological differences in upbringing and their consequences can be added to much stronger evidence about the material differences between classes. Poor people have to struggle with the personal consequences of material deprivation. In their locality they must endure higher stress from crime, traffic and dirt and their home conditions are more likely to be cramped. Their diet and physical health will be inferior to those further up the class scale. They will be vulnerable to unemployment more often and the jobs they obtain will lack a sense of personal control. All these factors will contribute to lower levels of self-worth and esteem. When they enter the patient role lower class patients are more likely to stay as in-patients for longer periods of time and thus become more severely disabled from re-entering society (Hardt and Feinhandler 1959).

The evidence from social psychiatric follow-ups of patients with diagnoses of schizophrenia shows that the more opportunities they have for employment the better their prognoses (Ciompi 1984; Warner 1985). Also, the point about esteem or relative self-worth has been confirmed in studies looking at quality of life in different classes. Whilst people in all classes have negative experiences, the proportion of these to positive experiences decreases with increasing class position. For instance, Phillips (1968) found no class differences in the reporting of negative experiences. There were, however, significant differences in the presence of *positive* experiences between high- and low-class respondents. The former were twice as likely as the latter to report feeling excited, proud or interested by an event during the last month than the latter. Phillips then concluded that lower-class people have fewer positive experiences to buffer themselves against life's stresses, which makes them more vulnerable to mental distress.

This is consistent with the findings of the longitudinal study of Myers (1974, 1975). It was found that, in all social classes, the greater the number of life events, both positive and negative, then the greater the probability of psychiatric symptoms appearing. But non-lower-class people experienced a greater proportion of positive events and this led to them being buffered from symptom formation more often than lower-class people.

So, whilst it can be demonstrated unequivocally that social stress is correlated with social class, the evidence is still not clear about its causal role in schizophrenia. The epidemiological evidence from social psychiatry seems to point strongly at the role of social stress in recovery and relapse, but this is not the same as deducing that social stressors actually cause schizophrenia. As we will see later (Chapter 5), the clear traumatic stress of sexual abuse raises the probability of most forms of psychiatric morbidity except for the diagnosis of schizophrenia. This role of stress in relapse, rather than aetiology, may account for the prevalence of schizophrenia being affected by social stress (but not for the incidence of first episodes) and may explain why lower-class patients recover less frequently.

The relationship between poverty and mental health status

The discussion above seems to confirm the relationship between low social class and severe mental health problems. However, given that there is not a neat inverse relationship between social class and mental well-being, it may be more fruitful to examine mental health problems in the more focused context of poverty. This focus allows us to explore the interaction between disempowerment and material deprivation. For example, if depressed groups are studied, black people are more *severely* depressed than their white counterparts with low socio-economic status (Biafora 1995). This could be accounted for by the double impact of oppression in this group (being poor *and* black). However, this interaction effect on mental health status between poverty and race is not clear cut. The Biafora study just cited is at odds with some studies which show no differences in depression rates between white and black groups. In Britain, high rates of schizophrenia are diagnosed in Afro-Caribbean groups, compared to whites but this is not the case for Asians, even though the latter contain very poor subpopulations.

Notwithstanding this problem about the interaction effects of race and class, an analytical advantage of focusing on poverty, rather than class *per se*, is that it helps us to clarify a contradiction about mental health service utilization. Generally, in health care there is an 'inverse care law', that is, access to health care increases with increasing class status. However, the reverse appears to be the case in mental health care systems. Psychiatric services are dominated by patients from low social class backgrounds. Superficially this might suggest that those with the greatest need are being responded to. That is, given that poor people are more likely to be diagnosed as mentally ill, services are responding to their need. However, there is a problem with this logic. While most health care interventions are voluntary and ameliorative in intent in their response to the needs of sick people, in psychiatric services, involuntary detention and treatment are never far away. A proportion of patients are being forcibly detained and treated by the use of therapeutic law, some are notionally voluntary but *de facto* detainees, and others are genuinely voluntary but exist in a service context where the threat of coercion is ever present (Rogers 1993a).

In the light of these peculiar features about psychiatry, it might be more accurate to conceptualize mental health work as part of a wider state apparatus which controls the social problems associated with poverty (what has been increasingly called the 'underclass'). Once conceived in this way, it lowers our expectations that service contact should necessarily be about aiming for, or achieving, a gain in the mental health status of service recipients, given that the latent, and sometimes the explicit, function of psychiatry is that of successful coercive social control. The latter entails mental health services serving the interests of parties (such as relatives and strangers in the street) other than the patients they contain and treat.

Thus, poverty is an important focus for understanding the relationship between social class and mental health because it highlights the social control role of psychiatry in response to certain types of social crises and deviance. The social *consequences* of poverty become a dimension of understanding mental health in society. Poverty is also important in understanding the social *antecedents* of madness and psychological distress. These antecedents include interactions with other forms of oppression (such as racism discussed above), the stress of poor living conditions and the impact of labour market disadvantage.

Relative deprivation has a greater impact on morbidity and GP consultation for stress-related conditions such as depression, anxiety and headache/ migraine. For all these conditions, higher levels of self-reported morbidity and a greater probability of consulting the doctor are associated with a cluster of social disadvantages – living in rented accommodation, unemployment, younger age and lower educational status. Relative deprivation is also associated with poorer mental health for this population of mothers of young children (Baker and Taylor 1997).

Fryer (1995) reviewed the evidence on the impact of labour market disadvantage on mental health and found that unemployment has a predictable toll on both the unemployed individuals *and* their family members. For example, mental health problems and deterioration in school performance increase in probability in the children of those who become unemployed. Fryer also reviews the evidence on the mental health impact of the spouses of those becoming unemployed and notes that people in low paid and insecure employment have similar symptom profiles to those who are unemployed.

The shift from an employed to an unemployed status (and its threat to those in insecure work) is significantly associated with the risk of depression, alcohol dependence, anxiety states and psychosomatic reactions. Some of these effects may persevere even after re-employment or attendance at retraining schemes. The latter have a positive impact on self-esteem but they do not necessarily ameliorate mental health problems.

As well as reviewing the empirical evidence on the effects of labour market disadvantage, Fryer also outlines the causal factors which might account for the increased probability of mental health problems. These factors include: the direct stress of impoverishment; the loss of social status after being unemployed; and a consequent experience of having one's agency thwarted. The last factor is important because it illuminates the mediating role of a sense of purpose and self-esteem which are associated with wage earning and which are lost to the unemployed person. A thwarted sense of agency also might be a mediating factor in the raised rates of criminality, prostitution and illicit drug use in those who have never worked and see no prospect of salaried employment.

These examples of overlapping 'deviance' might be understood as meaningful alternative roles to those being denied to people excluded from long-term lawful employment. Fryer also emphasizes the partiality of a causal account which relies only on the subjective aspects of loss of agency in unemployment. The direct material impact of poverty can be pathogenic in itself and in combination with the subjectivity of loss and social exclusion. The list of possible causal factors offered by Fryer is similar to that discussed by the recent work of Brown and his colleagues when discussing depression in women (see Chapter 3).

There is clear evidence of the negative impact of unemployment but this does not always imply that work promotes well being. As well as unemployment and its threat having a negative mental health impact, the stress of employment itself has been documented. In Britain in the 1990s, this has become a particular focus of interest in relation to the stress of paid caring. The Department of Health set one of its Health of the Nation's targets as improving the mental health of the NHS workforce. Newnes (1995) set up a counselling service for NHS employees in 1991 and reported a 200 per cent increase in demand over a four-year period. The causal factors which link work stress to mental health problems are complex and might include some combination of: work load; task monotony; threat of unemployment; accident risks; sexual harassment; sexual discrimination; racial discrimination; discrimination on grounds of disability or sexuality; and dual role stress in working parents (Davidson and Earnshaw 1991). In low-paid workers, the above list would be set in a context of relative poverty and the direct stress this entails.

The second broad set of antecedent factors relates not to employment status but to accommodation. However, it is important to note that whilst these are discussed separately for convenience here from employment factors, they are co-present and additive in the lives of many poor people. There is evidence that poor accommodation produces stress reactions in inhabitants (Hunt 1990; Hyndman 1990). For those who are homeless, mental health problems have been constructed by many psychiatric researchers as primary (a cause of homelessness) rather than secondary (a consequence of poverty on the streets) (Whitely 1955; Bassuk *et al.* 1984; cf. Hamid 1991). Snow *et al.* (1986) undertook ethnographic fieldwork to assess the mental health status of homeless people and found, using standard diagnostic criteria, that only 15 per cent of a population of 991 were considered to be mentally ill.

The catastrophic discourse about de-institutionalisation in those lobbying to retain large scale hospitalization of psychiatric patients has over-emphasized prevalence in homeless populations. For example, one British pressure group in the early 1990s in favour of retaining the mass segregation of patients (*Concern*) argued that 40–50 per cent of the homeless population was mentally ill and, moreover, that prison populations had grown in response to hospital closure (see Page and Powell 1991 (eds) *Homelessness and Mental Illness: The Dark Side of Community Care*). The latter collection also contained articles emphasizing the need to retain the Victorian asylums and the highly dangerous nature of madness (Hollander 1991; Jacobs 1991).

Thus, it is difficult to develop a clear picture of the causal relationship between homelessness and poor mental health, whilst ever it is confounded by political lobbying to control and segregate those with a psychiatric diagnosis. Those in favour of de-segregation such as the National Association of Mental Health (MIND) argue that older patients who were contained in the Victorian asylums have not been at risk of homelessness but that 'the new mentally ill' (i.e. younger patients who have never been in the older hospitals but are revolving-door patients, in and out of acute psychiatric wards) are vulnerable to homelessness. However, they, like their opponents wanting to reverse de-segregation, argue from a starting point of preferred policy development. This shapes the research questions they pose and their data analysis.

A final aspect to note about accommodation and hospitalization is that the latter can *jeopardize* the former. Bean and Mounser (1993) found that becoming a psychiatric in-patient may bring with it a loss of tenancy rights. When this occurs, the person may be rendered homeless by entering, not by leaving, hospital (the argument of those like *Concern* above). The Bean and Mounser study also highlighted that hospital discharge needs to be placed in the context of both admission to hospital and the community context of patients, particularly those who have episodic service contact ('revolving-door patients').

Social class and mental health professionalism

In this section we address a set of factors which reinforce (rather than singularly create) class differences in mental health status. A number of studies have focused on the impact of the 'cultural gap' which can exist between clients and their treating mental health professionals (Horwitz 1983). The latter concept refers to more than class differences as it can implicate race and ethnicity as well as age, gender and sexuality. However, class is an important consideration when people with mental health problems engage with professional services. Poor patients are more likely to receive a diagnosis of schizophrenia than richer patients, who are more likely to receive a less stigmatizing neurotic label or be allotted one of affective disorder (depression, mania, or manic-depression). Poorer patients are more likely to receive biological treatments than psychological treatments. Poorer patients are less likely to be referred for psychotherapy, are rejected more often on assessment by specialists and drop out of treatment earlier (Pilgrim 1997a). Poorer patients are more likely to be treated coercively than voluntarily.

Some of this picture could be accounted for by the simple issue of raised incidence of severe mental health problems in poor populations – i.e. the more severe mental illness profile of the latter warrants greater levels of coercion and biological treatments in mental health service responses. Sedgwick (1982) warned of the dangers inherent in social constructivist arguments in this regard. He commented that some critics of psychiatry wanted it both ways: on the one hand they argued that adverse material conditions cause severe mental illness (warranting more psychiatric services), and, on the other, they deconstructed, and thereby undermined, the legitimacy of diagnostic data demonstrating this causal relationship. They also complained of the social control role of psychiatric professionals.

However, as we noted at the end of the previous chapter, constructivism and causationism can be reconciled. It is logically quite feasible that the material conditions of poverty raise the probability of mental distress in a population *and* that professional interests are at play and, within this, the role and 'world views' of psychiatric professionals. This might include the class and cognitive interests of mental health professionals operating, when they respond to low-class patients in contact with services and formulate this distress in biomedical terms or in the thinly veiled value judgements of psychological interpretations. For example, clinicians tend to interpret psychometric test responses from lower socio-economic groups as reflecting greater psychopathology than similar responses from middle-class clients. Also, growing conditions of poverty significantly affects how people perform on tests of abstract thinking, intelligence and academic achievement (Franks 1993). Taken together, these processes point to *both* causal *and* constructed influences upon poor clients in service contact.

Poverty and and other class-related phenomena remain neglected areas in the training of mental health professionals, with the latter not being exposed to the narratives of poverty, oppression and daily struggle which would sensitize them to the needs of their client group. Schnitzer (1996) suggests that mental health professionals typically question the responsibility, cognitive competence and moral sensitivity of poorer clients. This may reflect not just the secondary socialization (in their training) of mental health professionals but also their primary socialization (in their class of origin).

A number of commentators have pointed to the absence of notions of class and inequality in disciplinary knowledge which underpin mental health professionals' practice. For example, in mainstream psychiatry and psychology textbooks class, ethnic, and gender inequalities receive little attention. Power inequalities are then marginalized and are seen as having little to do with psychiatric vulnerability or psychiatric management more generally (Horsfall 1997). Ussher (1994) points to the narrow focus of mainstream clinical psychology models, such as behavioural and cognitive behaviour therapy, which ignore class both at the level of theory and practice.

Lay views about mental health and social class

Whilst there has been a social psychiatric epidemiology which maps the relationship between social variations and mental health, the views of people within different classes about the topic of mental health and social class has, until recently, been a relatively neglected area. As we have outlined above there is an extensive literature which maps and puts forward explanations for differences between groups in the population in terms of mental health status. Traditionally, there has been little interest in how people themselves construed their distress and oppression. However, more recently, there has been a growing interest in the understanding of lay knowledge. One of the arguments for this greater concentration is to augment gaps in professional knowledge about how ordinary people understand their health. Sociologists such as Blaxter (1990) have explored the views that people have about inequalities in health in general. In relation to mental health, a recent study showed that lay people tend to adopt a relative, rather than absolute, view of mental health and social causation (Rogers and Pilgrim 1997). People in all social classes tend to view money problems as a central feature of mental well-being – though those from more middle-class backgrounds identify it as being more of a problem for working-class families. Similarly, work stress and stress related to common life events, such as bereavement and birth, were considered by working-class respondents to affect people similarly, albeit in different ways.

Perceptions of lay knowledge about help-seeking are also important – 'expectations' shape demand for, and use of, formal services. For example, in primary care settings lay people provide accounts of help-seeking about mental health problems which are different from those offered by GPs (Pilgrim *et al.* 1997). Professionals emphasize diagnostic categories (like depression) based upon a symptom approach to presenting problems. By contrast, patients themselves understand their problems within a unique biographical context situated in time and place. These attributions within a life story include factors such as poverty, employment and unemployment, domestic violence and life events (like birth and death in the family).

Conceptual problems of psychiatric epidemiology

Some disease categories such as schizophrenia have been subjected to persuasive critical deconstruction. For example, this diagnosis has been criticized for its lack of aetiological specificity, its lack of predictive validity and its lack of inter-rater reliability (Bentall, Jackson and Pilgrim 1988). It is a 'disjunctive' diagnosis. That is, two patients called 'schizophrenic' may have no symptoms in common (Bannister 1968). Some historians of the concept (Boyle 1991) have even demonstrated that the symptom profiles recorded in the late nineteenth century, when Kraepelin and Bleuler constructed the disease entity, first called 'dementia praecox' and then 'schizophrenia', bear little relationship to the first rank symptoms which psychiatrists currently use in their diagnoses. In other words, the features of patients given the diagnosis of schizophrenia at its conceptual inception were not the same as those with the same label today. These conceptual problems with schizophrenia are raised in this chapter because the diagnosis has been at the heart of the case for a class gradient in mental health. If the concept of schizophrenia is discredited by the critiques outlined, does this undermine our confidence in social causationist claims from over 60 years of social psychiatric research?

Discussion

Finally, we need to be aware when examining the relationship between social class and mental health, that the concept has itself become increasingly problematized within sociology. With the decline in the centrality of Marxism within social theory and its replacement by a mixture of other currents including feminism and post-structuralism, social class appears less frequently in the literature or is problematized by non-Marxists when discussing social stratification and societal disadvantage (Runciman 1990; Evans 1992; Goldthorpe and Marshall 1992; Westergaard 1992; Pahl 1993). Reflecting this trend, in the first edition of this book we provided only a section, not a whole chapter, on the topic. Parker et al. (1995) in their post-structuralist critique of psychopathology point out that:

Although by its very nature a 'social' concept, implying a group, increasingly 'class' has been a term applied to individuals. Worse than this, classes are defined in the psychological literature, without any reference to the exploitation of labour, alienation or oppression. . . . Indeed class is heard of less and we now hear more of socio-economic status – an individualised variable. Pilgrim and Rogers' (1993) *A Sociology of Mental Health and Illness* includes chapters on gender, race and ethnicity and age but only a section on class.

(Parker et al. 1995: 46)

There is now a trend towards viewing social class as a complex mixture of discursive, material and psychological factors which interact to produce inequalities. This approach brings with it a stronger focus on the personal experience of relative deprivation for individual and collective identity and emphasizes how inequalities manifest themselves in everyday life. A focus on the social environment and its dynamics, by investigating indicators of income and material equality, social cohesion, self-efficacy and trust is likely to be the most fruitful way of progressing knowledge about health inequalities in mental health. Within this approach, it may be possible to link the nature and circumstances of service contact with wider factors affecting the types and experience of mental health inequalities.

Currently there is a split between one type of literature on inequalities in mental health status and another on the inequalities that service contact might perpetuate. However, as we have discussed earlier, there is evidence that service contact brings with it risks that can have a sustained negative impact on mental health. A better understanding of the relationship between service contact and its impact on quality of life and psychological distress would illuminate further our understanding of one aspect of the multi-factorial interaction noted above.

Apart from the displacement of Marxism as the central discursive focus of class within sociology, societal changes have brought with them difficulties in thinking simply about the concept and formulating and conducting empirical projects. For example, the traditional use of the Registrar General's classifications system has become less and less meaningful. Women can no longer be conceptualized as sharing their husband's class status – not just because this is now ideologically rejected in the wake of feminism but because marriage has declined in popularity (so it fails to capture the range of forms of interdependent cohabitation). Also women, not men, numerically now dominate the labour market. Moreover, the old pyramid notion of class structure has been replaced by one which is nearer to a diamond, as traditional blue collar factory production has been eroded but service industries have expanded. Consequently, white collar work covers a variety of status and salary levels (from clerical low pay to rich executive earnings) and at the bottom of the diamond is a group of dispossessed people who are excluded permanently or semi-permanently from the labour market. This exclusion can be reproduced over several generations. The notion of oppression, which was previously associated mainly, or singularly, with low social class within Marxian sociology, is now linked to other social groups independent of their class position – women, black people, people with physical disabilities, people with learning difficulties, gay people, older people and, of particular relevance to this book, people with mental health problems.

Given the conceptual problems within both psychiatric epidemiology, discussed above, and the contested concept of class within sociology, we can make only very broad confident statements about social class and mental health. For example, it is safe to say that poverty contains causal influences which both create and exacerbate mental health problems. We cannot say definitively, however, that 'poverty causes schizophrenia'. We can say that being or becoming unemployed or homeless increases the probability of mental health problem development, although we cannot, with certainty, argue that a *particular* individual's mental health problems (or their relative's) are caused by their unemployed or homeless status. We can say that the oppression and powerlessness, associated with low social class, disadvantage poor people during mental health service contact (they are more likely to have interventions imposed upon them and be treated with biological treatments than those in a higher class position), but we cannot say that these discriminatory service eventualities are *only* attributable to social class, because other variables, such as race or gender, might be alternative or coexisting determinants of professional action.

To conclude

This chapter has explored a range of sociological aspects of mental health and social class. It is clear that whatever conceptual problems exist about understanding mental illness in the same way as physical illness, the social impact of low social class (especially its associated poverty) is similar for each. Basically, poorer people are significantly less healthy, both physically and mentally, than richer people. It is, however, more problematic to argue that there are social causes of specific diagnosed conditions (like 'schizophrenia'). This says more about the poor concept validity of diagnoses used by psychiatry than it does about the stress created for people by socio-economic inequality.

Questions

1 Does poverty cause schizophrenia?

2 Why are richer people mentally healthier than poorer people?

3 Discuss the relationship between homelessness and mental health problems.

4 Discuss lay views about mental health and social class.

5 Have changes in sociological interest in social class produced changes in sociological work on mental health and illness?

6 How does social class influence the way in which psychiatric treatment is given?

For discussion

Think about people you know with mental health problems and discuss ways in which their social class background has affected their lives.

Further reading

Blaxter, M. (1990) *Health and Lifestyles*. London: Routledge.

Warner, R. (1985) *Recovery from Schizophrenia*. London: Routledge.

Warr, P. (1987) *Work, Unemployment and Mental Health*. Oxford: Oxford University Press.

Wilkinson, R.G. (1996) *Unhealthy Societies: The Afflictions of Inequality*. London: Routledge.

Williams, S.J. (1998) 'Capitalising' on emotions? Rethinking the inequalities in health debate, *Sociology* 32, 1: 121–140.

Chapter **3**

Gender

Chapter overview

Most of the discussion about mental health and gender has been about women. This chapter reflects this in both the sociological discourse and social-psychiatric research reported. In addition, the question of men and psychiatry is addressed.

The chapter will cover the following topics:

- The over-representation of women in mental health statistics

- Does society cause excessive female mental illness?

- Is female over-representation a measurement artefact?

- Are women labelled as mentally ill more often than men?

- Men and psychiatry

The over-representation of women in mental health statistics

Although most academic attention about the topic of this chapter has focused on women and mental health, the study of gender is a comparative exercise in which the relationship of men and women to psychiatry requires exploration. Another point to make at the outset about this topic is that whilst sociologists have taken an interest in women and mental health, the funding of clinical and service research has not been associated with considerations of gender (Page 1993). Within the routine collection of information about mental health services, it remains evident that more women than men are, or are diagnosed as being, mentally ill. This is especially the case for anxiety disorders and other neurotic conditions. Claims about the over-representation of women have been based on two sources of data.

1 The number of people admitted to hospital and using psychiatric services is one source. Official statistics from the Department of Health (Table 3.1) suggest that many more women than men are admitted to psychiatric facilities each year. This tells us the number of people who have been identified and treated as psychiatric patients or, from a labelling perspective, those who have successfully had a label applied to them and the type of label that has been applied. It can be seen, for example, that women are classified as suffering from 'affective psychosis' at twice the rate that men are, but that for 'schizophrenia' men are slightly over-represented compared with women. Estimates have been made that for every male diagnosed as depressed, there are between two and six times as many women (Weissman and Klerman 1977). Women are also diagnosed as suffering

Table 3.1   Rates of admission to hospitals in England in 1986 per 100,000 population by sex and diagnostic group

Diagnosis	Males	Females	Excess of female over male rate (%)
All diagnoses	364	468	+29
Schizophrenia	66	58	−12
Affective psychoses	35	68	+98
Other psychoses	32	44	+37
Senile and presenile dementia	33	55	+67
Alcohol psychoses and alcoholism	45	20	−55
Drug dependence	9	8	−11
Neurotic disorders	22	42	+91
Personality and behaviour disorders	28	32	+14
Other conditions[1]	89	142	+60
Rates for all· diagnoses (1986)	364	468	+29
Rates for all diagnoses (1976)	320	447	+40

[1] This category includes depression not classified elsewhere

from both mono-symptomatic phobias and agoraphobia more often than men (Lepine and Lellouch 1995). The difference indicated for senile dementia is attributable to the fact that currently women are, on average, living longer than men and consequently they have longer to develop dementia. Also the gap between overall diagnosis rates has closed during the ten years of data collection after 1986, with diagnoses for both groups increasing during the period. The reasons for this are currently unclear. It may reflect a more cautious approach from psychiatrists accused of sexist diagnostic bias. Alternatively, perhaps men are being referred to psychiatrists more readily than in the past.

Caution needs to be taken in generalizing about the ratio of mental disorder between the sexes from figures on hospital admissions and rates of formal diagnoses made by professionals. Use of services is not necessarily an accurate indicator of incidence, i.e. the occurrence of mental disorder amongst different groups living in the community. Another caution relates to cross-national differences. For example, in China (*contra* the western picture) women are diagnosed as suffering from mental illness more often than men but in a different way. The prevalence of depression and neurotic disorders is lower in Chinese than western women. However, the prevalence of the diagnosis of schizophrenia is significantly higher for women than men in China, which might be accounted for by the cultural tendency in that country for women to be disvalued and coercively controlled (Pearson 1995). Busfield (1996) also points to historical analysis which suggests that 'far from being a long-standing feature, the aggregate female predominance (in admissions) is relatively new'.

2 Community surveys. These aim to provide information by measuring levels of mental disorder in society at large, independently of any contact people might have had with services. The findings of these studies have also been used to suggest that women experience relatively high rates of depression and other psychiatric disorders compared with men. For example, Walter Gove and his colleagues, focusing on higher female rates among married women than men, claim that women experience psychological distress more than men. Blaxter (1990) also found that, throughout the life span, women report greater psychosocial malaise than men and the gap between the sexes increases in older people. Blaxter's self-reported factors included depression, worry, sleep disturbances and feelings of strain.

How, then, can this apparent excess of female over male 'mental illness' be explained? The reasons for the over-representation of women in mental health statistics are highly contested, with a number of competing explanations being evident in the literature. These explanations can be broadly categorized into three main perspectives:

• Social causation – does society cause excessive female mental illness?
• Artefact – is female over-representation a measurement artefact?
• Social labelling – are women labelled more often than men?

These three questions will now be explored.

Does society cause excessive female mental illness?

That mental illness is rooted in women's life experiences has been expounded by a number of commentators. Most of these explanations have focused on the link between the 'stress' of women's lives and mental disorder. Two examples illustrate this social causation perspective.

Gove (1984) and his colleagues (Gove and Geerken 1977), who have written and researched extensively in the area of women's mental health, claim that the amount and particular type of stress experienced by women results in higher rates of female psychiatric morbidity. In particular, they look to two aspects of women's societal role to explain why women experience more psychological distress than men. First, the lack of structure in women's roles (which tend to be domestic) makes them more vulnerable to mental distress because they have time to 'brood' over their problems. In contrast, men have relatively 'fixed' roles. According to Gove, this means that the necessity of responding to the immediate and highly structured demands of the workplace distracts men from their personal problems and this offers a degree of protection that is not available to women. Second, citing community studies, Gove points to evidence that poorer mental health is found in situations where women are more likely to occupy nurturant roles (e.g. divorced women who care for children have a higher incidence of mental distress than divorced men and women without children). It is hypothesized that the social demands and lack of privacy associated with this role may be a causal factor.

Evidence of social aetiology and depression amongst women comes from the research of Brown and Harris (1978), who identified different factors which together point to the social origins of depression. This picture of aetiology is sometimes referred to as a multifactorial social model, where a wide selection of factors interacting with each other may be necessary preconditions for developing a psychiatric condition.

Brown and Harris draw attention to three groups of aetiological factors that need to be understood as interacting with one another to produce depression (see Fig. 3.1).

Vulnerability factors

Such factors might make women more susceptible to depression during a time of loss or in the face of another major negative life event. These biographical events include:

1 Loss of mother before 11 years of age. Subsequent research linked this to the quality of care that followed this loss. Those with poor subsequent care were particularly vulnerable to depression (Brown *et al.* 1986).
2 The absence of a confiding relationship with a partner.
3 Lack of employment (full- or part-time) outside of the home.
4 Presence at home of three or more children under 15 years of age.

When the opposites of these factors were found to be present, for example high intimacy with a partner and the presence of a mother after the age of 11, they acted to 'protect' women against depression.

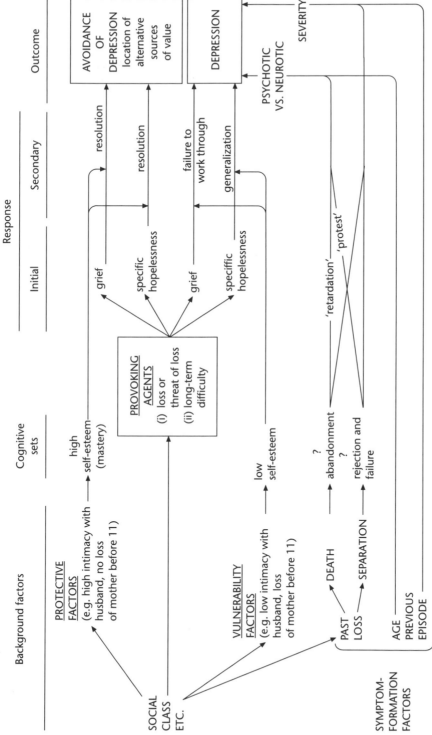

Figure 3.1 Brown and Harris's model of depression (from Brown and Harris 1978).

Provoking agents

These are factors operating in women's contemporary everyday lives, which may lead to depression, and include detrimental 'life events' such as loss through bereavement or marriage breakdown, or episodes of serious illness. Chronic difficulties as well as specific stressors are included here. The occurrence of these events determines when the depression will arise.

Symptom formation factors

These factors determine the severity and form of depression. In Brown and Harris's research, depression was found to be more severe if there had been previous depressive episodes and the woman was aged over 50. These social factors were linked together in Brown and Harris's research with psychological variables (cognitive sets). Women whose personalities were characterized by low self-esteem were more likely to experience the onset of depression than those who had high self-esteem.

The work of Brown and Harris in the 1970s has been extended in the interim. More data has been collected and, recently, more theoretical issues have been raised by Brown and his colleagues. Brown *et al.* (1995) compared clinical and non-clinical populations in Islington, north London. Drawing upon the work of Gilbert (1992) and Unger (1984), they elaborate their position about depression and the *experience* of life events. They conclude that the probability of depression increases not necessarily with loss or threatened loss *per se* but with the coexistence of humiliation and/or entrapment. Gilbert and Unger note that depression is commonly associated with feeling trapped and humiliated, such that there is an assault on the person's sense of self-worth *and* they have a blocked escape. The latter may then make the difference between a depressive and a non-depressive trajectory. For example, Brown *et al.* (1995) suggest that a woman being told that the paralyzed husband she is caring for will not recover might become depressed, but another, able to leave her violent or feckless partner, may feel liberated. Thus, being able to 'leave the field' may head off depression or reverse it in those already distressed.

The Islington study also highlighted more details about the risk factors associated with adverse childhood experiences. A third of the depressed women studied had experienced neglect or physical or sexual abuse in their childhoods. This subgroup had twice the chances of becoming depressed in one year, compared to those without such adverse antecedents (Bifulco *et al.* 1992). These childhood events also increase the probability of anxiety symptoms. Brown (1996) suggests that this might account for the common coexistence of anxiety and depression in adult patients.

Rigorous research such as that of Brown and his colleagues can tell us a great deal about the possible direct and indirect influence of social factors in the cause of female mental illness. However, the extent to which we can accept the conclusions of research that suggests that women experience more mental disorder than men rests on the way in which both mental health and gender are measured. The epidemiological work of this type rests on medical constructs (Brown and Harris accepted depression and other diagnoses measured by the Present State Examination). Likewise, work on prevention of mental health problems, in the wake of Brown and Harris's study, does not question psychiatric knowledge (e.g. Newton 1988). This is not the case with the next and subsequent positions.

Is female over-representation a measurement artefact?

The artefact explanation suggests that epidemiological measurement and its interpretation are faulty. From this point of view, some or all of the excess in psychiatric morbidity is not 'real', rather it is created by the design, assumptions and interpretations operating in social psychiatric research (using, for instance, the Present State Examination and the General Health Questionnaire).

As an example of a traditional causation study subjected to an artefact critique, we can take the work of Gove and his colleagues, which has been the centre of considerable debate (Busfield 1982; Gove 1984). This research focused on female psychiatric morbidity and marital status and claimed to demonstrate that married women have greater levels of mental distress than married men.

Gove and his co-workers take marital status as an accurate indicator for identifying differences in mental health between men and women. However, there are variations in marital relationships and the ways in which particular features of the relationship, such as the degree of role differentiation and shared power, act as a risk or a protective factor. Marital status does not lead to a unitary role outcome for men and women. For example, the notion of nurturant role assumes the presence of children in the marital relationship, yet it is also the case that 25 per cent of children in the UK are now born outside of wedlock. Similarly, a childless woman in full-time employment may have little in common in terms of role with another married woman, without employment outside of the home, who is also a mother.

The evidence of a link between gender and mental illness based on marital status may also be challenged if other comparisons are made. For example, there are larger discrepancies in mental ill health between single and married people than between married men and women. Busfield (1982) points out that single men are admitted to psychiatric hospital more often than married women. With regards to the explanatory links of different stressors associated with role, Gove does not explore why the same marital female roles seem to act as protective factors in physical illnesses. Whilst married women have higher rates of hospitalization for psychiatric illnesses, married men have higher rates of admission for non-psychiatric illness than married women.

Finally, the definition of mental illness used by Gove to support his hypothesis that women suffer from problems more than men has been subjected to the criticism that he focuses exclusively on certain types of mental disorder, such as depression and phobias. He excludes other types such as organic conditions and personality disorders (Dohrenwend and Dohrenwend 1977; Busfield 1982). A review of community studies carried out during the 1980s showed that although rates for the most common types of disorder are generally higher for women than men, rates reported by one epidemiological study (Regier et al. 1988) showed an almost equal sex ratio by including drug dependency and personality disorders.

These critiques seem to point to the possibility that an apparent excess of female mental disorder may be an artefact of the construction of epidemiological research. However, more recent research provides convincing evidence that undermines the artefact explanation and further supports the likelihood that women's greater risk of depression is a result of differences in roles and in their experience of life events. Nazroo *et al.* (1998) compared men's and women's experience of severe life events. Women were found to be at greater risk of depression than men when the event experienced involved children, housing and reproduction and where there was a clear distinction within households in roles between men and women. This suggests that women's increased risk of depression is a result of gendered role differences which are associated with differences in the type and experience of life events. Similarly, in relation to marital violence, gender differences in rates of anxiety (which are higher among women) have been attributed to the nature and meaning of physical abuse experienced by women (Nazroo 1995). Sociological research such as this, which focuses on the meaning and context of events provides us with a deeper understanding of the relationship between key variables identified by traditional social psychiatric epidemiology. Differences in the way in which men and women seek help from services may also account for their over-representation in mental health statistics.

Sex differences in help-seeking behaviour

There is not necessarily a direct relationship between experiencing symptoms and the decision to seek help. Symptoms are experienced more frequently than rates of medical consultation and admission to hospital suggest (the 'clinical iceberg', see Chapter 1). Patterns and processes of help-seeking are influenced by people's experience of illness, the way in which services and professionals have responded to people in the past and the levels of social support and alternative health care resources available to them in the community (Rogers *et al.* 1998). In the case of psychological symptoms, it is likely that the 'clinical iceberg' is larger than is the case with physical illness, because of the stigma of mental illness, the perceived ineffectiveness of medical interventions and a greater tendency to deny symptoms. Scambler *et al.* (1981) interviewed 74 working-class women and found that only 1 in 74 subjects who suffered 'nervous depression' or irritability consulted their GP, compared with 1 in 9 for sore throats. There is also some evidence to suggest that people with psychological symptoms delay seeking formal help for a long time. Rogers, Pilgrim and Lacey (1993) found that the time-lag between experiencing psychological symptoms and seeking professional help was more than 1 year for 20 per cent in their survey of 516 post-discharge psychiatric patients.

The relationship between experiencing symptoms is further complicated in psychological distress because of the high rates of formal referral by other people. In the study by Rogers *et al.* (1993), in nearly two-thirds of cases, help was sought by others or in conjunction with others. Thus, a decision to seek formal help in the case of psychological distress is a complex process dependent on both the incipient patient's and others' notions of mental health problems and the translation of the experience of these problems (e.g. tiredness, hallucinations, etc.) into a willingness to contact formal agencies.

At the community level, the relationship between gender and the 'real' rate of mental disorder may be distorted. Reported rates of symptoms in community studies may not be due to a greater incidence of mental disorder as measured by 'clinical symptoms', but a reflection of women's greater propensity to be disclosing about their symptoms. Self-reported morbidity is determined not only by the presence or absence of clinical symptoms but also by the perception and interpretation of symptoms by the person, together with their willingness to report illness in an interview situation. This entails a willingness to label/view problems in psychiatric terms and to seek help once a problem has been defined. Both these interlinked processes may be influenced by differences in attitudes, norms, values and expectations between men and women. Debating this issue in the 1970s, Dohrenwend and Dohrenwend (1977: 1338) asserted: 'Sex differences in the seeking of help correspond to attitudinal differences: women are more likely to admit distress . . . to define their problems in mental-health terms . . . and to have favourable attitudes towards psychiatric treatment.'

Women, then, may be more likely to recognize and label mental illness than men or, put another way, men may be less likely to view their problems as psychiatric ones. There certainly appears to have been an assumption on the part of researchers that women are more likely to be able and willing to talk about their mental health than men. This may, in turn, account for the female focus of much of mental health research, which we will discuss later. An example of how researchers operated such an assumption is in the cited community survey of Brown and Harris (1978), who are quite explicit that their choice of a female-only sample stemmed from a gender assumption: 'It also seemed likely that women, who are more often at home during the day, would be more willing to agree to see us for several hours . . . most of the women we approached were willing to talk to us at length about their lives and appeared to enjoy doing so' (Brown and Harris 1978: 22).

Women may also be more likely to act on their mental health symptoms than men by seeking professional help. It has been estimated that, in the US, women are approximately twice as likely as men to refer themselves for psychiatric treatment. Men, on the other hand, have been found more frequently to seek help on the advice of others (Kadushin 1969). Community studies suggest that, for those considered to be suffering from severe psychological distress (measured by the General Health Questionnaire) sex ratios for primary health care consultations are almost identical. However, in terms of overall rates of consultation with a GP, women appear to consult more than men (Williams *et al.* 1986; Rickwood and Braithwaite 1994).

It seems unlikely that this higher propensity to seek help is due to women having more spare time to visit the doctor than men. Women who combine maternal, domestic and employment roles have less time on their hands than employed men or housewives, and housewives work longer hours than employed men. However, Verbrugge and Wingard (1987) argue that women's roles, as part-time workers or housewives, may allow them greater flexibility (not time *per se*) to visit the doctor. Because of gendered assumptions about caring, women also make contact with GPs when taking their children to be seen for minor ailments. However, there is also some evidence to suggest that women with young children may put their children's health needs before their own and inhibits them entering the sick role (Brown and Harris 1978;

Rogers *et al.* 1999). Additionally, it may be that higher rates of consultation are not due only, or mainly, to the active help-seeking actions of women. Women's own accounts of stress, anxiety and depression seem to suggest that women normalize the mental health problems they report (Walters 1993) which is not commensurate with problem recognition associated with help-seeking from formal services. Moreover, a study of women's pathways to care in post-natal depression suggests that only one-third of women considered to be post-natally depressed by primary care professionals believed they were suffering from the condition. Over 80 per cent had not reported their symptoms to any health professional (Whitton *et al.* 1996). This suggests that contact with health services for other reasons, such as the seeking of health care for children, may allow for increased detection of problems which may contribute to seemingly higher consultation rates for female mental health problems.

Are women labelled as mentally ill more often than men?

A different explanation for female over-representation in mental health statistics is proposed by some feminist researchers, influenced both by labelling theory and constructivist frameworks. From this viewpoint, patriarchal authority, which seeks out and labels women as mad, is responsible for the over-representation. Women become vulnerable to being labelled mentally disordered when they fail to conform to stereotypical gender roles as mothers, housewives, etc., if they are too submissive, too aggressive or hostile to men.

Feminist writers argue that there is both a general cultural sexism, which renders women vulnerable to psychiatric labelling, and a specific sexism from professionals. Chesler (1972: 115) claims that, at a general societal level, there is a tendency to pathologize female behaviour: 'Women, by definition, are viewed as psychiatrically impaired – whether they accept or reject the female role – simply because they are women.'

Evidence for the pathologizing of women's behaviour by lay people can be detected in a study in which women were found to be more likely to come to the attention of a social worker for action under mental health legislation if they were married than if they were single. This confirms previous findings, which have shown that friends and relatives are crucial in applying labels at what Goffman (1961) refers to as the 'pre-patient' phase.

More specifically, medical discourse is deemed to be patriarchal and misogynistic. Here, Chesler's analysis has much in common with those of other feminist writers on health and illness who have viewed male doctors as defining illness with reference to women's emotions (e.g. English and Ehrenreich 1976). The profession of psychiatry is, according to Chesler, numerically male dominated and permeated by patriarchal stereotypes of female inferiority. This situation has arisen as a result of a historical legacy. As medicine, including psychiatry, successfully professionalized during the eighteenth and nineteenth centuries, so women healers became marginalized and excluded from positions of power. This male domination influences the way in which psychiatric diagnoses are applied to women as well as the types of diagnosis and the rates at which they are applied.

There is some evidence that these patriarchal assumptions are not confined to psychiatrists, but are operating in other parts of the mental health service. Barrett and Roberts (1978) found that male GPs construed their middle-aged female patients to be overly neurotic and requiring minor tranquillizers more than male patients. The doctors also often thought that the distressed women who worked would be better off resigning and they expressed a greater sympathy for male counterparts. Goldberg and Huxley (1980) also found that GPs are not as likely to identify a psychological problem if the patient is a man. Milliren (1977) studied older patients and found that male GPs diagnosed women as suffering from anxiety symptoms more often than men. When the latter were diagnosed they were offered minor tranquillizers less often than women by the GPs.

Sheppard (1991) provided further evidence that GPs discriminate against women. Doctors were found to be more likely to refer women as candidates for compulsory admission than men. According to Sheppard, this reflects the sexist practices of GPs, because their decisions were not always confirmed. That is, many of the female referrals were not subsequently deemed suitable for compulsory admission by Approved Social Workers (social workers specially trained in mental health law). Social work is a predominantly female profession. This was considered by Sheppard to be evidence of women workers being able to counteract the sexist practices of the predominantly male group of GPs.

However, others have found evidence of sexist stereotyping of female roles amongst social workers in relation to women with severe mental health problems (Davis et al. 1985). This suggests that having a predominantly female profession might not eliminate sexist practices. Similarly, Chesler's theoretical position rests on the premise that in the psychiatric profession women are massively outnumbered by men. Yet, statistics on the number of medical graduates embarking on psychiatry as a career suggests that psychiatry is rapidly becoming a less male-dominated system in terms of the ratio of male to female practitioners (Parkhouse 1991). This casts some doubt on the assumption that a numerically male-dominated psychiatric profession is solely responsible for sexist psychiatric practice.

It is likely that sexism in psychiatry has its roots in, and can be transmitted in, the type of knowledge, diagnostic categories and practices followed by the profession as well, which can still be called 'patriarchal' even when used by women doctors. Another dimension of feminist analysis has drawn attention to the assumptions inherent in the ideology of psychiatry. Disordered behaviour is defined according to what is considered normal or ordered mental health.

Research by Broverman et al. (1970) provides evidence of bias in the construction of notions of mental health and illness. This research showed that behaviour defined as 'male' is viewed by psychiatrists to be congruent with healthy behaviour, whilst behaviour defined as 'female' is not. Healthy women were in comparative terms considered to be more submissive, less independent and adventurous, more easily influenced, less aggressive, less competitive, more excitable in minor crises, seen as having their feelings more easily hurt, being more emotional, more narcissistic about their appearance and less objective than healthy men. Women were couched in primarily negative terms, even images of healthy women were perceived as less healthy than men.

Fabrikant (1974) reported that male therapists rated 70 per cent of 'female' concepts as negative, whereas they rated 71 per cent of 'male' concepts as positive. These recent examples of negative stereotyping can be found even in biographical forms of psychiatric knowledge, such as psychoanalysis. Masson's historical investigations of psychoanalysis reveal psychotherapists disbelieving reports from female patients of incestuous assaults on them, and compounding their distress through new abuse during treatment (Masson 1985, 1988a).

Gendered notions of mental health and illness seem to be prevalent amongst lay people as well as mental health professionals. Jones and Cochrane (1981) found from responses to a series of scales made up of terms depicting opposite personal characteristic (e.g. 'outgoing' versus 'withdrawn', 'sensitive' versus 'insensitive') that respondents clearly differentiated in the adjectives they chose to describe the differences between mentally ill men and women. In contrast, the terms used to describe normal women and mentally ill women were similar.

According to Showalter (1987), in her popular book *The Female Malady*, this feminized view of madness has its roots in the cultural representations of the nineteenth century. Images found in literature, legal and medical texts, as well as in visual imagery (paintings and photographs) of this period, suggest a connection between women and madness. This replaced the typical eighteenth-century cultural representation, which equated madness with the unruly and frenzied male. Societal ideas about femininity have, in turn, influenced psychiatric judgements and become established in psychiatric knowledge. Busfield (1982) has provided evidence of the sexism of contemporary diagnostic characteristics by examining psychiatric texts. She found that differentiation of types of disorder are ordered by sex-specific characteristics. For instance, in the case of the description of phobic disorders, abnormality and femininity converge, 'to the extent that women are expected and permitted to be more fearful and anxious than men' (Busfield 1982: 55).

So far, a picture has been presented of how others have sought to define mental illness in a feminized way. As well as professionals and lay people constructing problems in this manner, there are also indications that patients conceptualize their problems in a sex-specific way. Rogers *et al.* (1993) found that women were more likely to identify marital stress as the source of their difficulties. By contrast, men reported work stress to be of relevance three times more often than did women. This suggests that relationships in the domestic arena seem to take on a greater meaning for women than men. Women were also found to share their difficulties with others more readily than men. Women were more likely to choose their lay network of friends and neighbours as their first attempt to seek help.

There is some evidence to suggest that this willingness to disclose is reversed once contact has been made with professionals. A Dutch study (de Boer 1991) has claimed that problem formulation in therapeutic encounters is a product of the interaction of two different discourses – that of the therapist and that of the patient. Sex differences in 'problem formulation' were found in so far as men appeared to be more able to account for their problem in a therapeutic situation than women, who appeared to be more diffident. As a result, male influence on the definition and formulation of a problem at this stage may be greater than the influence of women.

A caution needs to be introduced about generalizing about the willingness of women to disclose and seek voluntary primary care or outpatient contact compared to men. This picture seems to hold true for white patients in European and North American clinical settings. However, the literature on ethnic minority women suggests a tendency for them to under-utilise such voluntary service contact opportunities (Padgett *et al.* 1994). The latter US study found that black and Hispanic women had a lower probability of accessing outpatient services than white women from similar class backgrounds. Overall, if race and class differences are ignored, women use out-patient mental health services more than men (Rhodes and Goering 1994) but within the female picture are racialized subgroups which are treated differently. For example, when young black women do have service contact they are offered less psychological treatment than white women (Cuffe *et al.* 1995).

There has been a tendency to view the social causation and the labelling explanation as contradictory, i.e. the over-representation of women is caused by either women's social situation making them sick or the pathologizing of women by a male-dominated mental health service (e.g. Allen 1986). However, Busfield (1988: 536–7) has suggested that these theories are not contradictory but complementary:

> To argue that the phenomena which have historically come to be constituted as mental illness have their roots in the difficulties of women's lives is not inconsistent with the view that the social nature and social consequences of defining a woman as mentally ill need to be emphasised. Neither is it inconsistent with the assertion that the label mental illness given current ideas and practices, often construes the phenomena in question in ways that are antithetical to a woman's needs and ignores the social conditions which give rise to their problems. Nor is it inconsistent with the suggestion that the identification of women's behaviour as pathological often involves the exercise of patriarchal power.

The effects of labelling secondary deviance – women and minor tranquillizers

In Chapter 1 we introduced the notions of primary and secondary deviance. Whatever the reasons why and how women enter the sick role in a psychiatric sense, a consequence is that they are subjected to more frequent medical and professional attention than men. They also tend to seek help and are diagnosed more frequently than men when suffering from problems that are dealt with by GPs. It is here that a recent controversy has arisen over the way in which women's problems are viewed and treated. In particular, attention has been directed towards the prescription of minor tranquillizers because of their addictive and dependency-inducing properties. Women consume psychotropic drugs in far greater quantities than men (Olfson and Pincus 1994). This is despite evidence which suggests that women express a strong antipathy to using drugs to solve their problems (Gabe and Lipshitsz Phillips 1982). By 1980, the excess of the female rate of consumption was estimated as 2:1, with four-fifths of this consumption being attributed to minor tranquillizers and sedative hypnotics (Cooperstock 1978). The date of this review might suggest that we should consider a lower estimate of minor tranquillizer prescription now. Table 3.2 indicates a steady decline in benzodiazepine

Table 3.2 Number of NHS prescriptions for benzodiazepines 1978–89 in Great Britain (millions)

	Year											
	1978	1979	1980	1981	1982	1983	1984	1985	1986	1987	1988	1989
Temazepam	0.3	0.7	1.3	2.1	3.1	3.6	4.2	6.3	7.2	7.8	7.7	7.1
Nitrazepam	10.2	10.1	9.0	8.4	7.9	7.0	6.4	6.0	5.5	5.2	4.6	4.2
Diazepam	11.1	10.5	8.8	8.0	7.1	6.2	5.4	5.4	5.2	5.1	4.5	4.1
Triazolam	–	0.2	0.5	1.0	1.1	1.1	1.3	1.6	2.0	2.2	2.2	2.1
Lorazepam	1.8	2.1	2.4	2.9	3.5	3.5	3.2	3.1	3.1	2.9	2.1	1.7
Chlordiazepoxide	2.9	2.6	2.2	2.0	1.8	1.6	1.3	1.2	1.1	1.0	0.9	0.8
Oxazepam	0.7	0.7	0.7	0.8	0.8	0.7	0.6	0.7	0.8	0.8	0.6	0.5
Lormetazepam	–	–	–	0.0*	0.2	0.4	0.5	0.1	0.2	0.2	0.2	0.2
Loprazolam	–	–	–	–	0.0	0.0	0.1	0.0	0.1	0.1	0.2	0.2
Clonazepam	0.0	0.0	0.0	0.1	0.1	0.1	0.1	0.1	0.1	0.1	0.1	0.1
Clobazam	–	0.1	0.3	0.4	0.5	0.5	0.5	0.1	0.0	0.0	0.1	0.1
Alprazolam	–	–	–	–	–	0.2	0.3	0.1**	–	–	–	–
Flurazepam	2.1	2.3	2.3	2.2	2.2	2.0	2.0	0.5	–	–	–	–
Clorazepate	1.0	1.0	1.2	1.1	1.2	1.2	1.3	0.3	–	–	–	–
Flunitrazepam	–	–	–	–	0.0	0.1	0.2	0.1	–	–	–	–
Bromazepam	–	–	–	–	0.0	0.1	0.2	0.0	–	–	–	–
Ketazolam	–	–	0.0	0.1	0.2	0.2	0.2	0.0	–	–	–	–
Medazepam	0.3	0.3	0.2	0.2	0.2	0.2	0.1	0.0	–	–	–	–
Prazepam	–	–	–	–	0.0	0.0	0.0	0.0	–	–	–	–
Total	30.6	30.9	29.1	29.5	29.7	28.7	28.0	25.7	25.3	25.5	23.2	22.1

* 0.0 = fewer than 50,000 prescriptions
** Limited list became effective, April 1985
Source: Hansard, 31 March 1988, cols 657–8w; 27 February 1990, 121–2w; 4 December 1990, 75–6w. Cited in Medawar (1992)

use during the 1980s. However, as can be seen from the totals at the end of the table, by the late 1980s the prescription rate was still over two-thirds of that a decade earlier, despite both litigation/campaigning from addicted users and cautions from professional bodies such as the Royal College of Psychiatrists (Medawar 1992). This limitation, rather than elimination, of benzodiazepine use suggests that women are still taking more psychotropic pills than men.

The prescription of minor tranquillizers can be seen as a medicalized response to personal troubles. From this vantage point the benefits of a medical response are to remove personal responsibility from the individual for their problems. For example, the guilt and unhappiness associated with depression can be dealt with simplistically if it is framed as an illness, which can be relieved by mood-altering drugs, rather than the responsibility of the individual's actions and their social circumstances.

However, from a different perspective, the prescription and use of such drugs are viewed as a means of 'social control' because they transform social problems into medical ones. The social effects of treating personal problems by medical sedation have been highlighted by Waldron (1977). She points out that the treatment of individual 'pathology' disguises its social causes and deflects attention from the need for political change to ameliorate the oppression of women.

Gabe and Thorogood (1986) found that women were most likely to find benzodiazepines to be a 'prop' in the absence of other means of support, such as paid work, adequate housing, leisure activities, and so on. This was particularly so in the case of middle-aged women, who were less likely than other women to have access to resources with which to manage their everyday lives. Women tended to express ambivalent views about taking minor tranquillizers: on the one hand, they expressed the view that they gave them 'peace of mind', and on the other, they emphasized the dangers and dependency-inducing aspects of taking these drugs.

Paradoxically, perhaps, in publicizing the dangers of addiction, women who have been prescribed such drugs have been subject to what labelling theorists refer to as 'deviance amplification'. The media, in taking up the problem of minor tranquillizer dependency, has tended to reinforce images of women as helpless, dependent and passive victims of addictive drugs (Bury and Gabe 1990). Not only did their original behaviour or primary deviance expose women more frequently to an addictive prescribed drug but the consequent addiction then became associated with their gender.

Does this additional labelling of women imply that they are subjected to medical control more frequently than men? Their greater contact with services and the minor tranquillizer problem being labelled as a 'women's problem' might imply that this is the case. Certainly feminist scholarship has been instrumental in gaining a wider recognition of the ways in which women have been oppressed by being labelled as mentally ill. This in turn has led to the setting up of alternative services. The Women's Therapy Centre in North London was set up with the explicit aim of providing feminist therapy that rejected patriarchal assumptions and was centred around enhancing individual woman's power and responsibility. According to Scambler (1998), the service also retained a collective notion and awareness of the social by providing group support aimed at re-socializing women to reject a subordinate position within domestic and social life. However, as Scambler points out, being outside of state-provided services means that access to the Centre may be denied to those in most need. Moreover, Pilgrim (1997a) has argued even feminist therapies retain the power discrepancies between therapists and patients inherent in all styles of psychotherapy and they retain many patriarchal elements intrinsic to the psychoanalytical legacy.

Men and psychiatry

As we noted in our interpretation of official statistics at the beginning of this chapter, it is not possible to make generalized claims about the overall predominance of mental disorder being an essentially male or female phenomenon. The nature and construction of mental health problems differ according to history, category and cultural context. However, the discussion of male mental disorder is, compared with the feminist literature on women and mental health, rare. This corresponds to a more generalized tendency in the sociology of health and illness in recent years to focus on female rather than male health disadvantage (Cameron and Bernardes 1998). An exception to this is research conducted into male unemployment and mental health. There is evidence to suggest that the experience of unemployment is detrimental to men's mental health because of the dissonance this gives rise to between a masculine self-image and social expectations of men being in full-time paid employment (Hayes and Nutman 1981). Studies have also taken as their focus the variation in male mental health according to wider economic and employment opportunities (Warner 1985). However, if we put to one side these studies looking at unemployment, the sociological discourse about gender and mental health is female dominated. Let us look at two examples of the different considerations given by both psychiatrists and sociologists to men and women with regard first to dangerousness and then to sexuality.

Gender and dangerousness

Men's behaviour is more frequently recognized as dangerous than women's. Indeed, men are violent more often than women in society, but consequently all men (including non-violent ones) may be subjected to stereotypical expectations. Comparisons are sometimes made between the statistics which show women to be over-represented in mental health populations whilst men predominate in criminal statistics. This may be related to the type of social judgement which is made about 'rule breaking'.

The recognition both of mental disorder and of criminality involve judgements being made about a person's state of mind and their conduct. In conditions such as depression, the judgement being made is more about a person's anguished and irrational state of mind, judged by their social withdrawal and 'motor retardation'. By contrast, a criminal act is more about a person's self-interested motivation, judged by the manifest gain made from their offence. However, both entail judgements about the relationship between mind and conduct – and weighing up the nature of this relationship decides whether the deviance ascribed is of a criminal or psychiatric type. As we noted in Chapter 1, these distinctions between rational or goal directed, and irrational or incomprehensible, rule breaking are not always clear-cut in the minds of either professionals or of lay people.

The connection between these considerations and gender is that men's conduct has been more associated with public antisocial acts, violent and sexual offences, drunken aggressive behaviour, etc., whereas women's behaviour has been associated more with private, self-damaging acts, where aggression is directed at the self rather than others, depression, parasuicide, eating disorders, self-mutilation, etc. Men are more likely to indulge in behaviour that is antisocial, and to be labelled as criminally deviant more than women. This is then reflected within psychiatry, in that men are more likely to have labels which refer to and incorporate the threat of their behaviour.

The notion of 'danger to others' is more frequently ascribed to male than female patients. The question of 'danger to self' is more complicated. Although women attempt suicide more frequently then men, the figures for actual suicide are consistently higher for men than women. However, a Finnish study of parasuicidal behaviour suggests that men make more gestures of suicide, as well as committing suicide more often (Ostamo and Lonnqvist 1992). Of course, suicidal and parasuicidal behaviours are ambiguous – they may be adjudged to be either self-injurious or antisocial or both. This may account for the prevalence being split between the two sexes and the contradictory findings about the ratio of such a split.

The affixing of diagnostic labels which imply 'dangerousness' and the focus on the behavioural consequences of a person's state of mind has corresponding implications. Female problems are more likely to be dealt with at the 'soft' end of psychiatry since, as we have already seen, they tend to be labelled with the type of problem that is usually dealt with in primary health care settings. Although such management is by no means always benign, as demonstrated by the negative effects of the reliance on minor tranquillizers discussed above, it more rarely requires compulsory admission. By contrast, men are more likely to be dealt with at the 'harsh' end of psychiatry.

Thus, once a label has been affixed, overall as a group, men are in some respects dealt with more punitively than women. This is especially the case at the interface between psychiatry and the criminal justice system. It is mainly men who are over-represented in the most stigmatized and policed part of the mental health system, the 'special hospitals'. Though many in these institutions are there for sex offences and other violent crime and their behaviour or threat to society might have warranted such a response, many have not been convicted of a criminal offence. The effect of such management can be seen not only in the negative media stereotypes portraying the inmates of such hospitals as 'animals', but also in recurrent government inquiries into the mistreatment of special hospital patients.

With regard to psychiatric referrals from the police, under section 136 of the Mental Health Act 1983 there is evidence to suggest that men are subject to arrest more frequently than women. Moreover, the police use handcuffs and detention cells more frequently for men than women (Rogers 1990).

Even where the differences in the rate at which a diagnostic label is attached is not great, the negative consequences of a label may be greater for
men than women. This can be seen in the case of schizophrenia in western
countries, where, overall, there is little difference in incidence between men
and women, as Table 3.1 shows, currently men are slightly over-represented.
There are, however, wide differences between the sexes in the incidence of
the illness at different ages. It has been estimated that the occurrence is twice
as great for men aged 15–24 than for women of the same age. For women
the peak age is between 25 and 34 (Warner 1985: 231). This may reflect
career and work related stress upon men at this stage in their lives.

Because men are diagnosed younger, when they are physically at their
strongest, this may induce more coercive actions from professionals during a
crisis. (We will return to the handling of aggression in black male patients in
Chapter 4.) Additionally, a greater prevalence of schizophrenia in males has
been reported for many developing countries. Just as the domestic role has
disadvantages associated with it, as pointed out in the study by Brown and
Harris, in other contexts it can be seen as a protective factor for women. One
possible implication of this is that as the proportion of women in the labour
force rises, so we can expect an increase in 'schizophrenia'.

The course of schizophrenia is also, in some ways, more benign for women
than men. Warner (1985: 142) reports that, historically, the proportion of
patients discharged as recovered is consistently higher for women. Differences in prognosis have also been noted. In the World Health Organization
(WHO 1979) international study of schizophrenia, proportionally fewer
women were in the worst outcome group at follow-up, and more were in the
best outcome category. In industrial countries women tend to have shorter
episodes of schizophrenia.

If we look at other disease categories, then the male/female distinction
drawn by feminist analysis above is only applicable to a western social context. In other places, men do worse than women. For example, cross-cultural
studies of depression show a slightly higher proportion of men than women
suffering from depression (Carstairs and Kapur 1976). Whilst women take
sick leave for minor psychiatric problems more often than men, the latter
tend to be off work for longer periods (Hensing *et al.* 1996). In relation to
domestic roles, women are more likely to be the victims of domestic violence
than their male partners, leading some analysts to argue that this might
account for raised primary care consultations and psychotropic drug use in
female patients (Mazza and Dennerstein 1996). These studies suggest that it
is the roles and context of people's situations that influence the type and
rate of mental distress, rather than anything intrinsic or constant about
being a man or woman. In some contexts, work outside the home can be a
threat to mental health, just as the domestic environment can. If domestic
violence were to equalize between men and women or be inverted then men
might well have raised levels of primary care diagnosis and prescribed
psychotropic drugs.

Gender and sexuality

The psychiatric response to homosexuality in one sense differs from responses to other types of 'problem' behaviour. Whilst today homosexuality

is designated as problematic by psychiatrists, in the nineteenth century its assumed biological determination led not to active physical intervention (as was the case with madness) but with a fatalism which prompted little therapeutic interest (Bullough 1987). It was only when psychoanalytical and then behavioural therapeutic methods were introduced, during the twentieth century, that psychiatrists began to interfere with homosexuality and aspire to 'cure' the condition.

The very optimism encouraged by these newer environmental/psychological theories of mental disorder prompted professionals to be more interventionist with homosexuals. Moreover, both male and female homosexuality was problematized by psychiatry because it was problematized more widely in western society. As Al-Issa (1987: 155) notes: 'Deviation from gender role expectations is traditionally considered abnormal.' Whilst more recent diagnostic frameworks (e.g. DSM III) no longer include homosexuality, *per se*, as a form of psychiatric disorder, it is retained as 'ego-dystonic homosexuality', when the person is unhappy with themselves. Thus, homosexuals who are unhappy, even within DSM III, remain psychiatric 'cases'. Other roles, say being a musician, cannot become a psychiatric case with unhappiness, there is no 'ego-dystonic musicality'. One of the difficulties in discussing gender and sexuality is that the psychiatric interest in gay men and lesbians has tended to focus on pathologizing or normalizing their sexual orientation (i.e. for it to be cured, understood or tolerated). As Rothblum (1994) has pointed out, there is little research which has investigated the ways in which gay and lesbian identities and lifestyles pose a risk or buffer to mental health problems.

The question for us here is not about wider explanations for psychiatry's response to homosexuality but whether men and women have been treated equitably. Certainly differences in society are discernible. Since the nineteenth century, male not female homosexuality has been designated as criminal. In Great Britain it is no longer criminal but it has a higher age of consent than heterosexuality (21 not 16 years). In the Isle of Man and Northern Ireland it remains illegal and it remains a court martialling offence in the armed services.

Once more, as with dangerousness, differential legal and cultural assumptions about homosexuality seem to associate maleness and antisocial behaviour and lower such an expectation of women. This is also reflected in the therapeutic discourse on homosexuality. Whilst most therapeutic schools have clinical reports, and even research on treatment outcomes, for both gay men and lesbians, male problems are alluded to more frequently or given a greater priority.

This prioritization of men as suitable cases for treatment was at its most exaggerated in the late 1960s and early 1970s, when behaviour therapists attempted to 'cure' male homosexuals using electric shock aversion therapy. More benign behavioural methods were used for lesbian patients requesting reorientation (such as desensitization and assertiveness training) but men were singled out for the aversion treatment. The latter not only failed to induce a shift of sexual orientation in gay men, it merely induced phobic anxiety and impotence in some of its recipients (Diamont 1987).

Another way in which male homosexuals suffer especially restrictive or punitive attention from the mental health system links to the point made above about secure environments. Because there are more men than women in secure psychiatric provision, this means that there are more gay men than lesbians living in closed systems. In such systems, homosexual behaviour is constrained by the lack of privacy permitted for sexual contact. Thus, advocates of women's rights in secure provision understandably complain of the plight of those lesbians who are incarcerated at the 'harsh' end of psychiatry (Stevenson 1992). However, it is logical to deduce that the infringement of homosexual rights must occur with a greater regularity for men than women, as the latter are under-represented in secure provision.

However, the more frequent constraints on male, rather than female, homosexual rights in secure provision needs to be considered alongside the greater vulnerability of women, once they are in such environments. Those women who do find themselves in secure provision are more vulnerable than male patients to sexual harassment and assault, from both patients and staff. Such predatory attention from men is particularly relevant given the type of women appearing in conditions of maximum security. For instance, Potier (1992) reported that 34 out of the 40 female patients with a diagnosis of psychopathy at Ashworth Special Hospital had been sexually abused in childhood or adolescence.

Having addressed the question of dangerousness and sexuality, we can now see why men are treated more harshly than women by psychiatry more often, though the small ratio of women at the secure end of psychiatric services may suffer individually more than men. Thus the focus on the over-representation of women in psychiatric statistics and the relative absence of men from the sociological discourse may gloss over important questions of gender, which are about both women and men.

Discussion

We began the chapter by examining the evidence about women appearing in mental health statistics more often than men. Various possible reasons for this state of affairs were rehearsed. We then went on to examine men and mental disorder, noting that less academic attention had recently been devoted to this. The fact that men may be more inclined to criminal deviance than women, or labelled as such, was suggested as a reason for this. However, in exploring the issue of men and mental disorder further, it is apparent that many of the same arguments that have been made about women and mental disorder are also applicable to men. This can be seen in relation to the influence of social roles and expectations, and in relation to psychiatric knowledge in the gendered construction of psychiatric diagnoses. If women are seen prejudicially as being illogical, then men are seen stereotypically as dangerous.

The concentration on women and mental disorder is a relatively new phenomenon. Gove and Geerken (1977) found that of the 11 pre-Second World War studies reviewed, three showed higher rates of mental disorder for women, whilst eight showed higher rates for men. Following the Second World War, studies showed higher rates for women while none showed higher rates for men. Busfield (1982) notes that higher admission rates for women are a phenomenon of the twentieth but not the nineteenth century.

How might these changes be accounted for? They may be a result of changes in women's social situation and psychiatric practices as Busfield has argued. A further possibility is that feminist scholarship itself may be a factor in constructing women and mental health as an object of study. Put another way, the shift towards identifying higher rates of mental disorder in women may be the result of a change in discourse. As the discourse changes, so too do the objects of attention. Identifying women as an object of study, in itself may accentuate the 'female character' of mental ill-health, establishing it as an essentially women's problem. For example, the work of Brown and Harris is often cited in texts as evidence that depression is a female problem. From this it may be inferred that the same problems are not experienced by men. However, Brown and Harris did not set out to study men, who were excluded from the research design at the outset. Therefore, from this study we do not know anything about the nature of male depression. If research is directed at women, to the exclusion of men, it is likely to produce evidence that links depression to women's experiences and social roles. Also, in attempting to make women more visible, some feminist scholars may have made men relatively invisible. Showalter (1987) attempts to develop *a sui generis* argument about women and madness in the nineteenth century. In so doing, types of madness which were linked to men and masculinity are ignored, giving the impression that only women suffer from mental illness and they, not men, are subject to psychiatric oppression (Busfield 1991). Busfield notes that Showalter attended selectively to gendered images of the female lunatic, distorting the topic of madness into a focused patriarchal medical attack on women. As we noted above, men are treated coercively by psychiatric professionals more often than women. Showalter's historical reconstruction is repeated uncritically, without Busfield's caution, in texts on women and mental health (e.g. Barnes and Maple 1992) and so it remains an important part of feminist discourse.

Feminists make much of the social disadvantage under which women suffer. Indeed, socio-economic indicators do demonstrate unequivocally that, overall, women suffer greater material deprivation than men. Notwithstanding such evidence, it is clear that particular groups of men are also subject to social disadvantage. There may be substantial evidence that men make women mentally sick, by stressing and labelling them more often than vice versa. However, the existence of a large number of men who are mentally disordered and particularly disadvantaged means that an exclusive focus on women and mental health precludes a full picture of the relationship between gender and psychiatry.

Rather than focusing on men or women and psychiatry, comparative analyses of men and women along a range of dimensions, including treatment, behaviour and portrayal of images of abnormality, are needed. In addition to gender, other variables need to be taken into consideration in understanding the mental health of women and men. What is clear in understanding gender and mental disorder is the need to focus more on the context and meaning of the cause and experience of mental health problems. As we have argued elsewhere (Pilgrim and Rogers 1994), a close relationship with social psychiatry had created one form of sociological analysis, following Durkheim, of treating mental health problems as social facts. Useful as this may be at showing the social origins of mental health problems, an understanding of the relationship between agency and structure, when considering the gendered nature of mental health problems, is also required. A recognition of meaning and context is also relevant to responding to the differing needs of men and women using mental health services. We return to this issue in the chapter on treatment. As will be seen in the next two chapters, gender as a variable in mental health is overlain by age and race.

To conclude

Gender and mental health has been considered extensively by sociologists. However, there has been an overwhelming focus on women. Paradoxically, this may have contributed to a discourse linking women and psychological vulnerability. It also disguises an underlying set of processes which make some men particularly vulnerable to coercive psychiatric treatment. Despite the continuing interest in gender and mental health, there is still not a clear sociological account of *why* women are over-represented in the way they are in psychiatric populations. This chapter has rehearsed some factors which can be seen as additive or competing factors in this regard.

Questions

1 Which factors might explain why women are over-represented in mental health statistics?

2 Provide a critical account of *The Female Malady*.

3 Provide a socio-historical account of psychiatry's response to homo-sexuality.

4 What has the *Social Origins of Depression* taught us about gender and mental health?

5 Why do women take more psychiatric drugs than men?

6 Why have men been overlooked in sociological studies of mental health?

For discussion

Consider arguments for and against the notion that women are less mentally healthy than men.

Further reading

Barnes, M. and Maple, N. (1992) *Women and Mental Health: Challenging the Stereotypes*. Birmingham: Venture Press.

Busfield, J. (1996) *Men, Women and Madness: Understanding Gender and Mental Disorder*. London: Routledge.

Kaplan, M.S. and Marks, G. (1995) Appraisal of health risks: the roles of masculinity, femininity and sex, *Sociology of Health and Illness* 17, 2: 206–221.

Nazroo, J.Y., Edwards, A.C. and Brown, G.W. (1998) Gender differences in the prevalence of depression: artefact, alternative disorders, biology or roles? *Sociology of Health and Illness* 20, 3: 3112–330.

Chapter **4**

Race and ethnicity

Chapter overview

This chapter will examine investigations into the relationship between mental ill-health and race. We will focus on the psychiatric response to Afro-Caribbean, Asian and Irish people in Britain. As in the chapter on gender, evidence about higher recorded rates of psychopathology amongst black and ethnic minority groups can be considered by different types of analysis, which can be framed as a number of questions. For instance, in Britain are Afro-Caribbean people 'madder' than white people because of their 'culture' or extra social stress, or are they labelled as mad by indigenous white people without just cause? Alternatively, does the knowledge-base of psychiatry, which has sought to explain the high incidence of psychopathology amongst black and ethnic minority groups, tell us more about the way in which these people have been constructed as being 'vulnerable' to mental disorder?

The chapter will cover the following topics:

- Theoretical presuppositions about race

- Race and health

- Racialized psychiatric admissions

- What is the nature of contact with psychiatry?

- Asian women and the somatization thesis

- Irish people and psychiatry

Theoretical presuppositions about race

Until recently, many social scientists rejected the use of the concept of race altogether because of its association with a dubious anthropological tradition left over from the nineteenth century. This used the concept of race to make biological distinctions between groups, and assumed white supremacy. This can be seen in relation to eugenics, the 'science' of racial improvement, which was a backdrop to the development of both anthropology and psychiatry at the end of the last century and the first quarter of this one. In its most extreme form eugenics culminated in the mass extermination of 'racially inferior' groups in Nazi Germany, significantly, along with physically and mentally disabled people of any race (Meyer 1988). The sterilization of mental patients and the eventual killings were instigated by the German medical profession and endorsed by the Nazi Government. Thus, social policies influenced by eugenic principles have intertwined considerations of both race and mental illness.

As Fernando (1988) has pointed out, there has also been a strong medical tradition which has operated on the basis that the brains of black people are inferior to those of white people. So, the link between race and mental illness has historically been a close one and medical-scientific knowledge has been far from neutral about the assumed relationship. It has played a significant role in the perpetuation of pejorative theories and oppressive practices about certain racial groups.

The notion of race within the social sciences is now typically used to refer to 'race relations', which involves the relationship between a dominant community and minority groups. In contrast, socio-cultural differences between groups are usually referred to as 'ethnicity'. This term also usually connotes a collective identity, so it embraces a subjective element for a person. The ways of life of different ethnic groups depend on a combination of their inherited culture and their relations with other cultures. (For a discussion about the various ways contemporary sociologists have addressed the relationship between race and ethnicity see Anthias 1992.)

Much of the debate about minority ethnic groups and health has centred on cultural difference as a way of explaining the differential experience of groups within the community (differences in language, values, norms and beliefs). This type of analysis focuses on the individual, or their culture, and is concerned mainly with examining the role of prejudice and discrimination in determining differences in health behaviour and the use of services.

Within these debates, 'prejudice' implies a psychological concept in that it refers to a set of personal attitudes. Transcultural psychiatry, for example, is concerned with how different ethnic groups are treated by mental health workers socialized in the ways of the 'dominant' culture (Rack 1982). This position advocates initiatives aimed at challenging and changing prejudices through 'race awareness' training. This works on the premise of challenging the stereotypical and negative views about minority ethnic groups held by powerful individuals, like professionals. But what tends to be missing from analyses based on prejudice is a consideration of the impact of inequality – how the latter is manifested in 'mental illness' rates, services and professional responses to black and other minority groups.

In contrast to the prejudice focus, 'racism' implies a sociological rather than a psychological analysis. This concept implicates institutions, not only individuals, in perpetuating disadvantage. For this reason, some commentators have advocated anti-racism (rather than race awareness) as an active strategy to combat institutional racism (Denney 1992). Denney also notes that the term 'black' is ambiguous. For our purposes we will use it to mean people of African, Asian or Caribbean descent. We also recognize that to be seen as 'black' entails being treated differently from white people – it is an oppressed identity (Fevre 1984). In this chapter, racism rather than prejudice will be emphasized. Before we start our examination of race and mental ill-health by reviewing the evidence for the over-representation of certain racial groups in the psychiatric system, a note will be made about race and health.

Race and health

The general health of people from black and ethnic minorities in Britain is poorer than the indigenous white Anglo-Saxon group. It is tempting to explain this purely in terms of the impact of racism. However, a more comprehensive account which respects multi-factorial causality would go beyond the racism explanation. Smaje (1996) suggests that such a fuller account would need to take into consideration the following:

• *Genetics* Because of their eugenic associations social scientists have a tendency to avoid genetic explanations. Whilst most (75 per cent) of the genetic material of human beings is identical and most (85 per cent) of the genetic variation occurs between individuals not races, the latter do show some differences (about 7 per cent of variance). The upshot of this is that some racial groups are more genetically susceptible to certain disorders. For example, there are differential incidence rates of sickle cell disease and phenylketonuria in Africans and North Europeans.
• *Migration* This is a complex topic in itself. Migrants may encounter new health threats in their host country. Also the circumstances of migration may be traumatic both physically and psychologically (as in warfare). Alternatively, it may be linked to high expectations, achieved or dashed, when a migrant wants to move in order to make a new life. Economic motives for migration may lead to racialized patterns of living in the host country, when people of the same origin move to the same area to work in the same employment context. Low paid work in poor areas of inner cities, for example, may lead to health outcomes which affect not just the migrants but subsequent generations.
• *Material disadvantage* Whilst migrants may enhance their wealth by moving, they may at the same time be relatively deprived within their host country. Low pay, housing disadvantage and unemployment make migrants susceptible to the direct health impact of poverty.
• *Cultural factors* Lifestyle, social networks and kinship differences from the host culture may lead to health losses and gains.
• *Racism* The health impact of racism is twofold. First, the direct effect is that racially victimized people are prone to stress, injury and death. Second,

the indirect effect is that racial discrimination in the housing and labour market produce lowered health outcomes.

With these general factors in mind we now turn to evidence about psychiatric admissions.

Racialized psychiatric admissions

Hospital admissions have been used as a measure of the incidence of mental illness amongst different racial and ethnic groups. Establishing a picture of admissions according to race or ethnicity is even more problematic than in relation to gender. Although some health authorities and social services have recently responded to calls for the introduction of 'ethnic monitoring', the presentation of statistical evidence by race or ethnicity is difficult to come by. The Department of Health does not routinely collect or issue data for the racial and ethnic origin of psychiatric patients.

Evidence about the racial and ethnic make up of psychiatric admissions to hospitals tends to be contradictory. Cochrane (1977), analysing 1971 psychiatric admissions, found that rates for Irish, Polish and Scottish immigrants to England and Wales were higher than for native-born people. Rates for those born in the Indian subcontinent were lower, whilst the rate for Caribbean immigrants was virtually the same as for the English-born. This contrasts with the findings of two other studies. Dean et al. (1981), examining first admissions to hospital in south-east England for 1976, found one and a half times the expected numbers for Afro-Caribbean-born people than for British-born people. Carpenter and Brockington (1980) recorded two and half times the rate of admission for Asian-born people and one and a half times the rate for Afro-Caribbean groups than for white British-born people.

There seems to be more consistent evidence for the over-representation of Afro-Caribbean groups in admissions than Asian groups. Of the studies conducted, only Cochrane's study seems to indicate lower rates for Afro-Caribbeans (Hemsi (1967); Rwegellera (1977); Carpenter and Brockington (1980); and Koffman et al. (1997) all found higher rates). For Asian groups the picture is much more variable. Although Carpenter and Brockington found higher rates for Asians overall, Hitch (1981) found higher rates for Pakistani-born people and lower rates for people born in India than native-born.

As well as providing a rather inconsistent picture, these studies suffer from a further methodological weakness. Although they tell us something about the rates of admissions amongst people entering Britain, they tell us little about admissions for different racial and ethnic groups within Britain as a whole. In using place of birth as an indicator of racial and ethnic origin, black people born in Britain are not counted with people entering the country from Africa and the Caribbean. (Currently, approximately 40 per cent of the black population in Britain was born here.) One recent study (McGovern and Cope 1987) attempted to deal with this shortcoming by recording ethnicity independently of place of birth, and found that more Afro-Caribbeans than expected, as measured against numbers in the general population, enter the in-patient system.

As we discussed in Chapter 3, hospital admission records are often incomplete and inaccurate. Consequently, they may be a poor indicator of the incidence and prevalence of mental disorder in the community. Few studies have set out to measure the rates of mental illness among different ethnic groups in ordinary populations. One study carried out in Nottingham did not confine itself to hospital admissions (Harrison *et al.* 1988) but included all patients in contact with psychiatric services over a two-year period. The researchers estimated that the incidence rate of schizophrenia for Afro-Caribbeans was 12 to 13 times higher than that of the general population.

In the psychiatric literature, two types of explanation predominate in attempting to explain the apparent over-representation of Afro-Caribbeans with schizophrenia and the under-representation of Asian groups. The first tends to look for reasons at the level of 'cultural difference'. For example, it has been suggested that the relatively low number of admissions for Asian groups is an accurate reflection of low rates of distress because of psychological robustness or fatalistic attitudes. It has also been suggested that there may be a tendency to avoid contact with services in the Asian community because of the stigma attached to psychiatric conditions or because of the inappropriateness of existing services which results in low uptake. A particular controversy which surrounds the discussion of Asian mental health relates to the adequacy of western psychiatric research to respect diverse meanings of distress (see later discussion).

The second type of explanation in addition to this cultural consideration, suggests a vulnerability to distress related to an adverse environment. That is, social deprivation and unfavourable conditions, such as financial difficulties, racial harassment and discrimination over housing, are implicated. However, since few studies have systematically investigated the impact of external stressors on the mental health of black people, the consequences of racism in employment, housing and education have not been assessed adequately. None the less, black mental health groups themselves describe diverse forms of stress derived from racism, which affect their mental health.

In one study, Afro-Caribbean users identified a variety of factors to explain their mental health problems. These included: problems of coping with adolescence and the education system, which builds up and then dashes expectations; growing up in a hostile environment with few positive images of black people; and parental and British white cultural input leading to confusion and conflict over identity (Frederick 1991). Another study has illuminated how Asian women tended to identify isolation and cultural differences as the root of their problems (Fenton and Sadiq 1991) whilst Asian men identified feelings of powerlessness as a result of unemployment or racism (Beliappa 1991).

It would seem that a simple social stress hypothesis, with poverty and racism predominating as causal variables, cannot be sufficient to account for the data available on psychiatric morbidity. After all, in poor inner city areas, Asian people as well as Afro-Caribbean people suffer recurrent racism. And yet, overall, the evidence seems to point to only the latter being over-represented in psychiatric records, not the former. This is not to argue that different racial and ethnic groups do not experience peculiar stressors, which lead to mental health problems emerging in particular individuals. But it would seem that such external stress is not a strong enough unitary explanation to account for the group data on over-representation amongst Afro-Caribbeans (or the Irish, as we will see later).

Community studies, as well as those that have examined admissions to hospital, have been criticized on methodological grounds, casting considerable doubt on the validity of their conclusions. Such criticisms include the unreliability of the diagnosis of schizophrenia, which means that data about ethnic groups is subject to a large margin of error (Sashidaran 1993). In the case of the Harrison study above, for example, it has been noted that: 'If one case was misclassified a 4 per cent change in incidence would be recorded. Likewise, if they [the researchers] had under-counted the number of people in the population deemed at risk by 200 the incidence recorded would be reduced by 40 per cent' (Francis *et al.* 1989: 161). Fernando (1988) has also pointed out that because these studies tend to be suffused with cultural stereotypes, it is difficult to make accurate estimates about 'true rates' of mental illness amongst different groups. He cites the example of a study by Bebbington *et al.* (1981), which attempted to explain the lower levels of minor psychiatric disorders, such as depression amongst Caribbean-born people, by their tendency to respond to adversity with 'cheery denial'.

In addition to explanations which focus on 'cultural' differences, or vulnerability to mental distress according to ethnicity, a third possible explanation lies with the way in which others involved with psychiatric practice respond to black people. This issue will be considered in relation to initial service contact and subsequent treatment.

Afro-Caribbean people are much more likely than white people to make contact with psychiatry via the police, courts and prison. In Britain, the police have specific powers under section 136 of the Mental Health Act 1983 to detain persons for up to 72 hours, in 'a place of safety', if they are considered to be mentally disordered and a danger to themselves or other people. Recent research on section 136 has shown rates of detention for Afro-Caribbean people to be up to two and a half times the rate of white people compared with the numbers living in the locality. The Afro-Caribbean people detained by the police also tend to be young and male (Bean *et al.* 1991).

Part III of the Mental Health Act 1983 also makes provision for dealing with patients concerned in criminal proceedings or serving a prison sentence ('mentally disordered offenders'). Here too, young black men are much more likely to come into contact with forensic psychiatry than white equivalents. Migrant and British-born second generation Afro-Caribbean men have been found to be referred 29 times more frequently than their white counterparts (McGovern and Cope 1987; Cope 1989). Although there has been no investigation of black people admitted to the Special Hospitals (maximum security hospitals), one study which looked at those discharged from them (Norris 1984) found higher than expected numbers of 'non-white' men compared with the proportion in the general population. Also, the 'non-white' group had committed less serious offences prior to admission. At each point of the processing of the criminal justice and mental health systems there appears to be a staged increase in discrimination. For example a report found black defendants, deemed to be mentally vulnerable, less likely than white defendants to be given bail and more likely to receive court orders involving compulsory psychiatric treatment (Browne 1990). At the other end of the spectrum from coercive psychiatry, there is evidence to suggest that black people are

under-represented in outpatient and self-referred services (Littlewood and
Cross 1980) and are less likely than other groups to be referred by general
practitioners (Hitch and Clegg 1980).

Why is it that black people come into contact with psychiatry in this way?
A number of interrelated factors appear to be implicated. There have been
suggestions that the culture of black people makes them more susceptible to
being identified by lay people and the police. The crux of this type of argument is that black people express their distress in a culturally idiosyncratic
way (Littlewood and Lipsedge 1982). It has been suggested, for example, that
the manifestation of 'mental illness' predisposes Afro-Caribbeans towards
police arrest because they present in a particularly disturbed or violent way
(Rwegellera 1977; Hitch and Clegg 1980; Harrison *et al.* 1988). More recent
evidence points to both a relative low registration with primary care services
on the part of Afro-Caribbean people who are subsequently admitted to
hospital (Koffman *et al.* 1997) and lower rates of treatment for depression
compared to other ethnic groups when they are in contact with these services (Nazroo 1997). The place where this behaviour takes place is also thought
to be significant. According to Bean (1986) if a greater part of young Afro-
Caribbean social life takes place in public, then 'mad' behaviour is more
likely to be detected and dealt with by agents, such as the police, than is the
case of white people, who have more of an 'indoor culture'.

As was mentioned in the previous section, explanations which emphasize
cultural difference have been criticized because they tend to make stereotypical generalizations about behaviour which may be erroneous. They also
incline towards identifying the problem as being situated in the person's
own culture, viewing it as pathological. One of the logical conclusions of
this approach is that to avoid detection as mentally ill, black people should
adopt white ways of behaving (such as staying off the streets). Holding the
individual's culture responsible for what resides in the racism of others, in
this way, has been described as 'victim-blaming'.

Other theories have emphasized the part played by other people in react-
ing to ethnic difference. Horwitz (1983) has noted that the tendency to label
a person mentally ill increases with the cultural distance between the labeller
and labelled. In other words, members of minority ethnic groups are more
likely to be labelled mentally ill than dominant indigenous groups. This may
lead to a predisposition on the part of white people in Britain to interpret
black people's behaviour as signs of insanity and danger. One study found
that lay people were more responsible for initiating police action than police
officers themselves. Afro-Caribbean people were also found to be less frequently
referred by their relatives or neighbours and more frequently by strangers
and passers-by than other ethnic groups (Rogers 1990). Thus, perhaps black
people's behaviour is interpreted in a more negative light by the lay (white)
public than is white people's behaviour.

The way in which black people's behaviour is viewed, together with the
high number of black police referrals, implies a process of 'transmitted discrimination' (Reiner 1986). This entails the police acting as a 'conveyor belt'
for community prejudices about black people's behaviour constituting a threat
to public law and order. This transmitted prejudice is then compounded by
other factors: a general conflictual relationship between young black men
and the police has tended to emerge; intensive policing strategies on inner

city housing estates with large numbers of black people have been implemented in recent times. These factors contribute to raised levels of police detention of all forms of deviance, including mental disorder.

The relationships that black people and the police have with other agencies are also relevant. The policies and reactions of the local courts and psychiatric services have been found to be influential in how the police react when detaining someone they believe to be mentally disordered. A study conducted for the National Association for the Care and Resettlement of Offenders (NACRO) found that the large rate of psychiatric referrals may have been due to the sentencing attitudes of magistrates. Decision-makers tended to err on the side of caution with black defendants considered to be mentally vulnerable. They had an elevated perception of dangerousness amongst this group (Browne 1990).

The ways in which black people perceive and utilize more traditional routes to the psychiatric services are also important. It has been suggested that Afro-Caribbeans are not as likely as other groups to be referred from GPs. The black respondents in one study were found not to have sought help of their own volition (Frederick 1991). Another study found that Afro-Caribbean women tended to be more critical of GPs and more proactive in moving from one doctor to another than their white counterparts. This was attributed to a number of possible factors. Black people may be distrustful of services to their group. They may also be cynical because of their first-hand knowledge of service quality. Many black people work in the NHS. Also, in the West Indies there is a cultural legacy of a fee for service model, which implies 'shopping around'.

The pathways by which black people come to the attention of mental health services have led some commentators to view psychiatry as part of a larger social control apparatus which regulates and oversees the lives of black people (Mercer 1986; Francis 1989). That black people, and in particular young black men, are also over-represented in all parts of the criminal justice system suggests indeed that both the 'criminalization' and 'medicalization' of black people are closely connected processes.

According to Francis (1989), higher rates of entering the psychiatric system via the criminal justice system indicate a coalescence of the criminalization and medicalization of black people. He argues for a much wider definition of what constitutes the psychiatric system to be adopted, which views it as an extended network of scientific expertise and professional practice. This would necessitate the position and management of black people being considered across a number of related state institutions, including schools, hospitals, social services, the courts and prisons. Francis suggests that this would highlight common practices and processes and bring together issues which have hitherto been analysed separately, such as the IQ testing of black children, which has led to high numbers being classified as 'educationally subnormal'. In theory, admission to hospital and service use serves the function of responding to mental health need. A complementary theoretical position to that provided by Francis (ibid.) has been suggested by Smaje (1996) and Nazroo (1998) when explaining ethic inequalities in mental and physical health. Their analysis involves abandoning an emphasis on a-historical and de-contextualized genetic and cultural factors, which has found favour in previous epidemiological work, and replacing them with a structural approach, which considers the fine-grain aspects of disadvantage faced by black people in society. The latter includes the experience of racism, ethnic identity and the relevance of 'group affiliation and culture while acknowledging the contingent and contextual nature of ethnicity' (Nazroo 1998: 710).

What is the nature of contact with psychiatry?

Type of admission

As important as the route of referral in determining the way in which black people are disadvantaged by the psychiatric system, is the nature of contact with psychiatry. Most patients admitted to psychiatric facilities enter as informal patients. Whether or not this is always the equivalent of people entering under their own volition without persuasion from professional and other people is a moot point (see Chapter 9). But informal patients have, theoretically at least, the right to refuse medication and the right to discharge themselves from hospital whenever they wish. Certain groups of black people enter hospital informally less often than white people. During the 1980s, around 8 per cent of all admissions to hospital, according to official statistics held by the Department of Health, were compulsory. However, 20–30 per cent of Afro-Caribbean patients are detained involuntarily (Cope 1989). The rate is even higher for young Afro-Caribbean migrants. One study monitored detention rates over a four-year period and found this group to be compulsorily admitted at 17 times the rate for compulsory admissions made from the community and, under admissions via the criminal justice system, 25 times more frequently (Cope 1989). This pattern has been confirmed by a recent point-prevalence study which found that black people were over-represented in admissions to psychiatric hospitals. They are also more likely to be admitted compulsorily and to be placed in locked wards (Koffman *et al.* 1997). Despite the widespread evidence of continuing over-representation of black people in compulsory admissions, these findings have not 'influenced policy or led to a strategy to ensure that services appropriately meet the need of the culturally diverse population in this country' (Bhui *et al.* 1995). Despite the cultural importance currently attributed to 'evidence-based practice' within health services, in the case of black people and compulsory admission to hospital simply providing evidence of certain trends does not seem enough to impact on the structure and organization of services.

Diagnosis

All psychiatric labels tend to be stigmatizing because they implicate the negotiation of self. However, psychotic disorders are more stigmatizing than neurotic disorders. Afro-Caribbeans are over-represented in psychotic disorders and under-represented in neurotic ones. Although most of this evidence about schizophrenia has focused on Afro-Caribbeans, one study reports higher rates amongst Asian patients as well (Shaikh 1985). Young black men are also almost exclusively likely to receive a diagnosis of 'cannabis psychosis', even though such a concept is of dubious validity.

What is the reason for the high rates of black people who are labelled as psychotic? Three main explanations can be gleaned from the literature on the subject: black people are mentally ill more often than whites; black people are mentally ill more often but they are given the wrong diagnosis; psychiatric theory and practice is part of a wider racism. Let us look at these three accounts in a little more detail.

The labelling merely reflects actual incidence

High rates of schizophrenia have been cited as an explanatory factor for the high rates of civil compulsory detention of psychotic black patients (Cope 1989). In other words, it is argued, black people become schizophrenic more often than whites. However, methodological uncertainties about the data on ethnic monitoring mentioned earlier, together with uncertainties over the diagnosis and aetiology of schizophrenia in general, and amongst Afro-Caribbeans in particular, cast doubt on this as an adequate explanation. The uncertainty over the aetiology of this disease category is indicated at the end of a study on the subject by Harrison et al. (1988) who identify a multiplicity of possibilities: potential biological differences in terms of genetic factors, neurochemistry, pre- and perinatal trauma, virology, and immunology merit further investigation, as well as possible effects of living in decaying areas with high unemployment and poor housing.

A desirable precondition of diagnostic validity is that a disease has a known cause. Schizophrenia, as with some other purported diseases, has no known cause – it lacks 'aetiological specificity'. This adds to the other known difficulties of its diagnosis being both unreliable and not leading to any clear predictions about outcome (prognosis) (Bentall, Jackson and Pilgrim 1988; Boyle 1991). Thus the 'actual incidence' position about black people is extremely weak because the diagnostic category of schizophrenia is so problematic. Authors of those studies, which appeal to the evidence of over-representation being accounted for by the purported raised incidence of schizophrenia in black people, simply fail to engage with the problems of conceptual and empirical validity which attend the diagnosis. This represents a leap in faith rather than scientific medicine.

Misdiagnosis

An alternative viewpoint is that admission rates for schizophrenia and other psychoses do not necessarily reflect the incidence of these disorders in community populations. Instead, records may reflect biases in diagnostic practices. Fernando (1988) has suggested that it is the ethnocentric view of psychiatrists that has resulted in this misattribution of labels, such as schizophrenia, by imposing Western concepts with little regard for the cultures of non-western people. According to Littlewood and Lipsedge (1982), terms such as 'schizophrenia' and 'cannabis psychosis' are used when black people display disturbed behaviour, whereas conditions such as depression are under-diagnosed by psychiatry. Evidence for the difficulties that psychiatrists have in affixing appropriate labels is derived from the observation that many more black, than white patients, had their diagnosis changed over time.

The misdiagnosis hypothesis tends to leave unchallenged the fundamental assumption that high rates of psychopathology actually exist amongst black people. What is claimed instead is merely that the wrong label is being applied. For instance, from studying patients with 'religious delusions' Little-wood and Lipsedge suggest that patients with 'acute psychotic reactions' may be misdiagnosed as schizophrenic. This viewpoint does not challenge the validity of diagnostic categories themselves, nor the scientific status of psychiatric knowledge or practices. (Littlewood and Lipsedge are practising psychiatrists.) Transcultural psychiatry, of which the Littlewood and Lispsedge study is an example, has also been criticized on the grounds that it provides a simplistic notion of 'culture', which has been adopted by predominantly white psychiatrists about black client groups (Sashidharan 1986).

Fernando, Ndegwa and Wilson (1998) argue that the misdiagnosis hypo-thesis needs to be accepted only as a partial account of the data on Afro-Caribbean over-representation. In their view, in addition to the misdiagnosis hypothesis, other concurrent explanatory factors need to be taken into ac-count which include institutional racism and the conceptual inadequacy of psychiatric knowledge in its totality (cf. Littlewood and Lipsedge ibid.). Within such a wider critique of psychiatric theory and practice from Fernando *et al.* lies an account of why psychiatry is unjust and irrational, to some degree, not just about black patients but also about its whole client group.

Racist psychiatric constructs

Other commentators are more aligned with a 'social constructivist' position. Not only are the diagnostic practices of psychiatrists viewed as problematic, *vis-à-vis* their encounters with black patients, but so are the content and production of the psychiatric diagnostic categories themselves. From this perspective, the notion of psychiatry as a scientific discipline, which remains unaffected by social forces, is rejected. The way in which race and culture are inextricably bound up in the construction of disease categories is illustrated by a number of past and contemporary examples. For example, 'drapetomania' was defined by an American psychiatrist Cartwright in 1851, as a disease which made slaves run away: 'The cause in the most of cases, that induces the Negro to run away from service, is as much a disease of the mind as any other species of mental alienation, and much more curable, as a general rule' (quoted in Ranger 1989: 354). Fernando (1988) points out the rise in racist categories is bound up with the institution of slavery and social control. Examples which have more relevance to contemporary psychiatry and the social control of black people are the constructs of cannabis psychosis and schizophrenia.

Cannabis psychosis is a label attached selectively to Afro-Caribbean people when British psychiatrists are perplexed by their behaviour (Ranger 1989). Psychosis is defined by the Royal College of Psychiatrists as a mental illness which 'cannot be understood as an exaggeration of ordinary expression'. As discussed in the chapter on gender, the notion of 'ordinary' here is based on dominant groups in society in terms of numbers, status and power. Thus, in Britain, 'ordinary' implies having a white skin.

Others have pointed to the racist assumptions underlying the theoretical tradition of Kraepelin, the German psychiatrist responsible for the development of the category and classification of schizophrenia (which he dubbed 'dementia praecox'). Kraepelinian theorizing, which dominates post- as well as pre-War western psychiatry, points to a 'tainted' gene pool as a causal factor in schizophrenia. This pool is associated with other forms of disruptive and dangerous conduct. These suggestions neatly fit racist stereotypes held about black people (Francis 1989).

Certainly it is well documented that German eugenic medicine, which underpinned the Nazi programme of racial hygiene and evinced the degeneracy theory of disability and dangerousness, also gives western psychiatry many of its presuppositions. Indeed, most standard psychiatric textbooks documenting the evidence for the heritability of schizophrenia (e.g. Gottesman and Shields 1972) report uncritically the seminal genetic research of Rudin and Kallman during the Nazi period in Germany (Marshall 1990). Thus, assumptions about genetic inferiority and race are deeply ingrained in psychiatric theory.

The question of racist constructs relates to the wider question, which we raised earlier about the capacity of western psychiatric knowledge to respond adequately to cross-cultural differences. Thus, even when psychiatric knowledge is not implicitly or explicitly racist, it is inevitably a product of its time and place. At present this means the dominance of ideas derived from nineteenth-century Europe, particularly the work of Kraepelin and Bleuler, which has been modified by later Anglo-American psychiatrists. This has culminated in the production of several versions of the American Psychiatric Association's Diagnostic and Statistical Manual in the US and the International Classification of Diseases in Britain. Both of these are predicated on earlier notions derived from Germanic psychiatry.

Even when less biologically and diagnostically orientated mental health workers have developed therapeutic rationales, such as Sigmund Freud in Europe, or Carl Rogers in the US, they are clearly western in their assumptions (for example about individualism and mind). Despite this, these psychotherapeutic systems are offered as being trans-historically and transculturally valid by their founders and followers (Pilgrim 1997a). In this sense they are not different to the biomedical rationales offered by their competing colleagues in the mental health industry.

Treatment and management

Being referred in a criminalized manner, together with a predisposition towards receiving a diagnosis of psychosis, have certain attendant implications, which will affect black people more than white people. Basically, black people are treated in a more coercive and punitive way within the psychiatric system. Afro-Caribbeans are over-represented in locked wards, secure units and the Special Hospitals (Bolton 1984; Jones and Berry 1986; Mohan et al. 1997; Fernando, Ndegwa and Wilson 1998). They are more likely to receive physical treatments than whites. Two studies have indicated the over-use of ECT for Asian and Afro-Caribbean patients (Littlewood and Cross 1980; Shaikh 1985).

The study by Littlewood and Cross also found that black patients were more likely to receive major tranquillizers and intramuscular medication, and were more likely to be seen by junior medical staff. Chen, Harrison and Standen (1991) confirmed these findings, noting that whilst no differences between black and white patients in medication levels were evident at admission, over time the black group received higher levels and were more likely to be prescribed depot medication.

Some psychiatrists have argued that the stronger interventionism black people are subjected to is in response to them being more ill (McGovern and Cope 1987). That is, the reasoning goes, because black people are schizophrenic more often, then they are treated forcibly more often using major tranquillizers – because that is how acute schizophrenia 'has to be' treated. Earlier we noted the problems of psychiatric authors like this failing to engage with the problems of validity in their diagnostic categories. In the absence of such criticisms psychiatrists will be unaware of the vulnerability of relying on dubious categories like 'schizophrenia' when drawing their conclusions about incidence and 'need' for treatment. However, there are indications that factors other than diagnosis are also implicated. Littlewood and Lipsedge (1982), for example, found excessive West Indian detention to be independent of diagnosis, whilst Bolton (1984) found that black patients identified by staff as uncooperative, but not aggressive, were much more likely to be transferred to locked wards than white patients.

Likewise, Noble and Rodger (1989), who reported a longitudinal record of violent incidents in the Bethlem Royal and Maudsley hospitals in London, found that in their control group of non-violent patients, 50 per cent of Afro-Caribbeans in the sample were detained formally or on a locked ward, whereas only 15 per cent of non-violent whites were managed in the same way. Black patients were also recorded to be violent more often than white patients, raising the question (for us but not the investigators) about a 'spiral' of expectations, similar to that found in authoritarian penal regimes. That is, staff treat black people more coercively than they do whites and so black people react to a discriminatory regime in a more aggressive way. This then prompts staff to behave coercively more often to incidents involving black patients, and the spiral continues.

The bias against non-violent black patients recorded in this study shows that a discriminatory backdrop exists in the mental hospital. To imply, as Noble and Rodger do, that the records simply reflect the greater aggressiveness (or illness behaviour) of black patients is, however, only one interpretation of their data. Violent behaviour, as any other, can of course be reduced to the disposition of individuals. But situational or contextual factors, such as the racism evident in mental health systems, and demonstrated by the data in this study, need to be considered by sociologists.

In summary, the picture drawn above about mode of referral, diagnosis, compulsory admission and psychiatric management indicates that black people (particularly young black men) are subjected more to the harsh end of mental health services than white people. However, there are exceptions to this pattern, which we will consider later when examining the Irish in Britain. First, we turn to another ethnic group in a British context.

Asian women and the somatization thesis

The focus within the psychiatric literature on the madness of young Afro-Caribbean men masks an important, but lesser explored, question related to the misery of Asian women. The minority discourse from psychiatric researchers about this topic suggests that Asian women present their mental distress as bodily symptoms – the somatization thesis (Currer 1986). This provides a case for an apparently legitimate form of medical management, i.e. doctors need to diagnose and treat an underlying mental illness (depression) despite the patient's somatic presentation. However, there are problems with this somatization thesis. Fenton and Sadiq-Sangster (1996) point out that the presentation of bodily symptoms by Asian women is ambiguous for a number of reasons: 'It could mean several things: (a) a non-recognition of mental illness, so that ailments are always presented as somatic, (b) a non-recognition of the link between physical ailments and emotional states, (c) a presentation of ailments as somatic despite some recognition of mental distress, and (d) simply a non-presentation of mental symptoms to bio-medical doctors' (Fenton and Sadiq-Sangster ibid.: 69). Given this unexplored ambiguity, the psychiatric assumption of somatization in Asian women is a pre-emptive construction. The latter has a tendency to stereotype whole groups of people. Another example of this is in relation to the investigation itself of 'Asian' health. The attempt by medicine to seek a pattern of health in a variegated group of people from a large land mass (the Indian subcontinent) containing several countries, religions and nationalities reflects a homogenization stereotype. Also, as Watters (1996) has pointed out, Asian people may encounter different styles and qualities of mental health services in various parts of Britain. Despite this, the psychiatric literature studying differences in hospitalization rates in Asian people assumes that these exist as a result of patient variables. Watters (1996) criticizes researchers for a number of rash generalizations about Asian mental health. He includes the following examples: an uncritical acceptance of the somatization thesis; an assumption that Islam is a protective mental health factor but Hinduism is not; and the assumption that Indians have an easier migration experience than Pakistanis. Another example of pre-emptive stereotyping is the assumption that Asian culture fails to have a notion of psychological causation (Ineichen 1987).

A final point which the literature on Asian mental health highlights is the vulnerability of western medical knowledge. The somatization thesis implies that physical symptoms disguise a true mental illness. However, given the centrality of the heart in south Asian culture (Krause 1989; Fenton and Sadiq 1991), sadness is articulated readily as being in that area of the chest – the heart 'sinking' or 'falling' (*dil ghirda hai*). The sufferer is not 'disguising' depression but is simply experiencing their distress in that way. One analysis which seems to bridge the gap between cultural determinism and medical positivism can be found in a study of South Asian women's lay knowledge. Fenton and Sadiq-Sangster (1996), in a follow-up to their earlier research, found that women describe and express mental distress in a culturally specific way but their descriptions did correspond with a number of the features associated with the western psychiatric category of depression. A problem with western psychiatric positivism is that it assumes a neat division between mental and physical illness. It also assumes that the linguistic expression of emotions is transculturally stable. However, cross-cultural comparisons reveal large variations in the use of words to describe subjective states. For example, some cultures have no word for 'anxiety'. The current western notion of 'depression' is a contemporary convention which may change in the future and was certainly different in the past. In the nineteenth century it was not used. Instead lethargy, weakness and low mood were labelled as 'neurasthenia' and extreme sadness dubbed 'melancholia' by psychiatrists. In China, the former term is still favoured over 'depression' by lay people and doctors (Kleinman 1988). Thus, the somatization thesis about Asian women may reveal more about the epistemological weakness of western psychiatry than the subjective weakness of its diagnostic targets.

Irish people and psychiatry

Whilst most of the debates about psychiatry and race have centred on the diagnosis and treatment of black people, the smaller literature on Irish people in Britain points to factors other than skin colour in understanding over-representation in psychiatric records. (For a summary of this literature see Greenslade (1992) and Bracken *et al.* (1998).) If we take two broad measures of distress from official statistics (suicide and psychiatric admissions) we find that Irish people, despite their white skin, are over-represented. Table 4.1 shows the picture for self-induced deaths from suicides and non-accidental poisoning according to official statistics reported by Cochrane (1977) in England and Wales, by country of origin. People from the West Indies have a low rate, whereas the rate for Irish people is high. The even higher figures reported for Germans and Poles probably reflects the large proportion of Nazi death camp survivors or their families. The Scots too have a higher self-induced mortality rate than those indigenous to England and Wales. It is

Table 4.1   Non-indigenous self-induced death in England and Wales

Country of origin	Standardized mortality ratio	
	Men	*Women*
All countries	100	100
Poland	221	207
Germany	177	239
Ireland (North and South)	154	149
Scotland	138	145
USA	98	198
India and Pakistan	100	122
West Indies	85	60

Modified from Cochrane (1977)

Table 4.2 Psychiatric admissions of immigrants (16+) per 100,000 in England

Origin by birth	Male	Female	All
Eire	1054	1102	1080
Northern Ireland	793	880	838
Caribbean	565	532	548
England	418	583	504

Modified from Cochrane and Bal (1989)

important to note that Welsh data cannot be disaggregated as they are collected together with English data sets by central government, although recently some internal Welsh studies are emerging.

Turning to psychiatric admissions, Irish immigrants are more likely than Caribbean immigrants to enter hospital (Table 4.2). The diagnosis of schizophrenia is highest in Caribbean 'immigrants' (of all racial/ethnic groups). But Irish people going to the British mainland are significantly more likely to be labelled as schizophrenic than those born there. Previous studies suggested that the Irish are under-represented in records of schizophrenia in England (Clare 1974). The recorded incidence for schizophrenia is higher in Eire itself than in the rest of the British Isles.

The over-representation of Irish people in psychiatric populations has led some commentators to generate more questions than answers when proposing a multi-factorial research programme. This might require an understanding which would include Irish child-rearing practices, long-term effects of emigration, poverty, rates of obstetric complication, mental health service over-utilization, late male marriage age in rural communities and specific forms of personal alienation from the neighbouring ex-colonizer (Jones 1997).

The Irish on mainland Britain have the highest rate of diagnosis for most categories, including neurosis, personality disorder, depression, 'other' psychoses and alcohol abuse (Cochrane and Bal 1989). As a consequence of this overall over-representation, the Irish have the highest rate of admissions to in-patient facilities of all ethnic groups in Britain (Bracken *et al.* 1998). Unlike with the data on Afro-Caribbean people, the gender bias is less clear for the Irish, with a slight female, not male, preponderence. These figures indicate that race and ethnicity clearly are important, as far as mental ill-health and psychiatric services are concerned. But given that the Irish are white, how can we make sense of their shared features with some black groups?

Two broad groups of interweaving features probably make the Irish vulnerable to mental health problems, one material and the other cultural, which overlap with the research agenda offered by Jones (ibid.). The material factors relate to the legacy of socio-economic disruption: poverty; famine; the military suppression of rebellion and insurrection; forced migration; and economic reliance on a neighbouring colonial power.

The cultural concomitants of these colonial and post-colonial material forces have involved a series of identity crises and confusions. As well as the general history of the Celtic fringe of the British Isles being relevant – the suppression of language and religion by an occupying English colonial power, which for varying periods has been resisted – the *internal* ruling elites of Ireland have often been pro-English and have not always shared the same cultural identity of their subordinates in relation to language and religion (O'Mahony and Delanty 1998). The latter authors also point out that the political hegemony of the Catholic Church has been linked to a conservative clerical nationalism, as well as an imposed civil culture which has: quashed intellectual dissent; been sexually repressive; subordinated women via familism; and engendered a strict child-rearing style, both in the home and in an educational system under its monopoly control. Additionally, the clerical adjudication over sin by celibates has operated as a ubiquitous social control mechanism over the Irish laiety creating mass self-doubt and guilt.

Some of the points made by O'Mahony and Delanty are also explored by Scheper-Hughes (1979) in her anthropological study of Irish mental health, although she traces ego-sapping child-rearing practices as much to the English colonial power as to the Church. The destructive cultural force of English colonialism and its possible mental health impact are also examined by Kenny (1985). Thus, Irish history is saturated, like other colonized countries, with an experience of exploitation, loss and separation from starvation and migration. But also there are peculiar religious and cultural forces which form a backdrop to Irish identity fragmentation. Together these may have been powerful historical sources of madness (and creativity) which cumulatively retain a contemporary resonance.

Discussion

There is an alternative way of viewing the debate on race and mental health, which goes beyond attempting to identify causal factors in the high incidence of mental illness amongst black and Irish people, or pinpointing prejudicial labelling practices. This focuses on the discourse of race and psychiatry.

As Foucault has argued, we live with an ingrained predisposition to view madness as essentially 'other' (Foucault 1965). The use of the Victorian asylums for warehousing the insane was a mechanism for bringing about a break in the dialogue between reason and unreason on the one hand, and society and the disturbed on the other. In the contemporary era, where mental hospitals are in decline, the narrative of loss and difference is preserved in the status of becoming a patient. This is clearly expressed by Barham and Hayward (1991: 2), who note that people who receive a diagnosis of schizophrenia tend to be viewed as 'lost to the disorder': 'Schizophrenia is more than an illness that one has; it is something a person is or may become. The person who has suffered a schizophrenic illness is someone in which a drastic rupture has been effected in the continuity of his or her biography . . . some schools of thought, we discover, do not accept there is an "after" with schizophrenia, only a "before".' This 'otherness' which characterizes the discourse on psychosis fits well with a new type of racism. This is preoccupied with who should be included or excluded from the mainstream of society: 'The new racism is primarily concerned with mechanisms of inclusion and exclusion. It specifies who may legitimately belong to the national community and simultaneously advances reasons for the segregation or banishment of those whose "origin, sentiment or citizenship" assigns them elsewhere' (Gilroy 1987: 45).

Within this discourse, people from black and ethnic minorities are identified as an alien force responsible for national decline and social disorder. Whilst the old racism, underpinned by eugenics, proposed sterilization and extermination, the new racism suggests banishment and exclusion. In the context of the British historical legacy of colonialism, the debate on race and madness may be seen as central to the inner workings of this 'new racism'. This chapter has reviewed the evidence on the mental ill-health of groups of people, who are the legacy of British colonialism as ex-slaves, servants, imported service labour and, in the case of the Irish, who are implicated in a postcolonial armed struggle.

Academic and psychiatric literature alluding to race accentuates those mental illnesses which imply a threatening and hostile alien presence. Professional and academic texts then become part of a wider discourse about a threat to a traditional social order. This threat includes: terrorism; non-Christian faiths; alien diet; arcane cultural norms; violent street crime; illicit drug use, etc. These images may then reinforce, or even be used to justify, English racism and endorse processes of segregation, exclusion or banishment.

The Mental Health Act 1983 and the Prevention of Terrorism Act 1978 may be conceptualized as being part of what Althusser (1971) called the 'repressive state apparatus', which allows for preventive detention without trial, and the segregation or exclusion of threatening or undesirable 'others'. Banishment and exclusion can be reinforced by powers under section 86 of the Mental Health Act 1983 to repatriate mentally ill aliens. Entry to the country on psychiatric grounds can also be banned under the Immigration Act 1971 (Rogers and Pilgrim 1989).

However, the legitimacy of repatriation has declined in a context where a growing proportion of black people are British-born. It has become logically untenable. British-born black people have no identifiable nation state to which they can be banished (whether it be to the Indian subcontinent or the Caribbean of their parents, suggested only now by neo-Nazi groups in Britain). Likewise, Europeanization has ensured that rights of residence will be protected for people from any part of the British Isles.

Coercive psychiatry, as part of the wider repressive state apparatus, offers itself as a postcolonial, Europeanized alternative to repatriation. Ideas about banishment to another country can be replaced by the mechanisms of exclusion and control afforded by the mental hospital, prison and physical treatments. Not only are black and Irish people more likely to be incarcerated in locked facilities, and restrained using physical treatments, they are concomitantly represented as the 'other' in the texts and practices of academics and mental health professionals.

Most of what is summarized in this chapter is part of a discourse in which threat predominates, not distress. For example, compared with the extensive psychiatric literature on compulsorily detained Afro-Caribbean men, there is relatively little to be found on the sadness and despair of Asian women living in the community (Beliappa 1991; Fenton and Sadiq 1991). Ironically, this picture of differential attention is reinforced by some critiques which concur with our points here about repressive control in a postcolonial context. For example, Fernando, Ndegwa and Wilson (1998) provide an elaborate and sophisticated critique of postcolonial psychiatry. However, whilst their book is entitled *Forensic Psychiatry, Race and Culture*, the great bulk of their analysis focuses singularly on Afro-Caribbean people. The Irish appear nowhere in the text, even though many of the authors' arguments would also apply powerfully to this ethnic group.

By posing questions and conducting research along a dualistic notion of 'black' and 'white', or (implicitly) ex-colonized and ex-colonizer, differences between these groups are accentuated and polarized, and the cause of the 'problem' is identified at the level of the pathology of individuals. Thus, we may find the reason that black and Irish people are 'madder' than whites in the discourse and practices of academic and clinical psychiatry (including reactive critiques), not in epidemiological studies, which try to measure the incidence of psychiatric morbidity amongst different ethnic groups. In addition to this discursive feature skewing our way of thinking about race and mental health, the impact of real historical colonial arrangements would appear to have a continuing negative impact on the overall mental health of recent generations of black and Irish people. It is little surprising that these current resonances can be found in the daily business of Anglo-American psychiatry (and the criminal justice system) given that the two countries were bound together in the past, socio-economically, not just linguistically, by the slave trade and colonialism. The present 'special relationship' between Britain and the US is based *inter alia* upon this legacy.

To conclude

This chapter has summarized arguments and evidence about the mental health of Afro-Caribbean, Asian and Irish people in Britain. It has drawn attention to methodological problems of interpreting evidence about over-representation and discussed the problems of Anglo-American psychiatry using a diagnostic approach which is ill-suited to people from black and ethnic minority populations. In the area of race, more than in others, the real causal impact of socio-economic disadvantage (not just discursive issues) requires particular sociological scrutiny.

Questions

1 What factors need to be considered when understanding the relationship between race and health?

2 Discuss the evidence about the psychiatric treatment of Afro-Caribbean people in Britain.

3 What factors might account for the over-representation of Irish people in psychiatric admissions?

4 What problems are highlighted for psychiatric knowledge by the 'somatization thesis'?

5 Discuss ways in which psychiatric services could improve their response to Asian people.

6 Discuss the role of racism in the creation of mental health problems and the character of psychiatric services.

For discussion

Consider the ways in which your background has influenced your views about mental health in your own racial group and in that of others.

Further reading

Brady, M. (1995) Culture in treatment, culture as treatment: a critical appraisal of developments in addiction programmes for indigenous North Americans and Australians, *Social Science and Medicine* 41: 1487–1498.

Fernando, S. (1995) *Mental Health in a Multi-Ethnic Society.* London: Routledge.

Halpern, D. (1993) Minorities and mental health, *Social Science and Medicine* 36(5): 597–607.

Smaje, C. (1996) The ethnic patterning of health: new directions for theory and research, *Sociology of Health and Illness* 18, 2: 139–171.

Chapter 5

Age

Chapter overview

The relationship between age and mental health has only occasionally been addressed directly by sociologists. This reflects the low status that children have had within mainstream sociology. As Mayall (1998: 269) has pointed out, they have been 'regarded unproblematically, as socialisation projects within the private domain'. It is only recently that a sociology of childhood has begun to be established, which focuses on understanding children's social position as a minority group and as 'embodied' health care actors and explores inter-generational relationships. To date, little of this type of socio-logical work has been undertaken in the area of mental health. Additionally, while there has been a growing interest in analyses which focus on changes in people's conception of health and illness through subjectively defined stages of the life course (Backett and Davison 1995) there has been little integration of the different dimensions of ageing within sociological thought (Arber and Ginn 1991). By comparison, socially-oriented psychoanalysts have explored the topic more thoroughly, as have developmental psychologists and child psychiatrists. In this chapter, the mental health implications of three phases of the life span will be examined under the following topic headings:

- Emotions and primary socialization

- Childhood sexual abuse and mental health problems

- Social competence in adulthood

- Biological decline and depression in older people.

Emotions and primary socialization

During childhood two factors become highly relevant to the question of mental health. The first is the emotional life of young people. The second is primary socialization – the ways in which newcomers learn how to become accepted and acceptable members of their parent society. Both of these factors are relevant for our purposes, because the field of mental health implicates distressed experiences and distressing conduct on the one hand and deviance from norms on the other.

As far as emotions are concerned, sociologists have drawn largely upon psychoanalysis. Freudianism has influenced a variety of social theories from structural functionalism to neo-Marxism (the 'Frankfurt School'). Psycho-analysis (see Chapter 1) offers a theory which connects the individual's inner life to their external social context. It provides an account of emotional life of individuals, whilst at the same time offering an explanation of how mental ill-health is determined by society. (For a wider discussion of the socio-logical status of psychoanalysis see Jacoby (1975); Holland (1978); Hirst and Wolley (1982); and Craib (1989).)

For Freud, civilization puts limits on the free expression and experience of emotions, particularly the instincts of sexual desire and murderous aggression. These limits lead to the need of the child to repress their antisocial feelings in exchange for family and societal acceptance. This battle between emotions and social conformity leads to the development of neurosis. However, Freud-ianism is a limited social theory. Freud's emphasis is on civilization (Freud 1930) leading to repression and neurosis. According to Freud, we are all neurotic (to some extent) for more or less the same reasons to do with balancing our instinctual needs with the constraints of reality made clear to us by our parents. Consequently, differences between social groups were not addressed systematically by his theory, although later analytically-oriented writers have explored women's issues (Mitchell 1974; Eichenbaum and Orbach 1982).

Freud offered an explanation for neurotic behaviour arising from anxiety. Later psychoanalysts also tried to address the question of depression (Bowlby) and psychosis (Winnicott and Laing) by looking at the impact of poor care and separation on the infant (from birth to two years). However, as an example of the divergent views within psychoanalysis, the influential work of Melanie Klein is distinctive because it focused on the pathogenic impact of the infant's inborn aggression (rather than poor care). By contrast, the work of Bowlby, Winnicott and Laing was heavily environmentally oriented – it emphasized parental privation and deprivation as the source of later mental health problems. Whereas Klein can be seen to blame the instincts for mental ill-health, the 'environmentalists' can be seen to point the finger at parents, particularly the mother.

Thus, variegated psychoanalytical accounts certainly emphasize a general social backdrop ('civilization') to emotional development, but the nuclear family then becomes its main frame of sociological reference. Mainstream clinical psychoanalysis tends to play down or ignore variables other than the family, such as the particular stresses associated with class, race, gender, age and sexuality. It also ignores the potentially powerful role of extra-familial social institutions, such as the school, in shaping the child's identity and their emotional life. Those psychoanalysts who have strayed into these wider areas of theorizing have tended to leave or be expelled from their professional culture (Reich 1942; Laing 1967; Masson 1990).

Psychoanalysis also assumes family relationships which are 'triangulated', that is, based on a set of tensions, which engender anxiety, created by children relating to a mother and a father. We now know that in many modern complex societies children grow up in contexts other than this, e.g. those with single or homosexual parents. (For an analysis of the social administrative role of psychoanalysis see Miller and Rose (1988).)

Turning to primary socialization, there is a strong consensus across theoretical positions in both sociology and psychology that childhood is a special part of the life span. It is a time when most of the rules and mores associated with the society and particular class and culture which the child inhabits are learned. It is also a time when gender-specific conduct is acquired. The child learns what is expected of him or her both at their current age and in the future, through their exposure to adult models of conduct. They learn gradually to control their body and their emotions in order to perform competently and efficiently in the presence of others. They learn the importance of a shared view of reality with their fellows in gaining security and in meriting credibility. All these learned capacities are also bound up with an increasingly elaborate and defined sense of identity. Thus, socialization is about learning how to behave in a context-appropriate way in society and it is about a person gaining a confident sense of who they are.

The relevance of socialization for mental health is that children learn to behave confidently and appropriately, following rules and complying with norms. This competence can fail if the person lacks the intellectual capacity to grasp what to do (currently this is termed a 'learning difficulty' and used to be called 'mental handicap' or 'mental subnormality'). It can also fail if the person lacks confidence in their performance as a social actor (this might be a way of thinking about 'phobic-anxiety') or if they are too sad to participate in everyday activities ('depression'). The competence can also be adjudged to have failed by others if the person fails to comply with everyday expectations of appropriate behaviour in context or they make idiosyncratic claims about reality. We will return to this below when discussing schizophrenia.

A final aspect of socialization relevant to understanding mental health is that children learn to control their emotions. The strong emotional expressions tolerated in childhood become less and less acceptable as the person matures into adulthood. Consequently, if an adult becomes more exuberant or sad than is deemed appropriate for the context by others, they may acquire the label of 'manic-depressive'. (For a sociological summary of the tasks of socialization in childhood see Dreitzel (1973).)

In modern industrial societies, which are regulated by versions of rationality, adult conduct is marked by a capacity to comply with both moral propriety and rational rules. By young adulthood, those of us who act either immorally, incompetently or irrationally will be deemed by others to be either bad or sick. Sometimes, which of these it is – badness or sickness – may be ambiguous both for lay onlookers and experts. As was noted in Chapter 1, mental illness can be understood as a particular form of deviancy which is not characterized by malice aforethought or motivated by personal gain or gratification, as is the case in criminal behaviour.

Part of our expectation of normality is that people will be competent in their social role and that their actions will be readily intelligible to us. So, if a person is so fearful or sad that their competence breaks down we may account for this in terms of mental ill-health. In everyday western terms they have had a 'nervous breakdown'. Likewise, if someone acts in a way which we cannot understand, we may account for this in terms of them suffering from mental illness. An example here would be a person talking to voices that no one else can hear. Either way, mental illness might be understood sociologically as failed or incomplete socialization.

Such a view is reinforced by the emphasis given by psychologists from different schools to the legacy of childhood on adult competence. Most psychologists assume that problems in childhood make the person susceptible to later mental health problems. Likewise, sociological models of depression in adulthood emphasize developmental vulnerability factors as well as current stressors (Brown and Harris 1978, discussed in Chapter 3). The social causationist model of depression from Brown and Harris involves a multifactorial approach. As far as childhood is concerned, a strong case has been recently made for a unifactorial causationist model, which links a variety of mental health problems to sexual abuse in childhood. Because of the strong evidence for this relationship, we will look at this in some detail.

Childhood sexual abuse and mental health problems

Whilst the connection between sexual abuse and distress can be viewed as a unifactorial relationship, this does not imply that there is a consistent outcome for all victims. Individuals do vary in their responses to similar abusive acts, and the severity of the abuse, its duration and the relation of the perpetrator to the victim have all been linked to variable outcomes (Finkelhor 1984). Another caution is that sexual victimization may be part of a wider picture of family disturbance which could be pathogenic. As Briere and Runtz (1987: 51) point out: 'Although symptomatology in adulthood may covary with early sexual abuse, in the absence of further data it is not clear whether the former is caused by the latter or whether both are actually a function of some third variable, such as dysfunctional family dynamics.' Notwithstanding this valid caution, reviews of the literature on the immediate and long-term effects of sexual abuse on child victims come to the conclusion that there is strong evidence that they are significantly more prone to mental distress than non-abused children (Wyatt and Powell 1988; Cahill et al. 1991). Not only is this evidence compelling, but it points to a wide range of effects which may account, in part at least, for the higher rate of reported mental health problems in women than men. Overall, girls are at greater risk than boys of sexual victimization. This is certainly true of intra-familial abuse (Rogers and Terry 1984) although there is some evidence that boys may be at greater risk from stranger-perpetrators (Abel et al. 1987). The large gap between male and female victims in terms of rates of abuse and rates of distressing consequences may be accounted for in part by the greater readiness of female victims to disclose on both counts (Finkelhor 1979). Also, as we pointed out in Chapter 3, the discourse on females has been more wide-reaching than

Table 5.1   Differences between sexually abused (AB) and non-abused (NAB) female attenders at a Canadian community health centre for crisis counselling (*n* = 152)

	% NAB	% AB	Sig. level
Current psychotropic medication	14.0	31.3	0.01
History of hospitalization	22.1	19.4	ns
History of attempted suicide	33.7	50.7	0.03
Battered as adult	17.6	48.9	0.0003
History of rape	8.3	17.7	ns
History of drug addiction	2.3	20.9	0.0005
History of alcoholism	10.5	26.9	0.02
Restless sleep	54.7	71.6	0.03
Nightmares	23.3	53.7	0.0001
Anxiety attacks	27.9	53.7	0.001
Trouble controlling temper	18.6	38.8	0.006
Desire to hurt self	18.6	31.3	0.07
Sexual problems	15.1	44.8	0.0001
Fear of men	15.1	47.8	0.0001
Fear of women	3.5	11.9	0.09
Derealization	10.5	32.8	0.0001
Out of body experiences	8.1	20.9	0.04
Chronic muscle tension	44.2	65.7	0.008

Modified from Briere and Runtz (1988)

that on males, with the bulk of the research on prevalence of abuse and its effects being focused on women not men (Becker 1988; Dimock 1988).

Sexual abuse makes child victims more likely than non-abused children to demonstrate the following:

1 Aggression.
2 Sexually inappropriate behaviour.
3 Sexual aggression.

Sexually inappropriate behaviour refers to the tendency of victims to become sexually interested in peers and adults in a way which is 'out of sync' with their age group. Sexual aggression refers to this process when it is associated with anger or violence. This trio of symptoms characterizing child victims of sexual abuse does not mean that they have only these problems. Other forms of distress reported include those suffered by non-abused psychiatric referrals (anxiety, depression, night terrors, language delay, hyperactivity, stealing, peer relationship difficulties, eating disorders, etc.). However, the trio does seem to mark sexual abuse victims off from non-abused children with emotional problems.

A number of epidemiological studies now indicate that these immediate externalizing effects in childhood translate into adult problems of both 'acting out' and of experienced distress. Studies of long-term effects have been on both clinical and community populations. Here we will give an example from each. Briere and Runtz (1988) examined the records of 152 consecutive women requesting appointments at the counselling department of an urban Canadian community health centre. Table 5.1 summarizes their results. The

Table 5.2 Lifetime prevalence of psychiatric problems in those sexually abused (AB) and those not (NA) in childhood (*n* = 3132)

	Men		Women	
	% NA	% AB	% NA	% AB
Alcohol abuse	23.2	35.7	4.1	20.8*
Drug abuse	7.8	44.9*	3.1	13.7*
Severe depression	3.9	13.8	5.5	21.9*
Phobic anxiety	7.0	6.5	12.5	34.2*
Any psychiatric diagnosis	34.0	71.2*	24.0	58.6*

* Significance level of 0.05. Figures summarized from Stein *et al.* (1988)

significant results in the far right column alert us to the symptom profile of the abused group. Notice the suicidal behaviour and the substance abuse, as well as the battered adult picture. This phenomenon of 're-victimization' is common in adult survivors of childhood abuse. There is some evidence that disproportionate numbers of victims are found working as prostitutes (Browne and Finkelhor 1986).

Other studies indicate that some victims also become perpetrators. Estimates of this vary. Longo (1982) reported that 47 per cent of male adolescent sexual offenders had been victims themselves. Becker (1988) reports a figure of 19 per cent in her adolescent sexual offenders clinic. The focus of the clinical discourse on sexual abuse is on male perpetrators and, with the exceptions just quoted, female victims. Recently, a minority interest in female perpetrators has emerged suggesting that they constitute between 1 per cent and 10 per cent of offenders. They appear to differ from their male counterparts in that they often act cooperatively with a male co-perpetrator; male offenders typically act alone. Given that the data reflects a preponderance of female victims and only a small minority of female perpetrators, it alerts us to the problems of accounting for sexual abuse simply in terms of adults repeating abusive relationships from childhood. The switching from victim to perpetrator is not inevitable, nor can it be invoked as a strong causal explanation of most abusive acts, as most victims of both sexes do not go on to become perpetrators.

Turning to an example of a community survey, Stein *et al.* (1988) interviewed 3132 adults in two Los Angeles areas – one predominantly white, the other Hispanic (Table 5.2). The symptom profile of victims is confirmed again in this study. Drug and alcohol abuse is evident, as are anxiety and depression. Significant differences do not appear in the groups in relation to diagnoses of schizophrenia, mania and obsessive-compulsive problems. The final column shows the consistent pattern of victims being more likely overall to receive a psychiatric diagnosis than non-victims. Elements in this range of adult personal difficulties seem to be more amplified in victims of intra-familial abuse than for those abused by non-relatives. Not only do they suffer the psychological impact of assault common to all victims, they also struggle with a particular sense of betrayal and stigma.

The stigma of the abused victim and the shame and criminality of the perpetrator make accurate estimates of child sexual abuse difficult. Baker and Duncan (1985) suggest child sexual abuse rates of 0.25 per cent for relative and 10 per cent (12 per cent female and 8 per cent male) for non-relative abuse in Britain. If these are accurate estimates, around 4.5 million British adults are victims of earlier sexual abuse. In the US, Russell (1983) reports much higher rates in her community survey of women – 38 per cent reporting one experience of sexual abuse before 18 with 4.5 per cent of the sample reporting abuse by their biological or stepfathers.

Prevalence rates of abuse victims of around 30 per cent are quoted by studies of psychiatric outpatient records (Gelinas 1983). This range of estimates poses a problem of interpretation. If Russell's estimates are correct, then it would appear that whilst the rates in the community of reported sexual abuse are high, this is not translating into a proportionate number of victims becoming psychiatric patients. What is implied instead, as with the Brown and Harris study of female depression in the community, is that there is a 'clinical iceberg' (see Chapter 1), with only some of the abuse victims presenting for professional help. By contrast, if the Baker and Duncan data is more accurate, then it would appear that sexual abuse during childhood is being reflected more closely in prevalence rates of psychiatric disorder.

Social competence in adulthood

One of the most controversial questions in current debates about mental health is the nature of schizophrenia (Bentall 1990: Boyle 1991). This diagnosis is the most common one given to those deemed to be suffering from a 'major mental illness'. It is also the one which is given most commonly in young adulthood. Orthodox psychiatric descriptions depict the schizophrenic as a person who is socially withdrawn and who suffers disturbances of cognition (thought disorder and delusions), perceptions (hallucinations) and emotions ('flat' or 'inappropriate' affect).

Psychiatrists are divided or uncertain about the cause or causes of such symptoms. Some argue that 'schizophrenia' is a genetically programmed 'time bomb' which explodes in adolescence, disturbing the functioning of the brain and the person. Others follow the view of Winnicott (1958) that it is an environmental disease, resulting from poor maternal care in the first year of life, leaving the person psychologically weak and without a secure sense of self. Adolescence marks a time when the person's sense of identity and capacity for independence is under scrutiny and strain, making them vulnerable to psychotic breakdown. Others have attempted to render schizophrenic behaviour intelligible within the confused and confusing communication pattern of the patient's family (Laing and Esterson 1964).

Because of weak aetiological agreement, schizophrenia is particularly vulnerable to labelling and constructivist critiques (Bentall *et al.* 1988; Boyle 1991). If the diagnosis is stigmatizing to its recipients, and of little use value to researchers, then such critiques become predictable. Boyle, for instance, notes that one of the conceptual weaknesses of the diagnosis is that it rests solely on symptoms, not signs. Consequently, it can never be validated in any way other than a circular fashion. Put simply, a person is deemed to be schizophrenic because of their oddity and they are deemed to be odd because they are suffering from schizophrenia. Boyle draws an analogy with diabetes. There, the subjective experience of fatigue can be checked against signs of hyperglycaemia in a blood test. Schizophrenia rests on value judgements about the person's unintelligible behaviour but has no equivalent of a blood test. This does not imply that diagnoses of physical illness cannot be deconstructed, nor that value judgements are absent in physical diagnoses. However, it does point to the particular construct validity problems of a diagnosis of schizophrenia and other 'functional' psychiatric disorders.

The questions begged for sociologists about schizophrenia are thus mainly about how it is negotiated or ascribed. This tack has been taken most systematically by Coulter (1973). He argues that focusing on debates about aetiology obscures the ways in which madness emerges, first through social negotiation in the lay area and then in professional confirmation (a diagnosis). Coulter focuses on everyday expectations of normality and competence. For instance, in relation to hallucinations he argues that to maintain our credibility in a social group there has to be a consensus about what our senses detect around us. In most contexts, if a person sees or hears something which others do not, then their credibility, and therefore their social group membership, is jeopardized. However, it is possible in certain contexts that such idiosyncratic capacities might strengthen rather than weaken their credibility and group status. The Christian mystic and some African medicine men are expected to have extraordinary visions. Indeed, their social credibility may rest on having these abnormal experiences.

In some cultures where hallucinations are valued positively, the bodily circumstances which increase the probability of their occurrence (fasting, fatigue, drug-taking, etc.) are often contrived deliberately. Al-Issa (1977) notes that, in western society, hallucinations offend rationality. Most of us suppress idiosyncratic perceptions because we learn that they are valued negatively. The 'schizophrenic' in contrast makes the mistake of, or is driven to, acting upon their idiosyncratic experiences. Community surveys indeed point to estimates of between 10 per cent and 50 per cent of the 'normal' population who hallucinate (Bentall and Slade 1985).

Thus, atypical idiosyncratic perceptions are not intrinsically pathological (although most western psychiatrists may insist that this is the case). Whether hallucinations are deemed to indicate a gift or a defect depends on the roles people occupy in particular cultures. Likewise, weird speech patterns are highly valued in those Christian sects which respect the ability to 'speak in tongues' (or 'glossolalia') (Szasz 1992; Bentall and Pilgrim 1993). Outside of these sects, in everyday western life, they may be taken to be an offence to rational discourse and so encourage attributions of mad talk from their fellows. Later these may be reframed as evidence of schizophrenic thought disorder by a psychiatrist.

Psychiatrists have tended to conceive of thought disorder as a stable set of cognitive idiosyncrasies or failures: woolly thinking, vagueness, bizarre content, neologisms (invented new words), poverty of thought, fixed and rigid or repetitive expressions. However, this list is extracted from the contexts in which judgements are made about social competence. Coulter emphasizes that, in fact, people may be judged sane by their fellows and yet often manifest such cognitive failures. Following Coulter, what matters are the circumstances in which in one social setting such speech oddities are judged or are valued to indicate madness (by lay people) and confirmed subsequently as schizophrenic illness by psychiatrists. When we discussed labelling theory earlier in Chapter 1 this was described in terms of 'contingencies'.

For Coulter, there are no abstract defining qualities of schizophrenic thought, but there are social settings in which the thoughts of some people are judged to be meaningless or illegitimate. These settings, and the decisions associated with them, involve family members and neighbours at home, or strangers in public places, who appeal for the attendance of psychiatric professionals to deal with a discomforting situation. In other words, madness, like the sanity with which it is contrasted, is socially negotiated. Consequently the best that sociologists can do is describe the particular contexts in particular cultures in which ascriptions of madness are made. To do this, knowledge of norms and competence are vital for the investigator. The latter is really studying a moral order and the way in which social actors attempt to maintain its stability by correcting or removing offending group members.

Whilst most cultures across time and place have some notion of oddity or madness, because norms of sanity vary, this notion is not constant. Nor is there a transcultural or tran-historical consensus on what causes oddity or how to respond to it when it emerges (Sedgwick 1982; Horwitz 1983). Each culture may have a notion of what it means to lose one's reason but these notions vary across time and place and so undermine the claims of modern western psychiatry that 'schizophrenia' and its symptoms are a stable set of factors to be studied.

When we considered labelling theory earlier, the work of Scheff was noted. For Scheff (1966) mental disorder is 'residual deviance', i.e. left over after criminality and other bad conduct is considered, but not attributed, by observers. 'Schizophrenia' for Scheff was then the 'residue of the residue' – a catchall ascription of madness, when other forms of mental disorder had been considered and rejected.

The diagnosis of schizophrenia predominates in young adulthood because that is when role expectations based on rational rule-following and goal orientation are highlighted. It is the age when the rationality of work and parenting are demanded of, and by, those involved. The schizophrenic defies or violates these expectations.

Biological decline and depression in older people

It is commonly assumed that, in old age, biological determinants take on a greater significance in accounting for deterioration in social competence, in conditions described collectively as the 'senile dementias'. Currently around half a million people in the UK suffer from the most common of these (Alzheimer's disease), a figure projected to rise to a prevalence of 750,000 over the next 25 years (Alzheimer's Disease Report 1992).

However, the salience of dementia and its purported biological causes in older people may be exaggerated. As well as people with dementia needing social support to maximize their quality of life and avoid physical jeopardy, there are many more older people with cognitive problems who have no proven neurological condition. Kitwood (1988) points out that Alzheimer's dementia can only be properly diagnosed post-mortem. Moreover, some people who are clearly confused and suffering impaired memory show no post-mortem neurological signs, whereas others who are not demented may show neurological deterioration. The loss of personhood which accompanies the progression of dementia has also been linked to the notion of 'social death'. Those who are close to the sufferer come to believe, and sometimes act as if, the person was already dead (Sweeting and Gilhooly 1997). Another point to note about dementia is that whilst it is mainly a problem of old age, it can occur, albeit more rarely, in middle age (pre-senile dementia). An example of an even younger population being affected is the small but increasing incidence in CJD amongst teenagers and those in their 20s, which appears to be causally related to eating products of cattle infected with BSE during the 1980s.

There is a secondary mental health impact of dementia – it affects informal carers (Morris, Morris and Britton 1988). Stress reactions are common in this group of carers, although some other studies highlight positive as well as negative psychological features of the caring role (Orbell, Hopkins and Gillies 1993). In Chapter 10 we examine the problematic status of the concept of 'carer'. However, here we will note that, in those with advanced dementia, direct physical care is demanded in a way which is usually not implied in younger patients with diagnoses such as schizophrenia.

Whilst dementia may have become a dominant modern culture image of becoming elderly, depression is actually more prevalent. Whereas the prevalence of dementia is about 5 per cent in the over-65s, rising to just under 20 per cent for those over 80, depression is much more common in the younger age band of older people. In Britain, community surveys indicate prevalence rates for depression of between 5 per cent in Edinburgh (Maule *et al.* 1984) and 26 per cent in Newcastle (Kay *et al.* 1964) for people over 65. Other studies more typically quote rates of 11 per cent to 15 per cent (Copeland *et al.* 1987).

About 2 per cent of the UK population of over-65s are in residential care. In this particular population, the prevalence of depression rises dramatically. A London survey of 12 old people's homes revealed that 38 per cent of the residents were depressed (Mann *et al.* 1984). Similar surveys in Sydney, Australia (Snowden and Donnelly 1986) found one-third of the residents depressed and a similar survey finding was reported from Milan, Italy (Spagnoli *et al.* 1986). Mild depression is more common in older women than men and it is also more prevalent in those suffering from physical illnesses (Brayne and Ames 1988).

The extent of the association of depression and physical ill-health is shown by a study of 100 patients referred over a 30-month period to a psychogeriatric service with depression (Dover and McWilliam 1992). The authors found that only 3 per cent of the men and 20 per cent of the women patients were physically well. The rest had a variety of serious complaints including cancer, cardiovascular disease, arthritis, deafness and respiratory problems. Sixty-five per cent of the sample had 'multiple illness'. Moreover, many of the drug treatments for some of these physical disorders are known to cause or

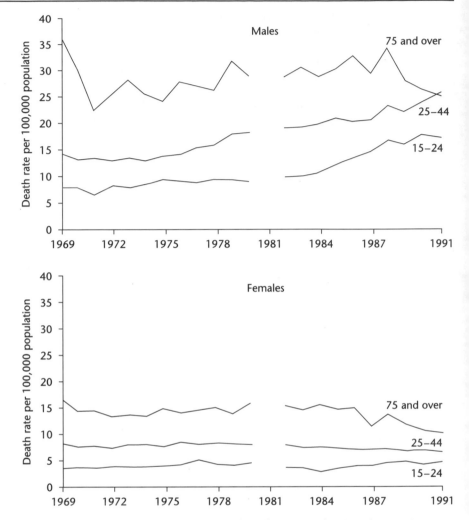

Figure 5.1   Death rates for suicide and undetermined injury by age in England 1969–91 (from HMSO 1992).

amplify depressed mood, suggesting an iatrogenic component in this group of depressed physically ill patients. The association of depression with physical illness in old age is highlighted by a recent review of several studies of medical (i.e. not psychiatric) in-patients which concludes that only one in five recover from their lowered mood state before death (Cole and Bellavance 1997). Suicide rates also increase in the older age group, and this is mainly accounted for by the high rates of male deaths. Twenty per 100,000 men over 65 commit suicide, three times the rate of men in the 15 to 24 age band (OPCS 1977). More recent official statistics indicate that suicide rates in the younger male group rose sharply during the 1980s (Figure 5.1).

What are the social implications of the data from psychiatric epidemiology of depression in older people? Starting with the very high rates of depression in residential homes, there are three explanations for these prevalence rates, which are not mutually exclusive:

1 It could be that those selected to enter these homes have been adjudged by relatives or professionals already to be in poor mental health, or vulnerable because of their lonely and under-supported home conditions (hence their referral to the homes).
2 The under-stimulating environment of these homes may induce apathy and morbid introspection (in the jargon of psychiatry 'dysphoria'). This has led some psychiatrists of old age to speculate that the homes may contain a number of people who are not 'clinically depressed' but who, instead, suffer from environmentally induced dysphoria, which may dissipate with a more stimulating care regime (Pitt 1988). Such a construction on the data of course assumes that there are clear demarcations to be made between clinical descriptions of 'true' depression and other experiences, such as apathy, anomie, listlessness, sad brooding, etc. Some other psychogeriatricians have pointed out that, in fact, it is not easy in the bulk of cases of sad old people to pigeonhole them as being 'ill' or 'not ill' (Murphy 1988).
3 A third consideration is that being moved to a residential facility is disruptive, entails a loss of previous surroundings and may mark a loss of personal control or autonomy. This imposed disruption and loss may have a depressing toll on the old person.

Turning to the community data on depression in old age, there are other explanations that could be offered for depression in old people, who are not in residential care:

1 The first, already noted, is that the probability of physical illness increases with age and this in turn makes older people vulnerable to depression (Post 1969). However, Blaxter (1990), studying the self-reported physical and mental well-being of people across the life-span, found that overall psychosocial well-being improves relatively in old age. This could be partially accounted for by the lower expectations of life quality in old age leading to an under-reporting of distress. Another factor is the dramatic improvement in the self-reported psychosocial well-being of richer people living in more comfortable surroundings (see below). An implication of the association of physical illness and depression is that good and effective physical care of depressed, poorer older people may have an ameliorative impact. Murphy (1988) suggests that the provision of aids for associated disability and other practical help to lessen the dependency of older physically ill people on their relatives may raise morale in the family system and thereby help lift depression.
2 The second incontestable fact about ageing is that relationships that have accumulated during the life-span are lost. Spouses, friends and siblings die off around a surviving older person, making that person prone to the aggregating effect of grief. Depression in old age may be understandable in whole or part as cumulative grief.
3 A third social vulnerability factor is that of material adversity. In a community study of life events preceding depression in old age, Murphy (1982)

found that poorer people who had experienced housing and financial difficulties were more prone to depression (of both mild and severe proportions) than better-off older people. Blaxter (1990) found that the psychosocial well-being of older people varied significantly with social class. Social classes 1 and 2 improved with age overall but those in social classes 4 and 5 deteriorated. (For a discussion of class and other variables affecting social support see Wenger (1989).)

4 A fourth consideration is the role of supportive and confiding relationships. Lowenthal (1965) found, like Brown and Harris (1978) in their study of younger women, that the presence of a stable confiding relationship was a protective factor against depression in old age. She also found that those most vulnerable are old people who try to form relationships and fail, rather than people who have coped throughout life alone. Murphy (1982) found in her community survey that 30 per cent of those reporting the lack of a confiding relationship were depressed. Given that 70 per cent of this group were not depressed, a multifactorial model of vulnerability and protective factors seems to be indicated (as with Brown and Harris (1978).)

5 A fifth factor which needs to be considered is that of abuse in old age. Eastman (1984) suggested that estimates of abused older people in the US vary from 600,000 to over a million. As with the abuse of children, prevalence and incidence are difficult to investigate accurately, given that abusers will typically deny the act. When the abuse occurs at the hands of paid carers, their job is at stake, as well as their reputation. Estimates of elder abuse rates in Scandinavia vary from 8 per cent to 17 per cent of older victims across Denmark, Sweden and Finland. In one of the Swedish samples 12 per cent of relatives admitted violence (Hydle 1993). Some authors extend the notion of elder abuse to medical neglect and iatrogenic disease in hospitalized older people (Gorbien, Bishop and Beers 1992). They include here: poor skin care; poor infection control; failure to make accurate physical diagnoses; leaving frail elders to risk falls; and inadequate dietary provision (as a cost-cutting method). The immediate and long-term negative psychological effects of abuse are difficult to ascertain. It is self-evident that sexual or emotional abuse or physical violence against, or neglect of, old people will not enhance their mental health. A complicating factor is that confused older people who suffer from dementia are prone to violence themselves at times which may trigger reactive aggression in some of their care givers. In one study (Paveza et al. 1992) it was found that in the year following a diagnosis of Alzheimer's Disease, 15.8 per cent of patients and 5.4 per cent of their carers were violent. Usually, age as a perpetrator risk factor for violence is linked to youth, but dementia raises the probability of violent acts in (one group) of older people.

Discussion

The sociological consideration of the life-span and mental health is clearly uneven. At the start of life, socialization is considered to be important and there is certainly no shortage of interest in this arena of social determinism.

Indeed, the consensus is very strong within social science that upbringing, acculturation and rule-learning are all necessary considerations about societal functioning and the relationship between the individual and the collective. Admittedly, some have complained that this theorizing has been exaggerated (Wrong 1961) but generally primary socialization is given a privileged position in a variety of sociological (and psychological) theories.

Psychoanalysis, a form of socialization theory itself derived from the psychological treatment of people with mental health problems, seems to have had a pervasive influence on different types of sociology. As far as childhood is concerned, sociological interest thus far has been theory-dominated. Despite this wide-ranging theoretical discourse about socialization, few sociologists have done empirical work on childhood and its problems (although there is the work of Russell and Finkelhor in the area of child sexual abuse and James and Prout (1990) who have studied 'normal' children). The evidence of child sexual abuse we reviewed has, ironically, posed particular problems for clinical psychoanalysis. This theoretical framework, which has appealed so strongly to so many sociologists, has found itself accused of a central cultural role in suppressing evidence of the sexual abuse of children. This is because of Freud's reversal of his theory in 1896. Prior to then, Freud tended to believe women patients' recollections of incest from childhood. After that time, Freud succumbed to the more comforting notion that these represented subjective fantasies on the part of patients. This then became the accepted 'wisdom' when dealing with patient-reported abuse by Freud's clinical followers (Masson 1985).

When we turn to the core of psychiatry interventions in young adulthood and beyond sociology became enmeshed with a social movement in the 1960s to challenge or discredit clinical theory and practice. As we noted in Chapter 1, Scheff's labelling theory and Goffman's critique of the asylum from within symbolic interactionism were associated with 'antipsychiatry'. The retreat from this association with political activism and 'counter-culture' was then reflected in the sociology of mental health. The latter became more theoretical with the emergence of poststructuralist appraisals of psychiatric discourse. This was, in part, a reaction against the humanism and civil libertarianism which had been associated with antipsychiatry. These post-1960s sociological approaches can be contrasted again historically with the earlier epidemiological tradition of the social causationists. The latter have not disappeared from the map of the sociology of mental health, given the community survey approaches of, for instance, Brown and Harris and Murphy in the 1970s and 1980s.

The main sociological deductions about mental health problems in older people have, mostly, to be made from clinical researchers (social psychiatrists like Murphy). Consequently, harder data is considered from epidemiological surveys at the expense of sociological theorizing. Whereas sociologists have theorized childhood extensively, but done little empirical work, they have done little in either realm as far as old people and their mental health problems are concerned. What theory does exist about later life has come from depth psychologists and has been poorly tested empirically (e.g. Erik Erikson's life-stage theory) or is from a position that emphatically privileges the individual over society (e.g. that of Carl Jung). This relative absence of sociological work on the mental health of older people may reflect a lesser valued group of people who are consequently as readily ignored by sociologists as they are by other people of employable age. This leaves older people being studied in the main by clinicians or by those who have taken a particular interest in social policy rather than social theory (e.g. Walker 1980; Townsend 1981; Wenger 1989). 'Gerontology' as a hybrid academic discipline overlaps with, but is not a subdiscipline of, sociology. Whilst sociologists have contributed substantially to gerontology (Fennell, *et al.* 1988; Jefferys 1989) the specific issue of mental health remains largely absent from their ambit of interest.

Thus, there are three main questions for sociologists given the above summary. First, should they now immerse themselves more in empirical research about childhood and mental health? Given that so many articles of faith have been linked to the theoretical assumptions of this period, for instance that the events of the formative years are predictive of adult personal functioning, sociologists could test their theoretical assumptions against longitudinal investigations. Second, will psychiatric professionals and their diagnostic and treatment activities be the continued focus of interest for the examination of adult mental health or will sociologists seek out new topics and dimensions of inquiry? Third, will sociologists be able to apply their liking for theorizing to the grey topic of older people, or will the latter continue to be scrutinized mainly by clinicians and social policy researchers?

To conclude

This chapter has taken three periods in the life-span (childhood, young adulthood and old age) and examined their implications for mental health. The importance of socialization has been emphasized and disputes about its meaning and relevance discussed. Adulthood brings with it expectations of role-rule consistency which mentally ill people challenge in their functioning. The social factors discussed in old age draw our attention to the importance of depression, not just dementia. They also highlight that ageism is present in sociological interest in mental health.

Questions

1 Why has the concept of primary socialization been so important in social science?

2 What is the relevance of primary socialization for adult mental health?

3 Discuss the impact of childhood sexual abuse on adult mental health.

4 What does the diagnosis of schizophrenia tell us about social norms?

5 What social factors influence the mental health of older people?

6 The sociology of mental health and illness is ageist – discuss.

> ## For discussion
>
> Think about your own family and others you know and consider the link between age and mental health within their relationships.

Further reading

Bifulco, A. and Moran, A. (1998) *Wednesday's Child: Research into Women's Experience of Neglect and Abuse in Childhood and Adult Depression*. London: Routledge.

Bright, R. (1997) *Wholeness in Later Life*. London: Jessica Kingsley Publishers.

Coulter, J. (1973) *Approaches to Insanity*. New York: Wiley.

Gearing, B., Johnson, M. and Heller, T. (eds) (1988) *Mental Health Problems in Old Age*. London: Wiley.

Kitwood, T. and Bredin, K. (1992) Towards a theory of dementia care: personhood and well-being, *Ageing and Society*, 10: 177–196.

Chapter 6

The mental health professions

Chapter overview

The questionable legitimacy of categories of mental illness (discussed in Chapter 1) extends to the roles, identities and functions of mental health workers. The explicit control function of mental health professionals, alongside their role as paid carers, has meant that they have been scrutinized in a more critical light than other groups of health professionals. This chapter will cover:

- Theoretical frameworks in the sociology of the professions
- Mental health professionals and other social actors
- Sociology and the mental health professions

Theoretical frameworks in the sociology of the professions

When sociologists first began to investigate professionals they provided a set of rather flattering descriptions. This was because, by and large, they were prepared to accept definitions provided by professionals themselves. These tended to emphasize that practitioners have unique skills, which are put altruistically at the service of the public. In recent times, this positive view has been altered substantially and in some cases virtually inverted. Illich (1977a) talks of medicine being a 'threat to health' and of welfare professionals being 'disabling' (Illich 1977b). Others reviewing the rise of the new middle class accuse welfare professionals of manipulating both the rich and poor in society for their own interests, as both providers and users of services (Gould 1981). Gouldner (1979) goes as far as speculating that professionals are coming to dominate not just public services but industrial, and even military, life. Despite these criticisms (ironically by and large from professional academics), for ordinary people the word 'professional' tends to imply both special skills and ethical propriety. It implies competence, efficiency, altruism and integrity. Hence, the converse of this is the everyday notion of what it means to be 'unprofessional' – to behave incompetently, inefficiently or unethically. As for contemporary sociologists, they largely agree on some basic characteristics of professionals:

1 Professionals have grown in importance over the past 200 years and expanded massively in number during this century.
2 Professionals are concerned with providing services to people rather than producing inanimate goods.
3 Though salaried or self-employed, professionals have a higher social status than manual workers.
4 This status tends to increase as a function of length of training required to practise.
5 Generally, professionals claim a specialist knowledge about the service they provide and expect to define and control that knowledge.
6 Credentials gain professionals a particular credibility in the eyes of public and government alike.

However, beyond this rough consensus, there is much debate about how professions might be understood sociologically. Here we will look at some of the main frameworks used within sociology to understand professions.

The neo-Durkheimian framework

Overviewers of the field of the sociology of the professions (Saks 1983; Abel 1988) emphasize a certain progression of events. At first, as has been mentioned, sociologists tended to simply categorize the professions and describe their work uncritically. Claims of special knowledge and altruism were taken at face value. This early sociological depiction of positive qualities was dubbed the 'trait' approach to the professions. A parallel and equally uncritical approach to the professions was provided by the structural functionalist accounts, which saw the professions as a static or stable social stratum which offered a socially cohesive role (Parsons 1939; Goode 1957). Durkheim saw professions as providing a disinterested integrative social function. They were one of the social forces which counterbalanced the tendency of egotistical individuals to fragment society. For the Durkheimian tradition, professions are a source of community for one another and stability for the wider society they serve. They regulate their own practitioners, ensuring good practice by establishing codes of conduct and punishing errant colleagues. They regulate their clients in their interest and in the interest of their host society.

The neo-Weberian framework

Those in the Weberian tradition (Freidson 1970; Abel 1988) emphasize that the professions develop strategies to: advance their own social status, persuade clients and potential clients about the need for the service they offer, and corner the market in that service and exclude competitors. Two notions in particular emerge from this picture for those following Weber.

Social closure

Collective social advancement rests upon social closure. By cornering the market, professionals offer a service which is closed off from others. A monopoly is gained to work in a specialized way with a particular group of clients (e.g. medical practitioners treating sick people) so that other occupational groups seeking a similar role are excluded. This closing off also means that only those inside the boundaries of the profession can scrutinize its practices – others are denied access and are kept in a state of ignorance. In order for professionals to maintain their social status they must convince those on the outside of their boundaries that they are offering a unique service and so they develop various rhetorical devices to persuade the world at large of their special qualities. To do this they must justify a peculiar knowledge-base that has a technical or scientific rationality on the one hand, but that, on the other, is not so easy to understand that anybody can use it. Medicine as a whole can be seen to provide such accounts to the world. However, this persuasion is precarious. The growth of alternative medicine (Saks 1992) is testimony to this, as are the doubts about the coherence and credibility of psychiatric knowledge which we examined in Chapter 1.

Professional dominance

The second main feature of this Weberian picture is that of professional dominance. Professionals exercise power over others in three senses:

1 They have power over their clients. The latter, convinced of the need for the service they are offered or seek, are dependent on professionals. An imbalance of specialized knowledge keeps the client in a state of ignorance, insecurity and vulnerability. This power imbalance is reinforced if the

professional operates on their own territory rather than that of their client, for instance by treating people in hospital rather than their own home.

2 Professionals exercise power over their new recruits. Thus, a dominance hierarchy is common in professions, with senior practitioners and trainers exercising control and discipline over their juniors. Power enjoyed in the upper ranks of a profession can only be secured by submission and deference in earlier junior days, as trainees are dependent on their superiors for career progression.

3 Professionals seek to establish a dominant relationship over other occupational groups working with the same clients. Professionals may seek to exclude existing equal competitors or they may seek to usurp the role of existing superiors. In medicine, in addition to excluding competitors (e.g. orthopaedic specialists who have kept chiropractors and osteopaths out of official health service practice) they also subordinate them (obstetricians directing the work of midwives) or limit their therapeutic powers to one part of the body (e.g. dentistry and optometry).

Thus, power relationships are of central importance to neo-Weberians. These are about gaining and retaining power over clients, new entrants and other occupational groups working with those clients. One way of thinking about the neo-Weberian focus is in terms of horizontal relationships between professionals and those they work with, as colleagues or clients, in order to sustain or extend the material advantages, status and comforts of middle-class life in society.

The neo-Marxian framework

When we look to the Marxian tradition, power relationships are also important, but now the focus is on vertical structural relationships. The question to be answered by neo-Marxians is 'Where do professionals fit into a social structure which is characterized by two main groups: those who work to produce wealth (surplus value) in society (the working class or proletariat) and those who own the means of production and exploit these workers and expropriate surplus value as profits (capitalists, the ruling class or the bourgeoisie)?' Marx gave scant attention to the third group of interest to us – those functionaries or 'white collar' workers who were neither exploitative capitalists who owned the means of production nor workers who produced goods and profits. Consequently, those sociologists upholding a Marxian tradition of analysis have had a number of conceptual difficulties with the professions.

Three positions have been taken up by neo-Marxians about the professions. The latter are deemed either to be part of the ruling class or part of the proletariat, or to constitute a separate and new social class holding contradictory qualities. The first type of claim is made by Navarro (1979) who argues that, for instance, the medical profession actually constitutes a part of the ruling class in capitalist society.

By contrast, Oppenheimer (1975) claims that the 'knowledge-based' professions have had control over their work eroded by the state bureaucracies which employ them (they have been subjected to 'bureaucratic subordination'). As a result, their control over their specialized skills has diminished ('deskilling') and consequently they have become part of the working class ('proletarianization'). Oppenheimer understands the collectivist strategies of professions as being no different from traditional trade union defences of working-class terms and conditions of employment. This contrasts with the neo-Weberians, who point to such collective action as being about upward social mobility. Thus, the neo-Weberians are clearly much more critical of the professions than Oppenheimer, who treats them with the sympathy implied by their status as an exploited group of workers who are vulnerable to wage erosion and unemployment.

Clearly, Navarro and Oppenheimer cannot both be totally correct if they claim to operate within the same sociological tradition started by Marx. Their apparent opposition is rescued by a third group of neo-Marxians who argue that they are both partially correct. This group, exemplified by the work of Carchedi (1975), Johnson (1977) and Gough (1979), emphasizes the contradictory position of professionals in capitalist society. They are not capitalists but they serve the interests of the latter. They are not full members of the proletariat (as they do not produce goods and surplus value) but they are employees and so they share similar vulnerabilities and interests of the working class. For instance, mental health workers would be seen in this contradictory position as being both agents of social control acting on behalf of the capitalist state and employees of that state and so vulnerable to the same problems of any other group of workers.

The picture is complicated further by many analysts of the professions drawing liberally on more than one tradition. For instance, Parry and Parry (1977), when discussing the rise of militant trade unionism within the junior ranks of the British medical profession in the 1970s, utilize Weber's notion of closure and Oppenheimer's proletarianization thesis. They go as far as arguing that Weber actually anticipated Oppenheimer's insights and thus they see no dispute between the Marxian and Weberian types of analysis about modern professions.

As we will see later in relation to the mental health professions, it is now common for sociologists to approach their work eclectically – they draw on more than one theoretical tradition. For some this has become an explicit prescription for analysis. For instance, Turner (1987: 140), when discussing health professions, comments that 'a satisfactory explanation of professionalization as an occupational strategy will come eventually to depend upon both Weberian and Marxian perspectives'.

The poststructuralist framework

Since the Second World War a new sort of sociological theory has emerged which builds on, but also departs from, the grander theory inherited from Durkheim, Marx and Weber. This has come to be known as poststructuralism because its focus is not upon social structures and their objective characteristics but on how society is described. One version of this approach treats everything as if it is a text (the 'textualism' of Derrida). This examines all social activity, including science and its applications, as if it were a literary genre. The second related version of poststructuralism, which is of most relevance to us here, is derived from the work of Foucault. His interest has been in the relationship between power and knowledge when regulating populations. For him, social analysis entails examining a: '. . . heterogenous ensemble consisting of discourses, institutions, architectural forms, regulatory decisions, laws, administrative measures, scientific statements, philosophical moral and philanthropic propositions – in short the said and the unsaid.' In particular, Foucault and his followers are concerned to map out discourses associated with particular social periods and places. This notion of discourse includes both forms of knowledge and the practices associated with that knowledge. For this reason, the notion of 'discursive practices' might connote more accurately the focus of the poststructuralists when discussing the professions.

The Foucauldians provide a different way of looking at applied knowledge in professional work. They have no notion of a clear or stable power discrepancy between professionals and clients or between dominant professions and subordinate ones. Power is dispersed, it cannot be simply and easily located in any elite group. Whilst it is certainly bound up with dominant discursive features of a particular time and place, these may change and they may be resisted. For Foucault and his followers, ways in which the person (the body and mind of the individual) is now described or constructed (measured, analysed and codified) are central features of contemporary society. Medicine and professions close to it have had a central role in this regard with their interests in diagnosis, testing, assessment and observation and the treatment, management and surveillance of sick and healthy bodies in society. However, in the poststructuralist account there is a failure to endorse the notion of self-conscious collective activity of professionals, to advance their own interests or to act on behalf of the capitalist state.

As we will see later, the mental health professions have been of particular interest to poststructuralists. This is probably because of the 'psy complex' having a chronic surveillance role in relation to mental patients and because it has been associated with two types of discourse. The first of these emphasized segregation and acting on the body (physical treatments) and the second emphasized the construction of the self via a set of psychological accounts (counselling and psychotherapy). The attack on the body and the construction of the self represent two key ways of understanding the activities of mental health professionals.

The above four general sociological frameworks have been the most influential in understanding the professions. As we will see below, in relation to mental health work, other sociological approaches have also been influential. These include symbolic interactionism, the sociology of knowledge, the sociology of deviance and feminist sociology. Before we discuss these let us look at the relationships which mental health workers have with other key social actors.

Mental health professionals and other social actors

A number of professional groups contribute to mental health work. The most obvious collection – psychiatrists, clinical psychologists, social workers, psychiatric nurses, occupational therapists, art therapists, counsellors and psychotherapists – is employed with the explicit assumption that mental health work is their main role. For this reason, they, or their practice and knowledge, are sometimes referred to as 'the psy complex' by poststructuralists (Ingleby 1983). One way of approaching the sociology of the mental health professions is in terms of seeking out examples within the above sociological frameworks which apply to mental health specialists. However, it would be misleading to give the impression that this core group in the mental health industry provides the only professional input in terms of contact with people entering the patient role or in terms of the negotiation of what constitutes a mental health problem. A variety of other personnel are also implicated, including general practitioners, the clergy, the police and social services care or case managers.

DeSwaan (1990) makes the point that members of the public are encouraged through personal contact with professionals and their clients, and through the media, to frame their personal difficulties in professional terms. He calls this process 'proto-professionalization'. For DeSwaan, what start as personal troubles or discomforts about a person's relationship with others can be framed as problems amenable to specialist help, even before contact with professionals occurs. Whilst DeSwaan focuses on the voluntary presentation to professions by those seeing themselves as suffering these difficulties, as we noted in Chapter 4, Coulter (1973) points out that members of the public also look to professions to rescue them from discomfort or threat caused by others whom they deem to have a mental health problem. Thus, the public are centrally involved in inserting mental health problems into the domain of professional activity in two senses. Sometimes they label themselves in advance as having a problem amenable to specialist help. At other times they look to professionals to help them cope with the distress, threat or anxiety which results from the conduct of others.

Thus, consideration of non-specialist professionals and lay people is important to understand how specialists obtain and retain their mandate of authority about mental health. We can think in terms of four groups of social actors who interact with one another to define the field of mental health problems:

1 The State (represented by politicians, civil servants and managers).
2 Mental health specialists.
3 Professionals who are implicated in mental health work some of the time (GPs, the police, the clergy) but who do not claim a specialist role.
4 That section of the general population that is already convinced of the need to frame their own distress or other people's troublesome conduct in professional terms – lay people who have been 'proto-professionalized'.

The increasing recognition of the coalescence of lay and professional perspectives and involvement in mental health, evident in the work of DeSwaan and Rose, highlights a parallel process of the changing knowledge-base and territory of mental health professional work. There has been a blurring of boundaries between mental and physical health work and models of health and illness. Disciplines across medicine and nursing have embraced the notion of 'holism'. Portmanteau models such as the 'biopsychosocial' model are gaining increasing popularity, particularly as a paradigm which challenges the reductionist and biomedical emphases of traditional health professionals (Dowrick *et al.* 1996). 'Emotional labour' has also become a focus of mental health specialist and generalist health workers alike as well as forming a focus of the analysis of work of non-professionals undertaking 'people work' (e.g. air hostesses) (Hochschild 1983).

The terrain of professional health work, particularly mental health work, has also changed. More work now takes place in the more 'open systems' of primary and community care. Institutionalized ways of responding and relating to patients inside organizations have given way to community-focused work. The need to obtain entry to patients' houses in order to carry out work has reduced the gap between professionals and patients – in so far as access becomes the object of negotiation between two parties, whereas in institutionalized settings it is frequently been taken for granted. 'Fringe work' which refers to a series of activities that professionals are not expected to do or 'supposed' to engage with (de la Cuesta 1993) assume a higher profile when professionals work increasingly in the community. The growing recognition of the mental health component of a wider range of health problems amongst different population groups and presented in primary care is evident in the rise in numbers of primary care counsellors employed to deal specifically with referrals from GPs and other primary care professionals.

Sociology and the mental health professions

Let us now return to the models described earlier within the sociology of the professions. The neo-Durkheimian approach is rarely visible in the contemporary sociological discourse about professional life although it can still be found in the writings of mental health professionals when they are generating a 'public relations' view of their own work. Examples of this can be found in relation to psychiatry (Clare 1976), and clinical psychology (Marzillier and Hall 1987).

Below, we start by acknowledging that many studies have drawn upon more than one theoretical framework. We then look at some purer sociological frameworks before addressing the influence of theoretical models from the study of deviancy, professional knowledge and patriarchy. The latter are important in addition to the work of the sociology of the professions because they come at the question of professional practice from a starting point other than the specialists themselves.

In regard to the other groups we have just noted (non-specialists and lay people), deviancy theorists are interested in the negotiation of deviant roles, like that of becoming a psychiatric patient. Whilst professionals are central to this, they are not the only group of social actors implicated. Likewise, sociological investigations of the transmission of knowledge start with an interest in knowledge but then look to how professionals are a vehicle for its reproduction, possession and modification. Feminists start from a wider interest in the male domination of women in society and then look to particular sites of this domination, like professional practice.

Eclecticism

Many of the attempts to understand mental health professionals have drawn upon more than one theoretical base. For instance, the extensive work of Andrew Scull on the development of psychiatry during and since the nineteenth century has, with some good reason, been described as a 'Marxist functionalist' model by Busfield (1986).

Certainly, as part of his analysis, Scull explains the rise and maintenance of psychiatry in terms of its functional value for economic order and efficiency under capitalism. The segregation of the mad and the delegation by the State of powers to doctors to keep madness under control are central to Scull's thesis. His emphasis is on the role of psychiatrists as agents of social control employed by the State to contain the threat of one section of a poor underclass – the mad. However, when explaining the finer dynamics of how doctors purged lay administrators from the asylums and sought upward social mobility for themselves, he uses a Weberian notion of 'closure', as in this example:

> Modern professions are not simply the *dominant* or most important providers of a particular service; instead they effectively *monopolize a service market* . . . During the nineteenth century, mad-doctors manoeuvred to secure such a position for themselves and acceptance of their particular view of the nature of madness, seeking to transform their existing foothold in the market place into a cognitive and practical monopoly of the field, and to acquire for those practising this line of work the status prerogatives 'owed' to professionals – most notably autonomous control by practitioners themselves over the condition and conduct of their work . . .
>
> (Scull 1979: 129)

Similarly, a work which builds heavily on the work of Scull is Baruch and Treacher's (1978) analysis of the functioning of psychiatry in Britain, which emphasizes the professional dominance of psychiatrists. Whilst Baruch and Treacher highlight the economic factors which both precipitate mental distress and are consequent upon a person entering the role of psychiatric patient, they also draw liberally for the latter purposes on the work of Parsons, albeit with critical reservations. They also refer positively to the post-Marxian social critic Illich, as well as to Scull, in their 'medicalization' thesis about the transformation of madness into mental illness by doctors. Indeed, whilst Baruch and Treacher, like Scull, could be labelled as 'Marxist-functionalists', they begin their book with a long quote from Illich's *Medical Nemesis*.

The medicalization of madness thesis and the emphasis on psychiatrists as agents of social control is by no means limited to neo-Marxians. Right-wing libertarian critics from within psychiatry have constructed social histories of their profession with these emphases as well. The best example of this is the work of Szasz (1971), who argues that psychiatrists are for the modern State what witch-finders were for the Church in mediaeval times. The work of Szasz also echoes some of the analysis of Foucault, which is described below.

In another analysis of twentieth-century psychiatry, Ramon (1985) looks at services and the professions of psychiatry, psychiatric nursing and psychology.

She dubs these for her purposes as the 'psy complex', echoing a post-structuralist term but at the same time firmly endorsing the political economy approach to welfare professionals given by the Marxist Gough (1979) we noted earlier (Ramon 1985: 21).

Turning to the analysis of a different profession, clinical psychology, eclecticism is evident again. Pilgrim and Treacher (1992) describe the historical development of the profession and its recent functioning. The profession in Britain has gone through four phases – psychometrics (1950s), behaviour therapy (1960s), therapeutic eclecticism (1970s) and managerialism (1980s). When theorizing the meaning of their description, Pilgrim and Treacher (1992) endorse the partial advantages of poststructuralist, neo-Weberian and neo-Marxian models for their data analysis. Psychologists have been mainly concerned with voluntary relationships (see discussion of poststructuralism below). They have tried to usurp the role of a dominant profession (psychiatry) to some extent and they have sought, via a campaign of registration, to attain a state-endorsed monopoly over psychological practice. Psychologists have demonstrably served the social administrative requirements of the capitalist state by seeking to regulate the behaviour of children and people with mental health problems and learning difficulties. In addition, Pilgrim and Treacher draw attention to questions of gender and race in understanding some of the features of the profession being white- and male-dominated (see below). These examples of eclecticism reflect that the earlier advice of Turner (1987) about the need to integrate Weberian and Marxian frameworks has been anticipated by a number of sociologists.

Poststructuralist accounts of the psy complex

Foucault's early writings on mental health began quite close to the Marxian emphasis on social control (Foucault 1961, 1965). However, he diverged from Scull's analysis on two counts even at this stage. First, he puts the beginnings of segregation at an earlier point, the 'great confinement' of the mid-seventeenth to mid-eighteenth century. Scull argues that most of the mad were still roaming free in society at the beginning of the nineteenth century and it was not until the mid-nineteenth century that the state asylum system was well established to segregate madness. Second, Foucault emphasized the moral, not the economic, order. Whereas Scull argued that psychiatry functioned to aid and abet economic efficiency, Foucault argued that psychiatry existed primarily to deal with those who offended bourgeois morality and rationality. For Foucault, segregative psychiatry was not concerned with either medical cure or economic efficiency *per se* but with moral regulation.

Miller (1986) notes that Foucault's work is essentially a 'prehistory' of psychiatry and it is then extended by Castel (1983) into the period when the profession became more firmly established in the nineteenth century. The moral regulation theme continues about the role of the alienist or psychiatrist. Madness now had to be dealt with within the rules of the emerging bourgeois 'contractual' society. During this period the psychiatric profession did not go unchallenged but it retained its central role in relation to the asylum.

The third phase of interest to poststructuralists has been the changes in psychiatry during the twentieth century (Castel *et al.* 1979; Armstrong 1980; Miller and Rose 1988). Here, four interweaving themes can be identified: (1) psychiatry as a professional enterprise is no longer restricted only to the asylum; (2) its practices are no longer only associated with coercive social control; (3) large bands of the population have been induced into an individualized state of psychological mindedness about their existence, via the media and education; and (4) following from the last two points, voluntary relationships involving lengthy conversations about the self are now sought out by the public and deployed by professionals (versions of counselling and psychotherapy) (Rose 1990).

The move beyond the asylum can be linked roughly to changes in practices during the First World War when the problem of shellshock required a new response to mental distress (Stone 1985). Psychotherapy began in earnest at this point: outpatient clinics were set up after the war and centres of excellence, like the Tavistock Clinic, which celebrated the legitimacy of psychoanalysis were established. Psychoanalysis had been attacked or ignored by psychiatrists before 1914. After the war, the Tavistock Clinic became associated with a wider cultural emphasis on the individual and the family, for instance, by promoting explanations of delinquency and mental distress, which were purported to arise from poor mothering.

Of central importance in this account is the rejection of the coercive social control emphasis of Scull and the 'antipsychiatrists'. For instance, Miller and Rose argue that the psy complex has increasingly emphasized voluntary relationship, which is sought out and appreciated by clients: 'We argue that it is more fruitful to consider the ways that regulatory systems have sought to promote subjectivity than to document ways in which they have crushed it' (Miller and Rose 1988: 174). DeSwaan's notion of 'proto-professionalization', mentioned earlier, also operates with a similar assumption about a cultural consensus between professionals and lay people that their everyday troubles can be solved by conversations (counselling and psychotherapy) which focus on, celebrate and construct, the 'self'.

However, the poststructuralist account still emphasizes the role of professionals in 'regulating' the everyday lives of their clients (Donzelot 1979). Abbott and Wallace (1990: 6) note that the caring professions:

> not only aim to change and control behaviour, but also help to structure the context of social and cultural life in a more general sense . . . [T]hey create both the object of intervention – the neglectful mother, the wayward teenager, the bad patient – and at the same time make these the targets of their intervention. Intervention is designed to normalize, to make subjects conform to the defined norms.

Thus, differences of opinion between sociologists about the regulatory role of professionals seem to hinge on differences of emphasis. The poststructuralists (and Parsons in his discussion of the sick role (1951)) emphasize a process of consensual decision-making wherein the client either comes to agree with, or already accepts, professional definitions of the nature of their problem. Social regulation occurs by agreement and with actual (or perceived) benefits to the client. By contrast, the Marxian tradition emphasizes the enforced imposition of a view on the client by professionals acting as agents of the state. The first of these suggests that the power to regulate emotional life and norms of conduct is diffuse or dispersed. Power cannot be located 'inside' any one particular group of social actors. Rather, it is understood as a relationship or discourse shared by several parties. The second account clearly locates power in the hands of professionals who dominate their clients at the behest of their state employers. Maybe both types of account are credible. Patients do seek out help in voluntary relationships. In addition, sometimes, professionals impose themselves on patients – they lock them up and give them treatments they do not consent to freely.

Because poststructuralist writers about mental health have tended to focus on twentieth-century developments, their emphasis has tended to be on the disciplinary, rather than repressive, power of psychiatric experts. This has led to a skewed poststructuralist interest, with Foucault's early concern with repressive power being replaced by an emphasis on psychological interventions which are 'anxiously sought and gratefully received' (Pilgrim and Rogers 1994). This shift emphasizes the role of the secularized confessional in modern society in Foucault's later writings:

> The confession has spread its effects far and wide. It plays a part in justice, medicine, education, family relationships, in love relations, in the most ordinary affairs of everyday life and in the most solemn rites: one confesses one's crimes, one's sins, one's thoughts and desires, one's illnesses and troubles; one goes about telling with the greatest precision whatever is most difficult to tell.
>
> (Foucault 1981: 59)

This role of the confessional is discussed in more detail in relation to mental health work by Rose (1990). He suggests a number of points in this regard:

1 Psychotherapeutic assumptions can be found to operate now in general medicine, education, advertising, and journalism and business management. They are not limited to the work of mental health experts.
2 A countervailing discourse has also emerged from some social critics about a 'modern obsession with the self' and a 'tyranny of intimacy in which narcissism is mobilised in social relations'.
3 Modern psychotherapeutic rituals mimic and displace the older emphasis on religious or spiritual pilgrimages. The growth of Protestantism with its emphasis on individual guilt and responsibility marked a bridge between mediaeval religion and the modern culture of the self and individualism. Alongside this emerged the 'civilizing process' (Elias 1978) in which self not State control became important – the growth in importance of etiquette and manners. Thus, a repressive State form of control was increasingly superseded by self-control.
4 New versions of the confession like counselling and the psychological therapies became means by which identities were inscribed upon their subjects. Mental health work produces 'the subjectification of work', 'the psychologization of the mundane', 'a therapeutics of finitude' and a 'neuroticization

of social intercourse'. What Rose points to in these phrases is the way in which work, common life transitions, disappointment, death and our intimate relationships are now framed within mental health discourses.

5 Following Foucault, Rose offers a triple aspect on psychological treatments. First there are *moral codes* in the language and ethical principles of therapy. These imply some notion of 'the good life' and are thus implicitly or explicitly normative. Second, there are *ethical scenarios* which are the sites or contexts in which the moral codes operate – social work practice, the courts, the private consulting room, etc. Third there are *techniques of the self*, which are developed to codify the exploration, definition and confrontation of the self in therapy (Foucault 1988). These techniques are not a unitary body of knowledge but a wide range of models which produce narratives of the self – heterogeneity of approach characterizes the psychological treatments.

6 These features of mental health work are not guided by the hidden hand of capital (cf. the neo-Marxian view of the professions) nor by the conscious collective self-interest pursued by professionals according to the neo-Weberians (see below). Instead, the main orientation of modern mental health work is one of reconciling or aligning the needs of individuals with the social, political or organizational goals which form the social context of therapists and their clients.

Having outlined the poststructuralist perspective of mental health work, we now turn to the application of an older sociological approach.

The neo-Weberian approach

This has already been mentioned in relation to clinical psychologists seeking a monopoly on psychological practice and on their boundary dispute with psychiatry (Pilgrim and Treacher 1992). It was also an important aspect of the study of a psychiatric unit by Baruch and Treacher (1978), in terms of the strategies which consultant psychiatrists used to maintain their dominant position in the mental health team working with in-patients.

In another study of psychiatrists, their relationship with the police has been analysed in terms of professional dominance. Rogers (1993c) studied the transactions that occurred between the two occupational groups when people deemed to be mentally disordered in public were taken for psychiatric assessment by police officers (under section 136 of the Mental Health Act 1983). Rogers found that psychiatrists operated a number of strategies to exert control over how the patient was dealt with. The technical knowledge of the profession was a focus for psychiatrists' dominance over police officers. Even though police officers identified mental disorder with the same technical efficiency as psychiatrists, the latter insisted on depicting the police as lacking in the credentials to understand or manage the client group. The police were not in fact interested in encroaching on the territory of psychiatric practice. None the less, psychiatrists acted to ward off a form of encroachment on their professional power that they perceived to be coming from police officers.

Sociologists who try to understand specific groups of professions usually find it necessary to appreciate how practitioners perceive their own role and that of others. The next wider sociological tradition to be discussed highlights this.

Symbolic interactionism

This approach can be found in Goffman's classic study of asylum life and of how the patient role is imposed on admitted psychiatric patients (Goffman 1961). What matters in this 'microsociology' are the meanings which are negotiated by various social actors involved in a drama or ritual. Goffman talks of 'degradation rituals', when the patient's identity is removed as they enter the psychiatric patient role (see below). This type of approach was extended by Braginsky et al. (1973) (discussed further in Chapter 7).

The symbolic interactionists can also be found in studies of how psychiatrists and other mental health workers see and justify their role. Goldie (1977) interviewed psychiatrists in order to understand the meanings they attached to their knowledge-base and their perceived superior status compared with non-medical staff. He also observed and took accounts from other members of mental health care teams about how they understood their particular expertise and powers. From this data he built up a picture of how psychiatrists maintain their mandate of authority in the field of mental health and how subordinate professions both challenge and maintain that mandate.

In another study of a psychiatric team using participant observation and interviews, Emerson and Pollner (1975) investigated the ways in which professionals classified their work with different types of patients. In particular, the investigators were interested in looking at how less acceptable work, such as the compulsory detention of patients in emergency duties, was conceived by workers. They found that this 'dirty work' or 'shit work' was accounted for by workers who preferred the morally superior role of being benign therapists. The dirty work conception derives from earlier work by Hughes (1971), who sees it as an aspect of all professional activity entailing a practitioner being obliged to 'play a role of which he thinks he ought to be a little ashamed of morally'. For Emerson and Pollner, the dirty work of acute psychiatry is that of social control – involuntary admission to hospital. In order to distance themselves from this explicit and morally dubious role, practitioners will point out that it is not really typical of their duties, that it is forced on them by circumstances or that they use the opportunity to help the patient as best they can.

The influence of the sociology of deviance

It is not surprising that some investigations of mental health work have started with the social negotiation of psychiatric patienthood, rather than looking at a particular profession. Coulter's work has already been noted (Coulter 1973). His concern was understanding how social crises in the domestic arena became reframed as psychiatric illnesses. A similar approach can be found in the work of Scott (1973), who tried to map out the powers available to professionals, prospective patients and significant others to establish or maintain the deviant role of mental patient.

Goffman's work has already been mentioned but it is important to note that his study of hospital life supplied us with important concepts related to the negotiation of deviance: 'the betrayal funnel' and the 'degradation ritual'. The former refers to the conspiratorial relationship which necessarily develops between relatives of identified patients who have been forcibly admitted to hospital and the receiving professionals. Goffman called this conspiracy 'the circuit of agents that participate fatefully in the passage from civilian to patient status'. The 'degradation ritual' refers to the removal by professionals of a person's everyday identity and a stripping away of their usual sense of self. They are labelled with a diagnosis and normal signals of their individuality (such as their own clothes) are removed.

This emphasis on the involvement of professionals in negotiating a deviant role can be found in Bean's study of psychiatrists, social workers and GPs who compulsorily detain patients (Bean 1980). In this study, Bean was testing the validity of claims arising from Lemert's (1974) work on group interaction, an extension of labelling theory about the treatment of one set of rule-breakers (criminals) and checking how this model applied to another group of rule-breakers (those diagnosed as being mentally ill). The principles of this model of deviancy are concerned with rules, their enforcement by parties (i.e. professionals) with designated powers, and how rule enforcement may or may not lead to an outcome which is intended. Bean's interest in testing the limits of this theory in the field of mental health work involved his observing the conduct and statements of professionals (the 'rule enforcers') in their work when admitting patients to hospital compulsorily.

The influence of the sociology of knowledge

Some sociologists have tried to understand the workings of particular professions in terms of the knowledge-base they employ. Within the neo-Weberian tradition this sociology of knowledge approach is evident in the work of Freidson (1970) when examining the general character of modern professional life. In relation to mental health workers, Sheppard (1990) has compared psychiatric nurses with social workers within such a framework. He takes the lead from Atkinson, who advocates the need to examine 'the relationship between education, practice and the organization of occupational groups' (Atkinson 1983). The rationale here is that a close look at that relationship will reveal how the assumptions about the knowledge will shape professional practice and illuminate how practitioners defend the legitimacy of their particular role. Following from this, empirical studies of professionals should attend to the meanings that practitioners attach to their work (in line with symbolic interactionism discussed above).

Sheppard (1990) suggests that social workers and community psychiatric nurses (CPNs) might in some respects overlap in the type of work they do with clients, but a closer look at the knowledge-base of each profession also points to differences. Social workers are influenced, albeit inconsistently, by social science. CPNs, in contrast, are preoccupied more by a focus on mental illness – how to account for it and how to respond to it. This means that practitioners accept psychiatric (i.e. medical) models of explanation and treatment or they react against them (i.e. take on board 'antipsychiatry' arguments). Their background is not within social science but is tied instead to a medical body of knowledge. Also, because of their role in relation to mental health law (social workers approved for this purpose are required to detain patients compulsorily), social workers may be more concerned with legal definitions of work rather than the nature of distress and its treatment.

The influence of feminist sociology

Feminist sociology has emphasized the subordinated role of women in three senses when discussing the caring professions (Gamarnikow 1978; Hearn 1982; Crompton 1987; Abbott and Wallace 1990; Witz 1990): (1) women are more likely to be subordinated as clients; (2) women on average occupy lower-status positions within professions; (3) those occupational groups which are numerically dominated by women (like nursing) are more likely to be subordinate to male-dominated professions (like medicine). However, because of the history of male asylum attendants being used to physically control lunatics in the nineteenth century, psychiatric nursing has been more male-dominated (and working class) than general nursing (Carpenter 1980).

Pilgrim and Treacher (1992) found that female clinical psychologists are less likely to occupy managerial and professional leadership positions than men. Moreover, they found that conservative male elements in the profession also lamented the greater proportion of women to men on the explicit grounds that this implies an inferior status and induces a decline in salary levels (Humphrey and Haward 1981; Crawford 1989). Feminism has also stimulated new forms of therapeutic practice which are tailored to women's needs (Eichenbaum and Orbach 1982).

Discussion

This chapter will end by drawing attention to the twin problems of uncertainty when discussing the mental health professions. The first problem is about the professions themselves. What are they up to? Are they concerned with ameliorating distress or with controlling deviant behaviour (or both)? To what degree are they effective in either of these roles? This question will be returned to when we discuss treatment in Chapter 7. In whose interests do they work – themselves, their clients, the general public, the state, patriarchy? What role does power play in their operations? Are they impartial benign practitioners or partisan oppressive enforcers of social conformity, deriving their role from wider inequalities of power (based on race, class and gender)? Do they crush individuality or celebrate and construct it? Any critical student of the mental health professions or critical practitioner within their ranks is drawn to these types of questions in one form or another.

The second problem relates to the lack of consensus on the part of sociologists when attempting to provide answers to these questions. Answers are provided but sometimes they concur with the work of others and sometimes they do not. The mental health professions represent a contested area of sociological inquiry which is rendered less contentious by eclecticism but remains contested nonetheless.

Both sides to this uncertainty characterize the discourse about mental health work at present. Two questions in particular will continue to tantalize social scientists for the foreseeable future. First, how do mental health professions with such a weak, controversial, contradictory and poorly credible body of knowledge (see Chapters 1 and 7) continue to maintain a mandate to regulate the lives of those they deem to be mentally unfit? Second, with the apparent mixture of coercive and non-coercive power operating in mental health work, how might the tensions and contradictions of the professions be understood?

The poststructuralists seem to come nearest to providing answers to these questions but they leave a number of loose ends. They notoriously ignore gender relationships (Rose 1990). They also understate the continuing role of coercive social control enjoyed by professionals and suffered by service users. Also, traditional epidemiological research seems to suggest that predictable inequalities in mental health derive from real differences between social groups, which are independent of a professional discourse or set of interventions. Arguably, professionals diagnose and respond to these differences, they do not simply create them in cahoots with other social actors. How then do we resolve questions about whether apparent differences in mental health between social groups are real outcomes of social inequality or constructed by-products of psychiatric discourse?

The work of mental health professionals is important to sociologists not only because of the character of their operations, strategies or practices. Professionals might also be deemed to account for the very existence of 'the mentally ill' in modern society on the one hand, or they might represent a set of occupations which respond to real socially determined forms of personal distress and social deviance defined by lay people on the other.

To conclude

This chapter has explored a variety of sociological approaches to mental health work. The diversity reflects wider unresolved disputes within the field of the sociology of the professions. In turn, these disputes are connected to divisions within social theory, with post-structuralism representing the most recent participant in debates about how health professionals are to be understood in society. As we note in the latter part of the chapter, sociological currents outside work on the professions have also been influential in some investigations of mental health work. The sociological perspective taken determines the reader's sympathy for, or criticism of, mental health workers.

Questions

1 Compare and contrast two perspectives from the sociology of the professions and apply them to mental health work.

2 'Mental health professionals and their patients are trapped in the same discourse' – discuss.

3 Are mental health workers agents of the State?

4 Whose interests are served by the work of psychiatric professionals?

5 What advantages are offered by sociological eclecticism when understanding the mental health professions?

6 Discuss the role of non-specialists in mental health work.

For discussion

Would you trust a mental health professional to help you if you were distressed? Consider this question by rehearsing what would encourage you to seek help and what would make you cautious about that approach.

Further reading

DeSwaan, A. (1990) *The Management of Normality*. London: Routledge.
Pilgrim, D. and Rogers, A. (1994) Something old, something new . . . sociology and the organisation of psychiatry, *Sociology*, 28, 2: 521–538.
Rose, N. (1990) *Governing the Soul*. London: Routledge.
Samson, C. (1995) The fracturing of medical dominance in British psychiatry, *Sociology of Health and Illness*, 17, 2: 245–268.

Chapter 7

Questions of treatment

Chapter overview

This chapter will examine the ways in which the treatment of people with mental health problems might be understood sociologically. In particular the two connotations of 'treatment' will be explored – one related to technical aspects of therapy, the other to do with the way in which people are treated as part of a moral order. The chapter will cover the following topics:

- Governmentality and therapy

- Therapeutics

- A brief social history of psychiatric treatment

- Criticisms of psychiatric treatment

- The moral sense of 'treatment'

- Who is psychiatry's client?

- The question of informed choice

- The social distribution of treatment

- The impact of evidence-based practice on treatment

- Mental health promotion versus treatment

Governmentality and therapy

Some sociologists have argued that we now live in a therapeutic society in which therapeutic ideas are not confined to clinical and hospital settings but permeate most areas of everyday life. 'Governmentality' in contemporary societies is achieved by the self-regulation of our activities through our own emotions and feelings and the internalization of psychological knowledge. The point is made by Rose:

> Through self-inspection, self-problematization, self-monitoring, and con-fession, we evaluate ourselves according to the criteria provided for use by others. Through self-reformation, therapy, techniques of body alteration, and the calculated reshaping of speech and emotion, we adjust ourselves by means of the techniques propounded by the experts of the soul.
>
> (Rose 1990: 10)

Notwithstanding the merit of this analysis for understanding cultural trends and the popularity of psychological ideas and therapies, in this chapter a more specific focus is taken of treatment. The term 'treatment' when used to refer to therapeutic procedures, itself presupposes that we share a view of people being ill. It assumes that we are trapped to some extent in a 'thera-peutic discourse'. In line with this, it is commonplace to accept the notions of 'talking treatments' or of 'drug treatments' or more specifically of 'electro-convulsive treatment' (ECT) (in the US this is called 'electroshock treatment' (EST)). We will, indeed, look at these procedures. We will also examine a broader notion of 'treatment'. How are people with mental health problems treated in the moral sense?

Therapeutics

This section will summarize the social history of psychiatric treatment before going on to examine recent criticisms of that legacy.

A brief social history of psychiatric treatment

Sedgwick (1982) notes that two broad responses to emotional problems are traceable as far back as Ancient Rome. On the one hand, attempts have been made to tamper with the bodies of people with emotional afflictions, for example douching them in water or drilling holes in their skulls to allow evil spirits to escape. On the other hand, in ancient times good counsel was also purported to be of help. Thus, it is possible to claim that there are certain stable trans-historical themes – one somatic (today's biological psychiatry) and the other conversational (today's psychological therapies).

In the twentieth century, western psychiatry has developed an eclectic mixture of these interventions. Those entering the role of psychiatric patient will be prescribed physical interventions (drugs or ECT) or some version of psychological treatment, or a combination of the two, with the former typically predominating. At the turn of the century this was not the case. Psychiatrists at that time had a narrow interest in lunatics in their asylums. These were assumed to have disordered brains and were therefore treated accordingly. Physical treatments were very limited and crude. By the 1930s, psychotic in-patients were being treated only with paraldehyde, chloral hydrate, laxatives and cold baths (Bean 1980). There was little or no interest in psychological treatments or in non-psychotic disorders until the First World War created a crisis of legitimacy for the dominant bio-determinist model of psychiatry. This was built on the assumption that lunacy alongside other forms of deviance like criminality and idiocy was a result of a 'tainted' gene pool. This hereditarian emphasis was formalized with the emergence of the pseudo-scientific discipline of eugenics. Eugenicists were convinced that racial improvement necessitated the resistance to external contamination by an alien racial stock and to the internal contamination by the tainted genes of the lower classes. The latter threat was amplified by their purported greater fertility.

With the First World War, 'England's finest blood' began to break down with 'shellshock', later called 'battle neurosis' and then 'post-traumatic stress disorder'. The officers and gentlemen and their lower-class volunteer subordinates could not be construed as being genetically inferior. Consequently, the tainted gene model of psychiatry virtually constituted a form of treason. To add to the problem for the hereditarian position, officers were breaking down at a higher rate than lower ranks. This crisis of legitimacy for the hereditarian model allowed in a newer discourse on mental disorder, largely rooted in psychoanalysis. Versions of psychotherapy were the stock-in-trade of the shellshock doctors of the time and in the treatment centres like the Tavistock Clinic, set up after the war, to treat compensation cases of the new disorder. A fuller version of this shift from biological to psychological approaches in treatment can be found in Stone (1985). Thus, by the end of the war, psychiatry began to become more eclectic, although a pattern was already discernible of neurosis being treated psychologically and madness being treated with physical means. The latter began to predominate again in the inter-war years, boosted in confidence by the appearance of insulin coma therapy in 1934, prefrontal leucotomy in 1935, and ECT in 1938.

Mainstream psychiatry after the Second World War marginalized the aetiological role of psychological factors and talking treatments. The main textbooks of that period, which were to dominate post-war psychiatric training, reasserted the Victorian biodeterminism of the profession's founders (Mayer-Gross *et al.* 1954). Once major tranquillizers were introduced in the mid-1950s, psychiatrists could begin to make the claim which is often repeated today that these drugs opened the doors of the hospitals and paved the way for community care. In fact, in-patient numbers were already dropping before the introduction of major tranquillizers and the reasons for deinstitutionalization are multiple (see Chapter 8). Whilst it is generally conceded by most commentators on psychiatry that it is now eclectic (Baruch and Treacher 1978; Ramon 1985; Busfield 1986) the bias towards physical treatments is still strong.

Also, despite the incorporation of social and psychological aetiological factors into modern psychiatry, there has been a tendency to reject the centrality of their relevance compared with purported biological causes (Royal

College of Psychiatrists 1973). Alternatively, they are given equal consideration but they still legitimize the disease model and the authoritative power
of medicine in the diagnosis and treatment of people with personal and
social problems. This revision of the medical model by Clare (1976) has been
described as a 'portmanteau model' by Baruch and Treacher (1978) to indicate that the disease formulation now takes more on board without being
undermined.

As well as psychiatry now offering a mixed therapeutic approach, albeit
biased towards drugs and ECT, other mental health professionals vary in
the types of treatment they offer. Psychiatric nurses might provide client-
centred counselling following the humanistic psychologist Carl Rogers or
psychoanalytically-oriented 'psychodynamic' psychotherapy, either individually or in groups. Some nurses are trained as specialists in behaviour therapy.
A similar eclectic mix can be found in the approach of clinical psychologists
to treatment (Pilgrim and Treacher 1992). In academic psychology the dominance of behaviourism broke down in the mid-1970s and was overtaken in
popularity by cognitivism. Therapists thereafter modified behaviour therapy
by treating cognitions as if they were behaviour – 'cognitive behaviour therapy'
thus evolved (see Chapter 1).

Criticisms of psychiatric treatment

Throughout medicine, therapeutic preferences are evident. Certain treatments
may predominate, but they coexist with lesser-used alternatives. They also
wax and wane in popularity with clinicians. In recent times they have also
been subjected to wider social and cultural influences. The media and 'public
opinion' have been influential in changing the regulatory frameworks and
provision of drugs. Mental health work is no different in this sense. However, the work of psychiatric therapists has been controversial for particular
reasons which go beyond the pattern of fads and fashions typical of wider
curative medicine.

1 Following Sedgwick's observation above, there is still a broad and unresolved
   tension between somatic and conversational modes of treatment. The dominance of the first of these has led to disaffection amongst service users.
2 Each of these therapeutic approaches has been attacked for its iatrogenic
   effects. Iatrogenic effects are those caused by the treatment itself. The term
   'side-effects' is a common version of this notion when talking about drug
   therapy. It is probably more precise to speak of 'unwanted effects' rather
   than 'side-effects'.
3 Each approach has been attacked for its ineffectiveness in ameliorating
   distress.

These three broad criticisms will now be elaborated.

Why do physical treatments predominate?

From a user's perspective, the fact that psychiatric treatments are biased
more towards drugs and ECT is indeed a problem. In one study, physical

treatments were given to 98 per cent of psychiatric patients whereas only 60 per cent gained access to some form of talking treatment (Rogers *et al.* 1993). The evidence on the clinical effectiveness (i.e. symptom reduction) is as powerful for drugs as it is for talking treatments (see later). User groups are generally more hostile to physical than psychological treatments. Moreover, the strong bias towards drugs reflects biomedical professional preferences at the expense of user choice.

Six mutually reinforcing contributory factors can be put forward to suggest why such a bias exists.

1 The medicalization of madness in the nineteenth century entailed a bio-logical emphasis. Scull (1979: 165) quotes the following from the *Journal of Mental Science* in 1858: 'Madness is purely a disease of the brain. The physician is the guardian of the lunatic and must ever remain so.' For doctors to ensure their jurisdiction over madness they had to assert or prove that it arises from some sort of physical pathology. Accordingly, the use of physical treatments is consistent with a biodeterministic aetiological theory. If such a position is not persuasive, then arguably mental illness is actually a sort of social, educational or existential, not physical, problem. As an indication of this, psychoanalysis, the prototype of the modern talking treatments, became divided in its early years about whether ana-lysts needed to be physicians.

2 During the 1960s, when large mental hospitals came under attack from a variety of sources, an opportunity was created for psychiatrists to shift their site of operation into mainstream medicine. Their preferred service delivery model was that of the District General Hospital psychiatric unit. Baruch and Treacher (1978) point out that this allowed psychiatrists to make a bid to rejoin mainstream medicine and thereby compensate for the low status traditionally enjoyed by their medical specialty. Whether this has actually led to an improving of their status within medicine is uncer-tain. However, aligning itself with general medicine was made more cred-ible by the content of its interventions being like other medical procedures (i.e. physical treatments; see Chapter 8). In the US Kleinman (1988) also noted that medication-use and the professional image of psychiatry as a poor relation trying to improve its medical reputation were intertwined.

3 Physical treatments are legitimized and encouraged by the profit motive. Drugs are a well known source of profits for their producers (Klass 1975). In addition to the profits accruing from the sale of psychotropic medication, these companies also sell drugs to offset the side effects of major tran-quillizers (e.g. induced Parkinson's disease). In 1984, MIND (the National Association of Mental Health) obtained and publicized information of the scale of public spending on psychiatric drugs, normally kept secret by the then Department of Health and Social Security. For instance, these drugs formed 17 per cent of NHS prescriptions and at that time £37 million per annum was being spent on minor tranquillizers alone. According to the government White Paper *The Health of the Nation*, by 1992 psychotropic drugs constituted 24 per cent of NHS scripts.

Drug companies promote their products through expensive advertising campaigns and sponsored events. Phillipson (1989) reported that by the late 1980s the drug companies were spending in the region of $2 million, just on advertising to American physicians working with elderly patients. In Britain, in 1981 one-third of the residents of old people's homes were receiving minor tranquillizers as night sedation (Morgan and Gilleard 1981).

4 Although millions in each international currency are spent yearly on psychotropic drugs, they are still arguably cheaper to deliver than labour-intensive talking treatments. For instance, minor tranquillizers (discussed in Chapter 3) are a cheap and quick way of disposing of emotional problems in the surgery. Likewise, a reliance on major tranquillizers to dampen down the agitation of psychotic patients, old people and those with learning difficulties has been a cheap alternative to crisis intervention, intensive family support and psychological programmes.

5 If psychiatry exists amongst other things, to control disruptive conduct, physical treatments are highly suited to this purpose because they can be imposed in the absence of cooperation. Medication, psychosurgery and ECT can, in certain circumstances, be imposed on people against their will, whereas it is very difficult to conduct talking treatments with resistant subjects. Indeed, most psychotherapists argue that consent is a necessary precondition for any form of their treatment and that this condition of free choice is clearly compromised by a client being captive (Pilgrim 1988). However, group therapy has been used inside secure psychiatric facilities. Indeed, the therapeutic community approach to treatment is arguably well suited for social control as it uses group pressure and conformity to realign deviant conduct.

6 Although discoveries about the behavioural impact of psychotropic drugs have often been a result of accident rather than design, once the effects are demonstrated and they are patented and marketed by drug companies, they provide a spurious illusion that biodeterminism has been proven (bringing us back to point 1 above). The drive for pharmaceutical companies to produce both innovative and 'me too' compounds for profit has entailed their stimulation of biological psychiatric research both directly via research funding and indirectly. In the latter regard, Healy (1997) has noted that even the patient who is drug 'treatment' resistant becomes a curious conundrum for neurospsychiatric researchers to solve using expensive medical technology to scan (live) and slice (dead) brains. The very use of that expensive technology then confirms the legitimacy of biological reductionism within psychiatry.

Minor tranquillizers

The benzodiazepines ('minor tranquillizers') have been discredited for their addictive qualities. They are only effective in symptom control for around ten days, with 58–77 per cent of recipients reporting sedation effects of the drugs (drowsiness, lethargy and memory disturbances). Thirty per cent of those taking these drugs for more than a few weeks will develop withdrawal symptoms, including panic attacks, insomnia, tremor, palpitations, sweating and muscle tension (Tyrer 1987). In a small percentage (under 5 per cent) more severe problems, including epileptic seizures and paranoid reactions, might occur. During the 1980s, the scale of iatrogenic addiction prompted a popular protest movement coordinated by MIND and the TV programme

That's Life, which led to litigation against the drug companies supplying minor tranquillizers (Lacey 1991). When they are used in older patients, minor tranquillizers can also lead to mental confusion and falls, necessitating emergency medical treatment. Learoyd (1980), studying medical emergencies in Australia, found that the psychotropic drugs were implicated in 16 per cent of the admissions to hospital of people over 65. Despite their dominant role in mental health services, professionals have failed to maintain a positive image of their prescribed minor tranquillizers.

Sociologists have illuminated the role and impact of wider social influences, institutions and processes on the use and acceptability of minor tranquillizers. Bury and Gabe (1990) have demonstrated the role of the media in legitimizing the social problem status of minor tranquillizers. More recently, they have presented an analysis of events surrounding the suspension of the licence, by the British Licensing Authority in 1991, for the widely used sleeping tablet Halcion (triazolam) (Gabe and Bury 1996). They identify four elements within these events – the claims-making activities of medical experts; legal challenges; the role of the media; and the response of the State. Together these have made a contribution to minor tranquillizers becoming a public and governmental issue rather than a purely clinical matter.

In relation to the same controversy about Halcion, micro-sociological factors within organizations like the Licensing Authority, have been offered as an alternative to the account by Gabe and Bury (Abraham and Sheppard 1998). These micro-factors include professional interests and the internal organizational arrangements and processes within institutions for reviewing and presenting data. Abraham and Sheppard suggest that these are more important than broader extra-organizational social influences in determining whether or not a drug remains widely available or is withdrawn from use (cf. Gabe and Bury). The authors claim that these micro-sociological factors are alternative explanations to those provided by Gabe and Bury (Abraham and Sheppard 1998). However, it seems more likely that social processes at *both* micro *and* macro levels are likely to sway the extent to which drugs are viewed as acceptable by authorizing bodies, the medical profession, the public and the State. It is also likely that in the future, trends, such as evidence-based practice (discussed below), and new organizational arrangements for regulating medical practice, such as clinical governance outlined in the NHS White Paper (England) (Secretary of State for Health 1998) will be a major influence on both clinical practice and public legitimacy in determining what is and what is not safe as a psychiatric treatment.

Major tranquillizers

The phenothiazine major tranquillizers, also called 'neuroleptics' and 'antipsychotics', create the iatrogenic problems of Parkinsonism (trembling), akithisia (inner restlesness) and tardive dyskinesia. The latter is a group of disabling and disfiguring movement disorders, including pronounced facial tics, tongue flicking and jerking limbs. Estimates of its prevalence in those prescribed major tranquillizers vary from 0.5 per cent to 50 per cent with a mean of 20 per cent (Brown and Funk 1986). The probability of the iatrogenic effect occurring increases the longer the drug is prescribed, the larger the dose and the more other drugs are given in a 'cocktail' (technically called 'polypharmacy') (Hemmenki 1977; Warner 1985). When larger doses are given ('megadosing') fatalities are also risked, warranting the invention of a new diagnosis for iatrogenic death from phenothiazines – the 'neuroleptic malignant syndrome' (Kellam 1987).

Given the serious dangers associated with neuroleptics, the degree of complacency about their use on the part of professionals has attracted particular sociological interest. Brown and Funk (1986) trace how the evidence about tardive dyskinesia was available to psychiatrists in the late 1960s. And yet, throughout the 1970s and 1980s major tranquillizer prescription rates were undiminished (they actually increased in frequency and in dose levels). Active and passive forms of professional resistance to the recognition of tardive dyskinesia as an iatrogenic epidemic were evident in this period. Some clinicians acknowledged its existence but challenged data on its claimed prevalence or argued that the therapeutic benefits outweighed the iatrogenic risks. Others simply failed to change their prescribing habits without comment.

Brown and Funk claim that two theories (professional dominance and labelling) have some merit in accounting for this professional resistance to change. Both acknowledge the importance of the powerless social position of patients. The labelling theory account suggests that the powerless position and low social status of psychiatric patients renders them both unimportant and invisible. Consequently, their treating psychiatrists do not take their complaints about 'side-effects', or their concerns about the debilitating effects of the drugs, seriously. Instead, doctors tend to be concerned only with the effectiveness of the drugs in symptom reduction (assessed by them, not the patients themselves).

The professional dominance theory focuses on the relationship between the status of psychiatry as a medical specialty and the role of physical treatment. We have raised this issue above in relation to the work of Baruch and Treacher in Britain. Brown and Funk endorse a similar picture in the US, with psychiatry tying itself to physical medicine and its attendant biological trappings. An over-reliance on drug treatment is inextricably linked to a professional strategy of collective upward mobility on the part of psychiatrists. Given this preoccupation with collective professional status, unfortunate consequences of biological treatment (like tardive dyskinesia) are ignored, denied or rationalized by clinicians. According to this theory, the needs of patients are ignored in favour of the political needs of their treating psychiatrists. A study of psychiatrists and recipient views of major tranquillizers (Finn et al. 1990) showed that both groups concur on the risks and 'bothersomeness' of side-effects. However, 'psychiatrists saw side-effects as significantly less bothersome than symptoms when considering costs to society' (Finn et al. 1990: 843).

It is, perhaps, not surprising that patients who experience the side-effects are often reluctant to comply with the regimen. What is, perhaps, more surprising is that given the range and severity of side-effects, non-adherence rates for major tranquillizers are the same as for other types of non-psychiatric medication. The problems associated with traditional major tranquillizers (the phenothiazine group of drugs) seem to apply less to a new generation of drugs, currently dubbed the 'new anti-psychotics'. Clinical trials suggest that they are more efficient at symptom reduction and that they are less liable to create movement disorders in patients. However, there is the risk of life-threatening blood disorders with some versions of the new anti-psychotics.

The sociological significance of the prescribing and compliance with anti-psychotics extends beyond the issue of the adverse effects and practices of the profession of psychiatry. Psychiatric patients' 'non-compliance' with medication has emerged as a significant social problem. Images of de-institutionalization, often promoted via the media, have become synonymous with the occurrence of socially unacceptable behaviour by ex-psychiatric patients living in the community. Within this recurringly publicized scenario, medication has been depicted as a valid means of managing and controlling people who are viewed as a potential threat to the social order. Compliance with these drugs has come to be seen as an indicator of the success or failure of a 'care in the community' mental health policy. In this sense, the need for patient compliance derives not only from public pressures about managing psychiatric patients appropriately but also it is a central tenet in the management of mental health problems more generally.

Both the closure of mental hospitals and caring for patients in the community has been predicated on the assumed effectiveness of major tranquillizers. The introduction during the late 1960s of depot medication can be seen as an early attempt to devise a strategy for the more efficient control of patients' behaviour in the community. (It involves patients being injected with long-acting drugs in their home or at a clinic.) Depot medication was uniquely marketed as a means of ensuring the receipt of medication which was not contingent on patients' consent to treatment on a daily basis or their daily self-administration of pills.

The effectiveness of neuroleptics has been assumed by professionals, politicians and relatives' groups who emphasize the importance of treatment compliance for discharged patients. This has extended to legal proposals to enforce medication compliance in community-based patients. However, a recent review of their effectiveness makes the following points (Fisher and Greenberg 1997):

• Only one in three medicated patients fails to relapse.
• Chronic use of the drugs leads to reductions in social functioning.
• To date, few researchers have attended to user views of being medicated.

The reviewer concludes that '. . . the overall usefulness [of neuroleptics] in the treatment of schizophrenia . . . is far from established' (Cohen 1997: 195). In relation to their iatrogenic effects Cohen (ibid.: 201) concludes that the 'neuroleptics' near-sacred reputation as "antipsychotics" is equalled only by their record as one of the most behaviouraly toxic classes of psychotropic drugs.'

Extending the point about assumed utility of the drugs, major tranquillizers have been viewed as the principal means of preventing 'the revolving-door patient' phenomena. They are a central plank of 'out reach' care, case management, the care programme approach, supervised discharge and the management of those with 'a severe and enduring mental illness'. However, the centrality of medication to mental health policy has not been unproblematic. The iatrogenic effects of medication have also become a focus of critical scrutiny and this has received greater publicity than at the time when Brown and Funk were discussing the topic in the 1980s.

The negative effects of major tranquillizers have been the focus of criticism from campaigning and mental health user organizations. Policy-makers are now faced with balancing the need to maintain medication-adherence, with the risks of iatrogenesis (Rogers and Pilgrim 1996). This dilemma has become increasingly difficult for policy-makers to manage in a cultural context of high sensitivity to risk, the emergence of a consumerist philosophy within the health service, and the growing acceptance of the legitimacy of lay perceptions and assessment of medicine within modern health care systems. The receipt of major tranquillizers occurs in a context of the wider meaning and symbolic significance that 'schizophrenia' has for patients in their every-day lives and of a policy context which stresses the need to survey and control the behaviour of people living in the community. For this reason, self-regulatory action in this group of patients has been found to be less evident, and the threat and application of external social control is greater than in relation to other groups of patients taking medication for chronic conditions (Rogers *et al.* 1998).

Antidepressants

Antidepressants have been associated with a number of disabling effects, including tiredness, dry mouth, loss of libido and impotence, blurred vision, constipation, weight gain and palpitations. The tricyclic version of this type of drug was implicated in around 10 per cent of deaths from self-poisoning in Britain in the early 1980s. Tricyclics have now been superseded by the selective serotonin re-uptake inhibitors (SSRIs), which are less toxic. However, the tricyclics are still widely prescribed. As well as the problem of self-poisoning, these drugs also amplify the side-effects of both minor and major tranquillizers when given in combination (Lacey 1991). Although the SSRIs are less toxic, initial claims of their non-dependency have recently been challenged, as withdrawal reactions have been notified to regulatory bodies (in Britain, the Medicines Control Agency). Reviews of studies of antidepressants versus psychological therapies in randomized controlled trials suggest that both are clinically effective in the short term, separately and combined, but no treatment is good at preventing long-term relapse in those who have had a depressive episode in their lives (Fisher and Greenberg 1997).

Psychological therapies

As far as the psychological therapies are concerned, it is not self-evident that they are benign simply because they are physically non-invasive. Two types of iatrogenic problems arise in psychotherapy. The first is the so-called 'deterioration effect' – where symptoms get worse during the normal course of therapy (Bergin 1971). Indeed, in psychoanalytical therapy one sign of its impact is the production of symptoms during a 'therapeutic regression'. Women are particularly prone to adverse effects when faced with male stereotypical expectations of mental health held by male therapists (Brodsky and Holdroyd 1975). Personal change is also paradoxically held back in some people entering therapy as this role reinforces passivity and dependency (Bakker 1975).

The second set of problems is to do with the personal abuse, suffered at the hands of unethical practitioners who exploit the power discrepancy existing, under conditions of privacy, to gain emotional or sexual gratification from their clients (Jehu 1995). A recent review of the latter problem noted that in the US over half of the malpractice suits taken out by people with mental health problems about their treatment at the hands of psychiatrists and clinical psychologists involve the distress created by sexual abuse by therapists (Schoener and Lupker 1996). Such has been the crisis of confidence thrown up by evidence of these iatrogenic effects of psychotherapy that some previously committed therapists have recommended the abandonment of therapy in favour of some type of self-help or have issued strong warnings to patients about the risks, as well as of the potential benefits, of psychotherapy (Masson 1988b; Smail 1996; Pilgrim 1997a).

None the less, users of in-patient services still ask for talking treatments, complaining that these are on offer less frequently from psychiatric services than physical treatments. Exclusion from such treatment seems to reflect a tendency to treat neurotic patients more readily in this way. There is mixed empirical evidence on this issue. On the one hand, psychotic patients seem to be more prone to deterioration effects than less disturbed patients (Bergin and Lambert 1978). On the other hand, there are claims of significant positive effects of psychotherapy with psychotic patients (allowing the latter also to avoid the problems associated with major tranquillizers) (Karon and VandenBos 1981).

Just as medication-use and the professionalization of psychiatry are interconnected (see earlier) professional questions also surround the differential use of psychological treatments. During the early professionalization of clinical psychology, its bid for therapeutic legitimacy centred on the behavioural treatment of neurosis. Psychologists tended to leave the treatment of madness to biological psychiatrists (Eysenck 1975). However, latterly psychologists have taken an increasing interest in the treatment of psychosis (Bentall 1990). As a consequence, the costs and benefits of physical and psychological treatments now need to be considered for all groups of patients as the unstable division of labour between psychiatrists and clinical psychologists has shifted.

Despite the user disaffection about biomedical treatments in psychiatry and an expressed preference for talking treatments, given the risks of the latter, it is not self-evident that they are more cost-effective than drugs and ECT. Indeed, it could be argued that in some ways drug regimes are more open to public accountability than are the talking treatments (Pilgrim 1997b). For example, provided that clinicians cooperate with them, drug protocols can make prescribing practices amenable to audit (by managers or even service users). By contrast, the effective elements of talking treatments largely relate to 'non-specific' effects of the therapist or therapist–client interaction. Good outcome in psychotherapy is not linked to particular models but to these benign, supportive or inspirational practitioner variables. It is much more difficult to operationalize and audit such factors than it is to set down guidelines about good drug prescribing practice. Also drug prescriptions are public and impersonal, whereas psychotherapy is private and personal. The

latter features seem to be linked to user preferences (to have their idiosyncratic experiences taken seriously). However, these are the very reasons why
talking treatments are liable to create deterioration effects because incompetent or abusive practitioners are shielded from public view.

Why is there a problem of legitimacy about the effectiveness of psychiatric treatment?

In addition to criticisms about the role of psychotropic drugs in sedating
disruptive individuals, drug treatments have been criticized for being ineffect-
ive at symptom control. Mention has already been made of the short-term
value of minor tranquillizers. Public knowledge about debates of the effectiveness of major tranquillizers is less evident. The psychiatric literature indeed
suggests that they are effective at reducing the probability of relapse (Hirsch
1986). However, the extent of this impact is quite modest according to one
oft-quoted study. Crow *et al.* (1986) reported that 58 per cent of patients
receiving the drugs were deemed to relapse within two years, compared to
78 per cent of a control group receiving a placebo. (In fact, there was only a
12 per cent difference between the two groups according to the original data,
which was corrected statistically but without explanation prior to publication
(Hennelly 1988).)
    We have already mentioned that there is mixed evidence about the effect-
iveness of psychotherapy. Behavioural critics of verbal psychotherapy have
maintained that spontaneous remission from symptoms accounts for positive change in two-thirds of neurotic patients (Eysenck 1952; Rachman 1971).
These doubts, plus those mentioned above from internal critics about deterioration effects, have certainly rendered psychotherapy problematic. Indeed,
the overall estimate of psychotherapy is that it is only of marginal (though
positive) utility because the gains it achieves are offset by deterioration
effects and spontaneous remission (Bergin and Lambert 1978).
    As for behavioural psychotherapy, this has been subjected to two types of
criticism. The first relates to the limited value of behavioural work for the
gamut of mental health problems referred to psychiatric services (Yates 1970).
The second criticism is that it slavishly adheres to, rather than challenges,
cultural norms. An example of this was the role taken up by behaviour
therapists in seeking to convert homosexual men into heterosexuals by using
electroshock aversion therapy (see Chapter 3).
    Thus, the legitimacy of psychiatric treatments is undermined by differ-
ent but interrelated dissatisfactions. First, there is the problem of effectiveness *per se* – no form of treatment claims startling improvement rates (let
alone 'cure') (Pilgrim 1997b). Second, given this poor showing in symptom
reduction, the iatrogenic effects of treatment become particularly salient.
'Side-effects' might be tolerated if significant therapeutic benefits were also
experienced by patients but with high iatrogenic effect rates and low symptom reduction rates, treatments become highly problematic (Breggin 1993).
Third, the use of treatments to ensure conformity (e.g. aversion therapy) and
quell disruptiveness (e.g. major tranquillizers) has highlighted, and stimulated opposition to, the normative and coercive role of psychiatric interventions (see Chapter 10). Fourth, currently there is a variable gap between the

evidence for effective interventions in clinical trials and these treatments being used effectively in actual services (see later discussion on evidence-based practice).

The moral sense of 'treatment'

In everyday parlance 'treatment' has moral as well as medical connotations. Certain medical specialties have been exposed to particular critical attention as far as this non-medical notion of treatment is concerned. One of these is gynaecology and the other is psychiatry. This might imply that certain aspects of the person need to be treated with particular sensitivity by medicine.

The final essay in Goffman's critique of the mental hospital, *Asylums* (1961), is subtitled, 'Some notes on the vicissitudes of the tinkering trades'. He analyses the mental hospital and the medical model of treatment as if it were a service industry directed towards the repair of damaged parts of society (psychiatric patients). If we accept Goffman's metaphor of psychiatry as a repair industry then we can examine how its 'customers' are treated.

To begin, the scope of psychiatry needs to be restated. At one end of a spectrum of psychiatric service provision is a picture of enforced detention and imposed treatments. In Britain we have the maximum security Special Hospitals, Regional Secure Units and in-patients detained under sections of the Mental Health Act 1983, in open hospitals or psychiatric units. At the other end of the spectrum are outpatients who attend voluntarily to see a therapist of their choosing in a variety of state-provided and private thera-peutic facilities. In between are patients who hover around a centre-ground of services, which contains a mixture of both voluntary and coercive prac-tices. Depending on their conduct, they may drift or be propelled suddenly towards one or other end of the spectrum.

What separates the two ends of the spectrum is essentially the question of free choice. If the mental health industry does indeed provide a service to its patients then we would expect it to manifest certain characteristics. Service industries provide options and opportunities for customers in pursuit of a product of their preference. Rotten products which customers found noxious or aversive would quickly disappear from the range of offers made by the industry. A person experiencing some form of self-defined psychological prob-lem or distress would have the resources (financial and cognitive) and the options to freely choose a form of amelioration. How does the mental health industry fare over this issue of free choice? We will explore this question by addressing two more which are begged: who is psychiatry's client? and what is the extent of informed consent given to patients?

Who is psychiatry's client?

One of the ambiguities which surrounds psychiatric work is whether or not the identified patient is the actual client of the service. Clearly, some party other than the patient is being served under those sections of the Mental Health Act which empower professionals to remove a person's liberty and/or impose treatment interventions against the patient's will. Coulter's work (described in Chapter 5) on decision-making about madness in the lay area traces such a process. Professionals are summoned in order to resolve a distressing drama to those around the patient. Similarly, when members of the public contact the police about a person acting bizarrely in the street it is clear that the client of the police-psychiatrist 'disposal' is not the patient, although quite who psychiatry is serving in this instance is ambiguous. Is it the distressed and perplexed member of public making the first police contact, is it the police themselves, or is it both?

Clearly, if a person is detained without trial, and they are interfered with without consent, then it is difficult to conceptualize them as 'customers' or 'clients' of psychiatry. Instead, the terminology favoured by the psychiatric service users' movement would seem to be more appropriate, of 'recipients' or 'survivors' (see Chapter 10). On the other hand, if a person chooses freely to make contact with a mental health worker, to seek help with a personal difficulty, in this instance they would seem to have a genuine 'client' status. However, even with this voluntary contact there is still a sense in which the client does not enjoy the same rights and privileges as other types of customers accessing a service industry.

The question of informed choice

This can be examined with reference to five criteria set out by Bean (1986). Bean suggests that to understand whether or not genuinely informed consent takes place in psychiatric services, we must ask the following questions:

1 Are the patients aware of themselves – are they competent at making judgements on their own behalf?
2 Do those who are assumed to be aware of themselves (relatives and professionals) use that awareness to act morally?
3 Do professionals supply comprehensive and comprehensible information to patients?
4 Are patients subjected to pressure or coercion when they are in receipt of psychiatric treatment?
5 Is consent to specifiable actions offered by professionals to patients?

Answers to these questions, suggested below, point towards psychiatric practice being problematic on all five counts:

Insight

Professionals may override the need to seek consent from patients about treatment if they believe that the patient is lacking in insight into their condition. However, three problems with the notion of insight can be noted:

1 Insight tends to be defined in a circular way. That is, insight means that a patient agrees with their psychiatrist. Sanity and madness are socially agreed notions and where agreement breaks down in a psychiatric encounter

between doctor and patient, then the more powerful party has their view upheld. Consequent upon this, the patient may lose their right to refuse treatment.

2 Even if we take it to be non-problematic on the first count, then mental illness is conceded by professionals to be episodic in nature. Given this consensus, how do psychiatrists know for sure when a person is aware and when they are not aware?

3 Given that professionals concede that psychotic patients who lack insight may be competent in certain regards (for instance the paranoid patient who can wash, dress and make money on the stock market) how can psychiatrists specify what insight actually means in terms of cognitive and social competence? Clearly, a patient may be aware of some things when they reflect on themselves but not on others; this is probably true of everybody. None of us can be aware of everything relevant to our existence all of the time. None of us can know our own minds for certain. (Indeed, if we are exposed to the tenet of psychoanalysis we are all encouraged to believe that the bulk of our mind is unconscious.) And yet, despite our ubiquitous failure to be fully self-aware, we get by most of the time in most of our lives.

Beck-Sander (1998) deconstructed psychiatric literature referring to insight and found it to have weak construct validity. She found that the concept was used by professionals to indicate four separate patient features:

1 Treatment compliance – when this is a defining feature of insight, then it is assumed that to resist treatment is necessarily irrational. This is a dubious assumption given the iatrogenic effects of psychiatric treatments discussed above. Indeed, if all patients were fully informed of these effects, treatment compliance would probably decrease generally.

2 Psychological mindedness – this can be found in the psychiatric literature as another proxy indicator of insight. It refers to insight as a reified defence operating inside patients which purportedly protects them from the pain of their illness. Thus, those with more insight are deemed to be more distressed, whereas those lacking insight are cut off from the pain of the purported disease process they are experiencing.

3 Prognosis is also used at times by psychiatrists as a circular indicator of insight. Those with more insight are deemed to have shorter periods of relapse into psychosis and the inverse is deemed to be true for those with less insight. This professional reasoning is *post hoc* and tautological. Moreover, given that prognosis is determined by a number of external, as well as patient characteristics, such as socio-economic opportunity and societal discrimination, then how can we ever know whether insight is a defining single feature when prognosis is good or bad for a particular patient?

4 Pathophysiology is offered at times by some psychiatrists as a correlate of insight. That is, purported neuropsychological dysfunction in psychosis is offered as an explanation for why psychotic patients lack insight into their condition. This is, of course, a possibility, much as cerebral bleeding accounts for the brain damage which affects the short-term memory and orientation in time and space of some dementing patients. The problem with this argument is that, by definition, the functional psychoses are *not*

organic conditions, at least they are not demonstrably so at present. They are defined by symptoms alone *because* biological markers (true signs) are absent, despite substantial biomedical and neuropsychological research into the psychoses.

Thus, the whole question of competence or self-awareness is problematic. Despite this, professionals have powers to treat patients without their consent and they do so using the notion of 'lack of insight' as if it were non-problematic. Moreover, this purported lack of competence on the part of psychiatric patients is the very rationale for why negotiation about consent is either deemed to be unnecessary or futile. Despite this, there is no evidence that psychiatric patients are actually less able than medical patients to understand what is told to them. Soskis (1978) found that, in fact, psychiatric patients knew more about the side-effects of drugs they were receiving than did medical patients. (Showing that if they are told they understand.) However, the psychiatric patients were less likely than the medical patients to be told why they were receiving the medication. This indicates that psychiatrists are less willing than physicians to discuss diagnosis and rationale for treatment with their patients.

The morality of others

The discussion above showed that, collectively, psychiatrists have not acted morally in relation to the needs and vulnerabilities of patients. Major tranquillizers are one of the main groups of treatments imposed on resistant recipients. Practitioners have also acted immorally in the case of the abuse of patients by psychotherapists. Thus, psychiatric therapists are prone to fail Bean's second criterion.

Comprehensive and comprehensible information

This question is the one most commonly addressed by disaffected users of services. Whether the disaffection is caused by drugs, ECT or psychotherapy, the recurrent complaint is that patients are not supplied with enough information about the advantages and disadvantages of the treatment offered or imposed. The minor tranquillizer campaign led to litigation against the drug companies and the prescribing doctors, which focused on both iatrogenic effects and the withholding of information at the time of prescription about these effects. The same has been true of litigation about major tranquillizers in the US (Brown and Funk 1986). Rogers *et al.* (1993) found that 60 per cent of a sample who had received major tranquillizers reported not being informed of their purpose, and that 70 per cent of this group were unhappy about the amount of information they had been given. Similar findings have been reported in studies in the US (Soskis 1978; Lidz *et al.* 1984). These complaints would indicate that psychiatry is found to be lacking according to Bean's third criterion.

Coercion

Given that in Britain a large minority of psychiatric patients are detained compulsorily, it is undeniable that in these cases coercion operates in psychiatry. Despite legal safeguards under the Mental Health Act 1983, these detained patients may be injected forcibly with drugs or given ECT or psychosurgery against their will. They can also be forced into isolation ('seclusion') without consent. The question begged is whether informal patients are genuinely in the patient role voluntarily. Rogers *et al.* (1993) compared those in their sample who felt their voluntary admission had been genuine with those who felt it to be not genuine. In the first group, 21 per cent reported some degree of coercion, whereas in the second group 80 per cent felt coerced into going into hospital. Similar evidence of coercion during 'voluntary' admission to psychiatric facilities has been found in the US (Klatte *et al.* 1969). Bean's fourth criterion is failed by psychiatry.

Specifiable actions

Bean points out that real informed consent cannot be consent to anything and everything. Instead, it must be consent to a specific action or circumscribed set of actions. If it were consent to anything then this would give arbitrary powers to professionals. Indeed, in secure psychiatric provision in particular it is commonplace for patients to be subject to the regime of what Goffman called a 'total institution' – all activities and interventions are determined by the regime of the hospital. When this is the case, patients have little or no moment-to-moment powers of decision-making. In effect, they abandon their right to agree or disagree to specifiable actions on admission or it is taken away from them.

Even in less coercive surroundings, if professionals do not give a full account, in advance, of what is to happen when a treatment is carried out, then they are not giving patients the right to agree to specifiable actions. For example, biological psychiatrists may be paternalistic about withholding information on major tranquillizers (in case it may worry the patient). Psychoanalysts may evade questions about their technique as part of their technique (to provide a blank screen for the patient's projections). Thus, for different reasons, both physical and psychological therapists may evade specifying their intended actions in relation to the patient they treat.

Having now discussed both the problems of identifying psychiatry's client and informed consent, let us return to Goffman's criteria of a good repair service industry. In essence he argues that such a service would have the following features:

1 The workshop of the industry would be benign and would prevent a deterioration in the condition that required repair.
2 Transporting the part in need of repair to the workshop would not introduce new forms of damage.
3 The damaged part is not linked inextricably to its possessor. That is, the owner can be separated from their damaged part for a defined period of time until it is repaired.

4 Those providing the service and those using it enter into the repair contract voluntarily and with mutual respect.

Psychiatry, at least in its hospital form, is clearly problematic on all four of
these counts. Reviewing the criteria one by one:

1 Psychiatry is clearly not always benign.
2 Entering the psychiatric regime itself is stigmatizing and can be distressing.
3 The damaged part and its possessor are one and the same. Mental illness is
   about a flawed or deviant self. This is why a psychiatric diagnosis has such
   profound implications, as a patient's credibility as a social actor or citizen
   is questioned, possibly for life.
4 Mental health law exists to enforce the relationship between service providers and service recipients (more will be said about this in Chapter 8).

The social distribution of treatment

One of the paradoxes of psychiatric treatment is that it inverts the 'inverse
care law'. The latter, which generally holds true for people with physical
health problems, refers to the phenomenon of those in the greatest need, as
a result of their socially-created illness, having the poorest access to the
health care system. Not only are richer people healthier than poorer people,
they also access better treatment from both publicly funded and private
health care systems. The opposite is true of mental health care systems at
least as far as in-patient care in Britain is concerned.

In the light of the stigma attached to mental health services and the role
of psychiatry, some of the time in the coercive control of socially disruptive
behaviour, then it is little surprising that some social groups are more vulnerable to service receipt than others:

1 Black and ethnic minority populations receive greater in-patient attention
   and physical treatments than white populations in Britain and the US.
2 In-patients are usually poor. They are often unemployed and unemployable.
3 Women are in receipt of more psychiatric treatment than men, although a
   caution here is that more men are treated coercively than women.

When we examine the research on receipt of voluntary outpatient attendance in mental health services, then a different picture emerges:

1 The utilization of long-term psychotherapy is inversely related to age (over
   65), (black) race and years of schooling (Olsen and Pincus 1994).
2 In the US black and Hispanic women utilize outpatient facilities less than
   white women (Padgett et al. 1994).
3 Black war veterans in the US receive less intensive treatment for post-
   traumatic stress problems than white veterans.
4 Black people drop out of outpatient family therapy earlier on average than
   whites (Kazdin et al. 1995). This finding needs to be seen in the context
   of the failure to incorporate cross-cultural counselling into mainstream
   services.

Thus, treatment is offered or imposed differentially in society in ways which reflect power relationships. This point is clearest in relation to social class, race and age but is more complex in relation to gender.

The impact of evidenced-based practice on treatment

A current development is the emergence of research knowledge and evidence as a means of controlling and improving the development and quality of health care services. The extent of its formal academic impact in the field of mental health is shown by the emergence in 1997 of a new dedicated journal *Evidence-Based Mental Health*.

The rising popularity of 'evidence-based practice' (EBP) is linked to the imperatives of health policy-makers to control service costs. It has also been overlain by a discourse on concern to assess the health benefits and risk of technology and treatments (Faulkner 1997). These concerns can be seen as rhetorical devices, which include the purported strengths of multidisciplinarity and benefits to users of cost-effective treatments. It is common now for all parties to accept in principle, evidence as a basis for clinically-effective and cost-effective interventions. The randomized control trial (RCT) remains the 'gold standard' of EBP, whilst evidence-based or lay knowledge and qualitative methods are afforded a lesser place. In the area of mental health there are particular problems in applying the experimental conditions of the RCT to services:

> In RCT's treatment fidelity is ensured, contaminating variables such as dropouts are eliminated and specific symptom reduction outcomes are investigated. In contrast in actual services, treatment fidelity cannot be assumed, people drop in and out of service contact and their presenting problems are often complex and not limited to specific symptoms . . .
> (Pilgrim 1997b: 569)

However, there have been specific aspects of treatments which have been evaluated along standardized criteria and guidelines in actual services. There is evidence too that the rhetorical devices of quality and evidence can be harnessed to empower mental health users to challenge mainstream psychiatric practices. Whilst this is very much a nascent and marginal trend, the insertion of criteria of quality into mental health services is likely to influence what comes to be acceptable knowledge about mental health service development. Two examples are given here of how a user, rather than professional, approach to treatment effectiveness can alter an evidence-based approach to service development.

Disputed evidence about ECT

First, the use of ECT, controversial since its inception, is an illustrative case study of the challenge of addressing patients' perspectives in the evaluation of health care technology. Despite widespread professional acceptance of

ECT, groups of former psychiatric patients have worked through the legal system to restrict or ban it as a treatment. This is an example of lay participation in the regulation of health care. It illustrates how differing conceptions of evidence can affect the evaluation of technology. This also provides an example of the value of a more complex definition of the significant outcomes of treatment and the growing practice of outcomes assessment and the way in which the outcome of treatment can also shape health policy (Heitman 1996). In other words, professional definitions of good outcomes and those offered by treatment recipients may not always coincide. Whilst some users' groups focus on ECT as an irredeemable barbarity perpetrated by professionals, some individual patients endorse it as a life saver, whilst others harbour life-long resentment about its use in their care (Rogers *et al.* 1993). Official professional accounts of ECT (Royal College of Psychiatrists 1995) give no hint of this mixed consumer perspective on the treatment and insist that it is safe and effective, even for children. With such discrepant views about outcomes between psychiatrists and their patients about ECT, services become a contested site for competing interest groups both in terms of viewpoints and evidence invoked within them.

Users' views as evidence in service research

Second, previous work on users' experience of mental health services with its roots in symbolic interactionism considered the experience of users as being worthwhile in its own right. This has been incorporated into a health outcomes approach to policy development, as has been pointed out by Godfrey and Wistow: 'The Department of Health has placed great importance on evidence-based purchasing rooted in the assessment and measurement of health outcome . . . We draw upon users' conceptions of acute mental health service to examine users' conceptions of outcomes . . .' (Godfrey and Wistow 1997: 326).

In a narrow policy approach, the accounts of users get transformed from narratives situated in their biographical context to a set of potential outcomes with which to measure the success, or otherwise, of a service. The knowledge base – qualitative methods transformed and presented as something 'new' – is a form of 'methodolatry' increasingly common in health service research which loses sight of social theory (Pilgrim and May 1998). A more holistic approach to outcomes would address a users' perspective which considers the entire course and experience of mental illness, i.e. the meanings of users and significant others of 'becoming' and 'being ill'.

The utility of a more holistic approach to outcome work was confirmed by Felton *et al.* (1995). Their study examined whether employing mental health consumers as peer specialists in an intensive case-management programme can enhance outcomes for clients with serious mental illness. They found that clients served by mental health teams with peer specialists demonstrated greater gains in several areas of quality of life and an overall reduction in the number of major life problems experienced. They also reported more frequent contact with their case managers and the largest gains of all three groups in the areas of self-image and outlook and social support.

Mental health promotion versus treatment

Historically, the types of psychiatric treatment discussed above have pre-dominated in the mental health field. However, a departure from a mental illness paradigm is evident in recent calls for the more active promotion of positive mental health. This trend in the mental health field reflects a shift evident more generally in health promotion and fits broadly within the contemporary and dominant approach to health promotion, which includes three areas – consumption, lifestyle, and risk. Burrows *et al.* (1995) describe the new paradigm thus:

> What is distinctive about health promotion is the attention that it gives to the facilitation of healthy lives: the idea that it is no good just tell-ing people that they should change their lifestyles without altering their social, economic and ecological environments. People must be able to live healthy lives. Health promotion aims to work not only at the level of the individual but at the level of socio-economic structures to encourage the creation and implementation of healthy public policies such as those concerned with transport, environment, agriculture and so on.
>
> (Burrows *et al.* 1995: 2)

The shift in the area of mental health can be seen in the expansive and holistic definition of health adopted by the World Health Organisation in the 1980s. 'By the year 2000, people should have the basic opportunity to develop and use their health potential to live socially and economically fulfilling lives' (WHO 1986). Recently, the active promotion of mental health has been evident in the government's approach to public health and health promotion. At the level of health policy too the recent Green Paper 'Our Healthier Nation' advocates a multi-sectoral approach to mental health prob-lems and advocates action to be taken at government, locality, and indi-vidual levels (DoH 1998).

Two features evident in this trend are the relocation of the epidemiology of mental illness away from a traditional psychiatric paradigm and the acknow-ledgement given to lay perceptions of positive mental health. With regard to the latter, sociologists have been party to this reorientation by engaging in a research agenda examining lay epidemiology (described in Chapter 1). This orientation has also placed a higher value on strategies for maintaining mental health.

Those who have researched in this area have identified both proactive and reactive lay action, self-reliance, cognitive strategies (taking up a particular psychological stance to everyday events), and stress-reducing activities, such as sport, as common mental health strategies (Rogers and Pilgrim 1996). The focus of the amelioration or management of mental health problems has also shifted. Lay management strategies of dealing with mental health prob-lems have been given a higher priority than previously in formal health promotion strategies, including those with professionals (Trent and Reed 1997).

Discussion

This chapter has looked at how patients are treated by the psychiatric service. The sociological discourse about this topic has tended, itself, to be divided between the poles of the spectrum of service delivery mentioned above. On the one hand, it has been concerned with critically exposing treatment as mystified coercive social control. On the other hand, it has become preoccupied with those psychological interventions which are 'anxiously sought and gratefully received'. Sociology is a mirror to the divided territory of psychiatry and, arguably, it contributes to that division.

Psychiatric treatment remains in a precarious state of legitimacy. This uncertainty is then amplified by the doubts about the effectiveness of both physical and psychological therapeutic approaches and the complaints that have accumulated about the iatrogenic effects of these treatments. The contradictory picture of psychiatry, mixing as it does both coercion and voluntarism, and an eclectic range of treatments from leucotomy to psychoanalysis, also increases the gap between expectation and reality. If patients entering the psychiatric system expect lengthy explorations of their biography and actually get a cursory interview, followed by a prescription for antidepressants, then the chances of disappointment are great. Likewise, if people look to psychiatry as a source of comfort during times of personal confusion and distress and actually encounter an impersonal controlling regime, with professionals who serve third parties rather than the patients they are supposedly treating, then disaffection is, again, likely.

The uncertainty surrounding the legitimacy of psychiatric treatment is also amplified by the structural inequalities in access to the range of its interventions. In other words, as we have explored elsewhere in the book, not all social groups are represented evenly throughout the spectrum of psychiatry. Some receive much harsher treatment than others. Black people are less likely to receive psychotherapy and more likely to receive medication and ECT. They are also more likely to be treated coercively than white people, with the exception of the Irish in Britain. Richer clients can afford to pick and choose between therapists in private practice, whereas poorer clients have to take what is given by state-employed professionals in their particular locality. Those diagnosed as being psychotic are less likely to receive psychological treatments than those who are diagnosed as being neurotic. Men are over-represented at the 'harsh' end of services, etc.

If entering the psychiatric system *ipso facto* entailed being treated well, then those groups which are over-represented (like black people) would view themselves as being in receipt of preferential treatment. The fact that over-representation is instead a source of concern and anger to these groups, reflects the suspicion with which psychiatry is viewed (as being an oppressive part of the extended state apparatus of control). Sociological investigations of how psychiatric patients are treated (in both senses of the word) may need to take on board this complexity and these contradictions. Up until now, two main 'camps' of sociology might be seen to have been warring about how to describe and understand psychiatric treatment. The humanistic bias of symbolic interactionism, exemplified in the work of Goffman, contributed to the notion of 'antipsychiatry' and focused on the degradation of the individual and their loss of citizenship. The anti-humanistic bias of the poststructuralists conceives only of discourses which patients and therapists contribute to (or are trapped in). According to this view, individuals are produced, rather than destroyed, by psychiatry.

The psychological technologies, like the psychotherapies, are indeed now deeply implicated in modern secular society, contributing to the regulation of a moral order and promoting the contemporary importance of the 'self'. Arguably, the same is true of an approach which emphasizes the promotion of positive mental health. The problem for the poststructuralist position is that the old humanistic, antipsychiatric arguments about the coercive power of the State are still highly pertinent to those groups which continue to be its particular target. It is not surprising that such groups remain hostile to psychiatry, rather than receiving it gratefully when contributing to 'productive power'. Sociology cannot ignore either the productive technologies of the self or the destructive potential of coercive psychiatry. Both have to be considered together.

To conclude

In this chapter we have covered a wide range of considerations about psychiatric treatment. This has included reviewing the literature on specific forms of treatment and the social forces which shape its production and maintenance. Sociologists have contributed to a critical discourse about treatment along with the 'anti-psychiatrists' and disaffected service users. At other times, sociologists have suggested that psychiatry is part of a wider set of processes of governmentality. Overall, sociological scrutiny (exemplified in the work of Goffman) has tended to expose the logical contradictions of treatment. At the same time, the influence of Foucault has focused more on productive power rather than the coercive role of psychiatry in society. For the foreseeable future, sociologists are likely to retain an interest in both of these aspects of professional mental health work.

Questions

1 Does psychiatry produce or crush subjectivity?

2 How can non-compliance with psychiatric treatment be understood?

3 Why does the 'inverse care law' not apply in psychiatric services?

4 What problems are associated with the concept of insight?

5 To what extent does Goffman's work on large mental hospital life still apply today?

6 Discuss the rationale for evidence-based mental health care and barriers to its success.

For discussion

Consider whether you would be prepared to volunteer for psychiatric treatment if you became psychologically distressed. What would be the pros and cons to consider in this decision?

Further reading

Breggin, P. (1993) *Toxic Psychiatry*. London: HarperCollins.

Gabe, J. and Bury, M. (1996) Halcion nights: a sociological account, *Sociology* 30, 3: 447–470.

Fisher, S. and Greenberg, R.P. (1997) *From Placebo to Panacea: Putting Psychiatric Drugs to the Test*. London: Wiley.

Romme, M. and Escher, S. (1993) *Accepting Voices*. London: Mind.

Trent, D.R. and Reed, C.A. (1997) *Promotion of Mental Health*. London: Ashgate.

Chapter **8**

The organization of psychiatry

Chapter overview

This chapter will explore the changing organizational form of mental health work under four main headings.

- The sociology of the hospital
- The rise of the asylum
- The crisis of the asylum
- Responses to the crisis

The sociology of the hospital

In modern western societies, the hospital has become the central institution for the delivery of health care, the training of health professionals and medical research. When analysing the organization, sociologists have tended to use as a working model the general hospital which deals with acute physical illness. The way in which the modern general hospital has been depicted provides a benchmark with which the mental hospital can be compared.

The modern hospital, with its high-technology equipment, elaborate procedures and specialized skills has frequently been viewed as an outcome of 'scientific developments' and medical progress over the last century (Tuckett 1976). This assumption has led a number of sociologists to comment that the modern hospital is an example of Max Weber's notion of a 'bureaucratic organization'. Sociologists of organizations have identified characteristics of the 'typical' modern hospital that have been influenced by Weber's ideal type. Perrow (1965), a systems analyst, examines three dominant features of general hospitals:

Complexity

Hospitals are complex organizations, which process inputs (patients) in a way which materially changes them (in this case cures them). Perrow identified three factors which determine the way in which organizations function:

1 The cultural system, which sets the legitimate or formal goals.
2 Technology, which is the means for achieving these goals (in the hospital this includes the types of therapeutic techniques in use).
3 The structure of the organization in which techniques are embedded and person-power organized as a means of achieving the set goals.

Hospitals, like other complex organizations, such as factories and schools, operate on the basis of an interdependence between technology and structure. Cost-effectiveness and the efficiency of providing and operating sophisticated technology may determine the type of hospital service. For instance, specialist radiography equipment may have been responsible for the demise of small cottage hospitals and the relocation of services and staff to centrally based larger general hospitals.

Specialized division of labour

Hospitals are characterized by a highly specialized division of health labour (what Durkheim termed 'organic solidarity'). This can be seen in hospital wards organized around the plethora of sub-specialties of medicine (e.g. ENT wards, radiology, orthopaedics, rheumatology, cardiac units, gynaecology and obstetrics, etc.) and the strict demarcations between the roles and tasks of different health occupations.

Structure and command system

The third characteristic of the modern hospital is its complex authority structure and command system. A system characterized by increased specialization, and the need to service patients round the clock every day of the year, necessitates a complex administrative structure. In Britain, the NHS has witnessed a struggle between bureaucratic and clinical authority in running hospitals. Weber's notion of the former refers to a system of officers in a hierarchical relationship and rationally organized by means of a system of rules and regulations. In contrast, clinical authority has tended to operate on the basis of the dominant professions, which usually means the autonomy of individual consultant medical practitioners. The problems encountered by administrative reorganizations of the NHS, which were aimed at achieving a more coherent and rational means of organizing and delivering health care, may well be due to a clash between these dual lines of authority. For example, in surgical services, clinical authority at a local level, with consultants deciding to do a large number of operations, may well subvert the long-term planning and budgetary arrangements set by non-clinical managers. One of the aims of the recent introduction of managerialism to the NHS was to overcome this dual authority. This was done by amalgamating the two strands, making clinical directors responsible for the management and delivery of health care. The introduction of clinical governance into the NHS in 1999 will strengthen this shift towards bringing the medical profession under managerial control.

Given this description of the general hospital, how does the psychiatric hospital look?

The rise of the asylum

The structure and organization of the large mental hospital did not fit the ideal type of the general hospital. Its architectural design and daily functions were organizationally incongruent in terms of therapy, structure and location. For example, whereas the general hospital is geographically located for easy access, many of the large Victorian asylums were deliberately built away from centres of populations.

The lack of fit between institutional forms inspired by thinking in the last century, and twentieth-century norms regarding health care delivery have led to a crisis within these organizations. This crisis has formed the focus of a critique of the institution, which has emanated from a number of sources. Tracing the creation of large institutions can help us understand their demise. (This is the assumption behind the work of critical social historians such as Michel Foucault and Andrew Scull.) There are two competing accounts giving differing interpretations of events and policy of the establishment of the asylum system. The first is a conventional account, sometimes referred to as a 'Whig', or from a feminist perspective a 'great man', version of history. This type of history is usually written by and for the confident and successful and it emphasizes the valiant deeds, altruism, and humanitarianism of key agencies and individuals. From such a perspective the asylum is viewed as part and parcel of medical progress and an increasingly humane way of dealing with 'mentally ill' people.

For instance, Jones (1960) stresses the humanitarianism behind the reform movement leading to the Lunatics Act 1845. This Act compelled county authorities to establish asylums and enforced their regulation via a centralized Lunacy Commission and a system of medical records. Much of Jones's account centres around the official reports of Metropolitan Commissioners between 1828 and 1845 and the role of government-appointed bodies (such as Parliamentary Select Committees), which drew public attention to the poor state of workhouses and private madhouses. The establishment of early institutions modelled on the moral treatment regime of the York Retreat is described as arising from 'the consciousness felt by a small group of citizens of an overwhelming social evil in their midst' (Jones 1960: 40). In fact, moral treatment failed to transfer from the early charity hospitals like the Retreat to the State-run asylums, although its image dominated the rhetoric of asylum reformers (Donnelly 1983). Jones (1960: 149) sees the implementation of the 1845 Act in a humanitarian light: 'Ashley and his colleagues had roused the conscience of mid-Victorian society, and had set a new standard of public morality by which the care of the helpless and degraded classes of the community was to be seen as a social responsibility.'

Critical historians reject this more conventional account of events. The incarceration of mad people in asylums is seen as inextricably linked to the wider-scale containment of social deviancy: the poor in workhouses and criminals in prisons. The accounts of alternative histories vary. Scull, a Marxist, suggests that mass confinement (of which the asylum system constituted an integral part) was a product of urbanization, industrialization, and professional forces during the first half of the nineteenth century. The development of capitalism, with its demand for wage labour, meant that the existing means of poor relief was ill-equipped to deal with social deviance produced by the new market economy. Thus, the old outdoor system of relief in operation since the Elizabethan Poor Law was replaced by mass incarceration in institutions.

From the beginning of the nineteenth century a gradual process of segregation took place. Poor, able-bodied people (that is those fit to work) were sent to workhouses, which were orientated towards instilling 'proper work habits'. These people were separated from those that could not work, which included those deemed insane and in need of incarceration in asylums. At the same time, ideas about madness were changing. It became recognized as a loss of self-control and not, as previously, a loss of humanity. These changing values were influenced by the exposure of the brutal treatment of those in madhouses. This encouraged the abandonment of mechanical restraints and it endorsed regimes, such as the York Retreat.

These new social values permitted a greater willingness to accept a medical view of madness, the ascendance of which Scull attributes to the entrepreneurial leanings of medical practitioners, who were at the same time making efforts to professionalize and expand. Lucrative pickings were to be had by the profession trying to capture the madhouses previously run by laymen. Rather than having to attract patients to them, the asylum provided them with a ready-made and captive clientele.

Unlike Jones or Scull, Foucault does not concern himself with the specifics of the history of institutions. He views the hôpital générale at the end of the seventeenth century (where at one time 1 per cent of Paris's population who were 'incapable' of productive work were incarcerated), as symbolizing a new concept of madness. The spirit of capitalism, which Foucault traces from the enlightenment onwards, promotes rationality, surveillance and discipline. Reason becomes separated from unreason. This separation out of unreason, whereby madness comes to be seen as the lack of the faculty of 'logos', is symbolized in the replacement of lepers by lunatics. The latter became the new 'race apart'; and their confinement followed.

Critical histories therefore challenge self-congratulatory versions of history, which tend to mask the interests of powerful sections of society, such as the psychiatric profession and the central capitalist State. However, Rothman (1983) suggests that there are problems with critical, as well as Whig, histories because in both accounts 'conception triumphs' over data'. According to Rothman, a focus on ideology, whether it is humanitarianism (Jones), capitalism (Scull) or surveillance (Foucault), can divert the historian's attention from the complex empirical reality of specific individual cases. For example, Scull's emphasis on the economic, Rothman claims, is overstated. The early American system of asylums appeared in the absence of a market economy. Ideas about madness, he suggests, can be influenced by idiosyncratic factors other than those associated with a capitalist mode of production (for example, ideals related to localized political activity and religious doctrine).

Sociologists in the 1960s were party to critical arguments about the dehumanizing effects of the asylum when the direction of mental health policy was clearly focused around whether or not to proceed with mass hospital closure. With the passage of time, when hospital closure and resettlement has become the norm, more recent sociologically informed commentary suggests that the history of the asylum is a contradictory one, particularly when seen in the context of the rise in new forms of surveillance, ways of dealing with psychiatric patients, and in a society which is arguably no more tolerant of psychiatric patients than previous generations. Gittens' (1998) socio-historical analysis of a large psychiatric hospital in Essex based on the biographical narratives of staff and patients who lived or worked in the hospital suggests contradictions and paradoxes about the way the asylums were. In relation to women patients it is clear for example that the hospital, based as it was on men- or women-only wards constituted a 'women-only space' and true asylum in a social context in which there was little such space in external community life. Moreover, the hardships and restriction of asylum life need to be balanced against the external social, economic and political conditions during the heyday of the asylum such as extreme poverty, unemployment and wars which affected people's abilities to cope with difficult material and personal situations. The ambiguous history of the asylum is captured in the conclusion to Gittens' book reporting her study:

There has been a tendency to see the old asylums as isolated, inward-looking institutions that may have benefited staff, but rarely patients, while 'community care' gives patients greater opportunities in the wider world. In closer scrutiny what I have found in this study, as in history – and life – generally, is a great deal of contradiction. In some ways, conditions have improved for those suffering mental illness, in other ways they have not. Some people have benefited enormously from changes over the past few decades, others have not.

(Gittens 1998: 220)

These different histories and interpretations point to the way in which accounts of psychiatric organizations are themselves socially constructed and influenced by the particular point in time in which they are written. We turn now to the processes underlying the dismantling of the asylum system. Again, competing explanations influenced by different perspectives and reading of events provides a complex and contested picture of the causes of hospital rundown and closure.

The crisis of the asylum

The asylum system was problematic from its inception. The ideals of 'moral treatment' were abandoned almost immediately. The system rapidly became overwhelmed by the numbers admitted with chronic conditions. Political pressures were encountered to keep costs down. Although the dominance of the institution began to wane from the 1930s onwards, with a gradual reduction in the number of asylum residents, it was not until the late 1950s and early 1960s that it was faced with a sustained analysis and critique. These criticisms will now be examined. Ronald Laing, David Cooper and Thomas Szasz were psychiatrists who challenged traditional professional theory and practice. (Collectively they were dubbed 'antipsychiatrists', although only Cooper conceded the label.) They were concerned to develop services to patients based on voluntary psychological approaches and consequently they attacked current coercive, biological and institutional psychiatry. Goffman (1961), in his seminal work *Asylums*, considered the mental hospital to be a 'total institution'. This he defined as a place of residence with a large number of people isolated from wider society, for lengthy periods of time, which runs according to an enclosed and formalized administrative regime. Goffman described four types of total institutions:

1 Those which care for the incapable and 'harmless' (such as nursing homes and hospices).
2 Those which provide for those who are perceived as an unwanted threat to the community (for example, sanatoriums for people who suffer from TB).
3 Those which cater for the intentionally dangerous where the welfare of the inmate is not paramount (for example gaol and prisoner of war camps).
4 Those that are designed for people who voluntarily decide to retreat from the world, for instance for religious purposes (monasteries and convents).

Mental hospitals are examples of the second type of total institution. Model (or Weber's 'ideal type' of) total institutions possess a number of characteristics. All aspects of life are conducted in the same place. Activities always take place in the presence of others and are strictly timetabled and geared towards fulfilling the official aims of the institution rather than the needs of individuals. A strict demarcation exists between 'inmates' and staff. In relation to the mental hospital the latter is characterized by narrow, hostile stereotypes. Patients are viewed by the staff as bitter, secretive and conspiratorial, whilst staff are viewed by patients as harsh and authoritarian.

On entering the mental hospital (the 'in-patient' phase of the patient's 'moral career') individuals undergo what Goffman refers to as the 'mortification of self'. 'Self' is not used to refer to a personal attribute, rather it is conceptualized as being constructed by the pattern of social control which exists in an institution. The mortification of self occurs as a result of two stages. On entering the hospital a person is deprived of their previous identity through regimentation. This entails stripping a person of their previous affirmation of self, movement is restricted, clothes worn on entry are replaced with pyjamas or hospital-owned clothing, and personal belongings such as money and jewellery are taken away. This manner of entering the hospital Goffman referred to as a 'degradation ceremony'. Once on the ward, inmates are invited to disown their former selves through a devaluing of past lives in 'confessionals' with staff and in ward groups. Daily life on the ward is also subjected to close and constant scrutiny, making privacy an impossibility.

Although Goffman's work was undertaken in an American context, similar analyses were being made of British mental hospitals. This British work was carried out by researchers who accepted psychiatric knowledge as being legitimate. Although their work was critical of custodial care, they need to be distinguished from the 'antipsychiatrists' (whom Wing went on to attack (Wing 1978)). Moreover, their work is more empirical in its methodology than Goffman's study, whose work can be dismissed or queried as being theoretically elegant but weak on substantive evidence, beyond his own participant observations.

Wing (1962) drew attention to the social withdrawal and passivity of hospitalized patients, which could be correlated with length of stay and was independent of clinical condition (i.e. psychotic symptoms). Wing and Freudenberg (1961) demonstrated how such signs of institutionally induced apathy could be quite rapidly reversed if chronic patients were placed in a stimulating work environment. Brown (1959) and Brown and Wing (1962) demonstrated the severe effects of institutionalization and showed that sustained efforts by clinicians to reverse these effects could be demonstrated by comparing hospitals with custodial and more therapeutic policies. None the less, the same pattern of withdrawal and apathy being correlated with length of stay was evident in all three hospitals. Brown and Wing cautioned that although enthusiastic medical leadership in the better hospitals could improve the functioning of chronic patients, these could be reversed by others later. Moreover, they commented, 'It is unlikely that the functions of an energetic reformer can be built in to the social structure of an institution' (p. 169).

Scott (1973) highlighted the passivity and symptom-inducing effects of the mental hospital and its attendant illness model, which he viewed as forming a 'treatment barrier' between professional and client. Russell Barton's *Institutional Neurosis* (1959) is traceable to his observations of Nazi concentration camp inmates. Inmates surrounded by corpses and excreta refused to move from the huts they were living in. Their bizarre attachment was compounded by stereotypical pacing. Barton noted the similar stereotypical behaviour in the closed and unstimulating environment of 'back ward' life in large mental hospitals.

This Anglo-American critique of the mental hospital from the 1960s was augmented by later work. Braginsky *et al.* (1973) found that acute patients wanted to leave hospital but that chronic patients took no interest in their clinical condition, instead they found ways of remaining invisible to staff, whilst maximizing the comforts they could find in the hospital. These patients actively wanted to stay in hospital in preference to the uncertainties of poverty on the outside.

A source of 'popular' criticism has emerged more recently from organizations representing the views of recipients of services, the media and policy campaigners (see Chapter 10). The mental health users' movement, which has emerged as a new social movement in a variety of countries during the 1970s and 1980s, views the asylum in negative terms. For instance, when asked about the closure of mental hospitals in a recent study, one key figure in the movement responded: 'Will Jews be homeless if the concentration camps close down? Should we have concentration camps for the homeless this is the question?' (quoted in Rogers and Pilgrim 1991: 135).

Because more ex-patients now live outside of hospital (either because they have been discharged from 'long stay' wards or use hospital facilities intermittently) they are more likely to frame demands around their civil status. Consequently, they hold up the old asylums as symbols of their oppression to be demolished.

An example of a later academic critique is provided by Martin's *Hospitals in Trouble* (1985), which highlights the failures of caring in British mental institutions between 1965 and 1983. During that period, ten inquiries of national significance took place into incidents and bad conditions within British mental illness and handicap hospitals. The problems forming the basis of complaints (which were often exposed by 'whistle-blowing' staff) ranged from inhumane, brutal and threatening behaviour by staff to lack of care through negligence and indifference. (Since the publication of Martin's work, mistreatment in large institutions continues to be exposed, for instance in Broadmoor and Ashworth Special Hospitals during the early 1990s.)

In attempting to analyse the origins of this endemic crisis, two questions were posed by Martin: how do trained carers come to behave contrary to professional standards? and how have hospitals been arranged in such a way that abuse and neglect have not been prevented? Martin found that some other organizational goal (such as staff convenience or public safety) had implicity usurped the goal of caring ('the subordination of care'). He also identified six types of isolation, which largely answered the second question. These were:

1 *Geographical isolation.* Most large institutions were situated out of main town centres, and even where they did not they were cut-off from local communities.
2 *Immediate isolation* referred to the fact that wards within hospitals were often isolated from one another and operated as little 'fiefdoms'. Martin found that it was only a small minority of wards within each hospital investigated which formed the basis of complaints.
3 *Personal isolation* referred to situations in which individuals were left in charge of large numbers of difficult to manage patients. Untrained and isolated staff were often left to cope with unbearable conditions.
4 *Consultant isolation.* The worst wards were found to be those rarely visited by the responsible consultant, with everyday management being left to junior medical staff. Thus, professional abdication of responsibility and lack of leadership was an important factor.

5 *Intellectual isolation* referred to a lack of professional stimulus, staff development, and access to training opportunities.

6 *Privacy* was a prerequisite for abuse; patients who were regularly visited by relatives were not usually the focus of complaints.

The structural nature of this isolation has led a number of social scientists to have a pessimistic stance towards the possibility of reforming the internal workings of large institutions. As we noted earlier, even those accepting the legitimacy of psychiatric theory and practice, such as Brown and Wing, questioned the reformability of psychiatric hospitals (even before the series of inquiries burgeoned after the mid-1960s). Whether or not all attempts at reform are futile is a moot point. However, what can be pointed out is that hospital scandals have continued in the 1980s and 1990s, unabated by attempts to introduce a watchdog role through visits by external organizations such as the Mental Health Act Commission and Health Advisory Service. This is discussed in greater detail in Chapter 9.

Responses to the crisis

Therapeutic communities – 'humanizing' the hospital?

Therapeutic communities (TCs) – small units or wards designed to make the social environment the main therapeutic tool – were pioneered in Britain during the Second World War by psychotherapeutically orientated psychiatrists. The number of soldier patients suffering from the stress of warfare meant that the individual model of therapy became untenable because of scarce staff resources. These army psychiatrists were encouraged to experiment with a variety of group methods to increase staff cost-effectiveness. The twofold objectives looked for in therapeutic communities were identified by Main in the 1940s (1946) as: the need to resocialize patients who had become dependent as a result of traditional hospital practices; and the use of the hospital environment as a therapeutic agent through establishing social participation. The latter was considered to be particularly valuable in treating people with neurotic conditions.

Inherent to the TC ideal was the belief that the social structure of the ward, group atmosphere, and ward morale were important elements in the therapeutic endeavour of psychiatry. Central to these objectives was the need for rapid change of the organization of the hospital, in order to make it more flexible and egalitarian. Attempts were made to break down the traditionally rigid and hierarchical role divisions between staff and patients, and decisions on the running of the TC were to be decided through group discussion. The latter measure was designed to promote communication between staff and patients.

TCs developed rapidly during the 1960s but soon after they became marginalized. Thus, their success in changing mainstream psychiatric theory and practice has been modest. The main weaknesses seem to stem from their organizational form. Perrow (1965) has pointed to the shortcomings of TCs as viable organizations. In particular, he points to the failure to change fundamentally the social structure of the organization, which he traces to the failure of the TCs' 'technology' (or the means used for reaching the set goals). The wider organization (the mental hospital), of which TCs formed only a small part, continued to operate custodial practices and the bureaucratic and professional structures remained relatively impervious to change. This limitation was clearly recognized in Italy, where TCs were seen as only a preliminary step towards the total dismantling of the asylum system, which came to be viewed as unreformable. In describing the psychiatric reforms in one Italian locality, Franco Basaglia states that they were: 'More akin to the political struggles which broke out in other areas of social life in the 1960s, breaking up established institutions and exposing their shortcomings, than to avant-garde psychiatric experiments like the therapeutic community in England or la psychiatric institutionelle in France' (Basaglia, in Ingleby 1981: 185).

The 'technology' for reaching the set goals of therapeutic communities was not enough to change custodial goals and existing structures. In other words, the group work and social environment was not effective in changing sets of superordinate institutional relationships. Certainly, the success of the therapeutic community, as an ideology or therapy, was limited in persuading British psychiatry to move away from a medical model, as indicated in an interview with Maxwell Jones, a pioneer of TCs, in 1984: 'For orthodox psychiatry it [the therapeutic community ideal] has provided a name to be wheeled out whenever it wants to defend Britain's reputation as the country which pioneered social psychiatry and to be conveniently forgotten otherwise' (*The Guardian*, August 1984).

An alternative to trying to humanize the institution is the run-down and closure of hospitals.

Deinstitutionalization

In the twentieth century many countries have followed a policy of hospital run-down and closure, often referred to as deinstitutionalization. In 1954 there were 154,000 residents in British mental hospitals. By 1982 this had fallen to 100,000. In other countries the degree of deinstitutionalization has been even greater. For example, in Italy between 1968 and 1978 the asylum population fell from 100,000 to 50,000.

Critiques in themselves may not lead to change. Scull comments that the work of social scientists on the disabling and custodial function of the asylum was not accompanied by evidence of greater public tolerance towards emotional deviance. The reasons thought to be responsible for deinstitutionalization are multiple and contested, and implicate a complex set of interrelationships between the medical profession, public morality, the State and political economy. A number of different accounts have been offered for deinstitutionalization policies, which we will consider in turn:

1 The 'pharmacological revolution'.
2 Economic determinism.
3 A shift to acute problems.
4 A shift in the psychiatric discourse.

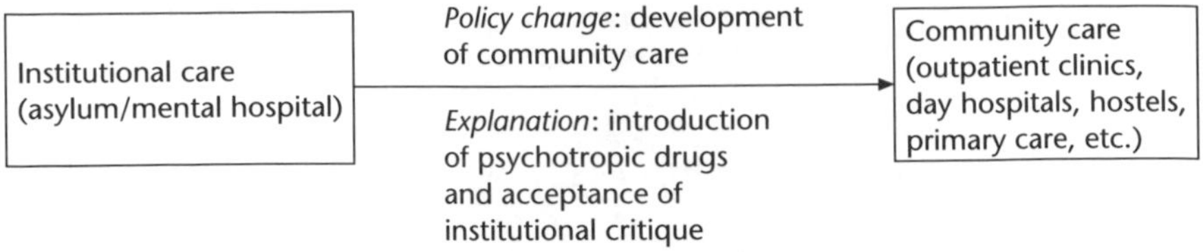

Institutional care (asylum/mental hospital)	*Policy change*: development of community care	Community care (outpatient clinics, day hospitals, hostels, primary care, etc.)
	Explanation: introduction of psychotropic drugs and acceptance of institutional critique	

Figure 8.1　The pharmacological revolution (from Busfield 1986).

The 'pharmacological revolution'

The most frequently cited 'official' explanation, simply put, suggests that advances in medical treatment of mental illness permitted patients to be discharged from institutions *en masse*. According to this view of change, the introduction of major tranquillizers enabled the alleviation of symptoms in psychotic patients, allowing large numbers of asylum residents to move into the community. Busfield (1986) summarizes this model diagrammatically in Figure 8.1.

However, this account of deinstitutionalization generates both theoretical and empirical difficulties. For example, it cannot explain why community care policies were applied to a range of care groups such as the mentally handicapped, who are not deemed to be able to benefit from such drug treatment. More importantly, a number of studies demonstrate that an increased pattern of discharges occurred prior to the widespread use of major tranquillizers. Nor did the introduction of psychotropic drugs appear to accelerate the rate of discharges. The pattern of the fall remained consistent with that preceding their widespread use.

The notion that medical intervention was principally responsible for 'decarceration' may have been deduced from a reading of the official statistics produced on mental hospital inmates of the time. However, Scull (1977: 83) points out that a reading of these sources of data may have led to erroneous interpretations being made, since they mask: '. . . earlier changes at the local level and obscure the degree to which the fall in overall numbers, when it did come, represents a continuation rather than a departure from preexisting trends.' Thus, according to Scull, whilst psychotropic medication has helped manage deviance post-deinstitutionalization (through the control rather than permanent alleviation of symptoms), they were not responsible for the genesis of this policy.

Other analyses of data sources indicate that organizational factors and social policy initiatives are responsible for changes in the location of psychiatric practice. Table 8.1 shows the growth in the number of psychiatric beds in a number of European countries post-Second World War, which ran counter to run-down in the UK and the US. Whilst the type of increased bed use varied from one country to another (in some it was short-term beds, in others new specialist facilities) the point is that in-patient care increased during a time when the major tranquillizers were widely and increasingly utilized.

Table 8.1 Post-war growth of psychiatric beds in Europe

Country	Year	No. psychiatric beds
Belgium	1951	19,841
	1970	26,553
Austria	1950	9,868
	1975	14,314
Italy	1954	88,241
	1961	113,040
Spain	1949	25,571
	1974	42,493
Federal German Republic	1953	86,640
	1975	112,791

Source: Adapted from World Health Organization Statistics Annuals

Economic determinism

Scull (1977: 1) provides an alternative explanation for 'decarceration', the term he uses to describe the '... State sponsored policy of closing down asylums', which he relates to changes in social control mechanisms. Scull contends that with the emergence of the welfare state, segregative control mechanisms became too costly and difficult to justify. The cost inflation of mental hospitals prior to, and after, the Second World War was brought about by the elimination of unpaid patient labour and increased cost of employees, as a result of the unionization of labour. The latter had the effect of contributing to the doubling of unit costs (because of the cost of a shorter working day and holiday entitlement). Busfield (1986) summarizes Scull's account of decarceration in Figure 8.2.

The maintenance of ex-patients on welfare payments and the 'neglecting' of community care becomes a more viable State policy. The reality of community habitation for ex-inmates, according to Scull, has been an unmitigated disaster for the majority. The inhumanity of the asylum has simply been replaced by the negligence of the community: 'the alternative to the institution has been to be herded into newly emerging "deviant ghettoes", sewers of human misery and which is conventionally defined as social pathology within which (largely hidden from outside inspection or even notice) society's refuse may be repressively tolerated' (Scull 1977: 153).

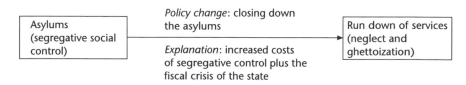

Figure 8.2 Decarceration (from Busfield 1986).

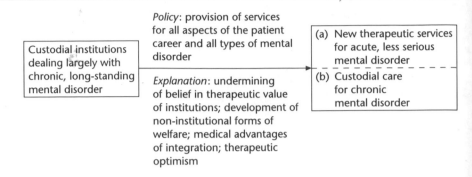

Figure 8.3 Busfield's account of institutional change (from Busfield, 1986).

A shift to acute problems

Scull's replacement of a technological determinist argument with an economic determinist one also gives rise to empirical and conceptual difficulties. In particular, his account has been deemed defective on the grounds of timing. Busfield points out that the State's fiscal crisis (which is the main reference point for Scull's thesis) characterizes the post-1970 eras. During the 1950s, when American deinstitutionalization policies developed rapidly, the economic growth which accompanied increases in public expenditure meant there was relatively little concern about the latter. Scull's explanation also fails to acknowledge the rise in expenditure, and development of mental health services outside the hospital sector. There have, for example, been large increases in psychiatric services in the area of primary care. Rather than the non-provision of services, Busfield has argued that community care has brought with it a shift in orientation from the chronic long-term patient towards those with acute or less serious problems. Her account of institutional change is shown in Figure 8.3.

A shift in the psychiatric discourse

A fourth position avoids both economic and technological determinism. Rather than attempting to identify causal mechanisms, the aim is to describe the object, ideology and organizational arrangements which constitute contemporary psychiatry. Prior (1991) argues that the target of psychiatric practice changes over time. Each new object is accompanied by a different type of clinical practice and organizational setting. For example, the nineteenth-century view of madness took as its focus the brain and forms of degeneracy, which demanded exclusion and control in the asylum. In contrast, the concepts of 'psyche' and 'the unconscious' in Freudian theory centred around the concept of 'mind'. The rising popularity of psychoanalytically informed ideas also started to cloud the distinction between normal and pathological behaviour which, according to Ramon (1985), helped destigmatize mental illness.

These new ideas required a socio-medical organization conducive to intimate therapeutic encounters between individual client and therapist. Prior argues that the lack of fit between modern psychiatric theories of the mind and madness necessitated the organizational change described as 'deinstitutionalization'. Prior perceives the 'therapeutics of mental illness at the end of the asylum age' as being widely dispersed. There is dual responsibility for mental health between medical and social services. The latter focus on aspects of patients' lives, such as 'social networks', employment and family relationships, the former is subdivided between nursing and medical input. Medical input takes as its focus the physical characteristics of the patient, diagnosis and physical therapies such as ECT and psychotropic drugs. The object of focus, for nursing in particular, centres around improving patient behaviour. However, such a focus on behaviour is not compatible with a hospital milieu since, by definition, it necessitates the patient's contact with society, both to test the patient's behavioural competence and extend their behavioural repertoire. The attendant therapeutic endeavours, which centre around such things as the 'normalization' of behaviour and the building of social networks, thus require a community environment rendering the hospital 'functionless'.

Prior's analysis avoids the assumptions inherent in the economic interest argument of Scull and the pharmacological revolution position of official accounts. However, a set of empirical questions which are important in assessing the merits of the different theoretical positions that have emerged around deinstitutionalization remain unanswered. For example, although there has been an expansion of psychodynamically informed therapies and a greater focus on the social relationships of patients, it is a moot point whether a biomedical hospital-centred psychiatric practice has actually been replaced with extra-hospital activities.

Community care or reinstitutionalization?

There remains substantial confusion surrounding the meaning of the term 'community care', which reflects a lack of clarity over the ultimate goals of such a policy. In practice, community care refers to mentally disordered people receiving 'care' in non-asylum settings. The main initiatives include the development of psychiatric units in District General Hospitals (DGH), psychiatric services in primary health care settings, the expanded use of community psychiatric nurses, the development of community mental health centres, the provision of domiciliary services, the development of residential and day care facilities, an increased emphasis of voluntary services and informal care by relatives and friends, and the relocation of mental health responsibilities from the secondary care sector to primary care.

There has been a rapid development of certain community resources. For example, between 1977 and 1987 Community Mental Health Centres in Britain expanded from one to 54 (Sayce 1989). Psychiatric services delivered via primary care are another area of expansion. However, it would be misleading to exaggerate the extent of reprovision from hospital-based services to the community. Mental health provision in Britain is still largely hospital-based. In the US, where a longer period has elapsed since the Community Mental Health Act 1963, than since the British NHS and Community Care

Act of 1990, the old, large State asylums have simply been replaced by a
network of smaller, private in-patient facilities. Even there, Community Mental
Health Centres were forced under fiscal pressure to shift to a custodial role
(Samson 1992).

Samson insists that the US has never had proper community care but that
instead a variety of economic and professional pressures have ensured a
policy of reinstitutionalization. Consequently, he argues that those who
attack the 'failure' of community care policies are actually attacking a straw
man, given that what has actually happened is deinstitutionalization followed by reinstitutionalization. Similarly in Britain, the theory of community living has often been replaced by the practice of deinstitutionalization.
The political objective of community care was first mentioned in the Mental
Treatment Act 1930 and, by the 1970s, there was a bipartisan political goal
of transferring people out of institutions. Yet, it was only in 1985 that the
first British mental hospital actually closed.

By the late 1980s, 85 per cent of resources spent on mental health by the
State were still bound up with hospitals (Sayce 1989). Data supplied by the
Department of Health in 1992, showed both numerical losses and gains to
hospital-based psychiatry. Although the number of psychiatric beds decreased,
from 193,000 in 1959 to 108,000 in 1985, by 1985 there had been a rise in
the number of small psychiatric hospital facilities from 303 to 492. And even
though hospital resident numbers dropped by 24 per cent between 1980 and
1990, psychiatric facilities still contained 36 per cent of all hospital beds by
the latter year. In 1990 there were more than 50,000 psychiatric in-patients
in England alone, at any one time. Moreover, despite a steady decline in the
number of people occupying hospital beds since the 1960s, short-stay admissions rose dramatically, creating 'revolving-door' hospital care, rather than
fully fledged care in the community.

Perhaps the pertinent question to pose is why did it take so long to translate the objective of community care into practice? The structure of two key
organizations (Community Mental Health Centres and DGH psychiatric units),
designed with the aim of making the asylum redundant, illustrates the con-
trasting nature of provision incorporated under the heading of 'community
care'.

Community Mental Health Centres (CMHCs) are a non-hospital-based
provision that appeared on the British mental health scene in the 1970s.
According to Sayce (1989), this service can be defined as 'a multi-professional
non-hospital-based centre, offering an easily accessible service including
sessional therapy/support/treatment with individuals or groups'. Within this
broad definition Sayce has outlined four main models of CMHC, which she
dubs: (1) 'comprehensive local mental health services'; (2) 'low key sessional
model'; (3) 'day care model'; and (4) 'community development' model. The
first involves psychiatrists usually in a director role, offering a range of treatments and assessments. In the second, the centres are only open part of the
week and have programmes based on therapeutic group work and an emphasis
on outreach work, using the centre as a base. The final model rarely includes
psychiatrists and concentrates on mental health promotion and preventive
work. The 'client' in this model is the whole 'community'. Sayce's research
showed that by 1987 there were 49 CMHCs in existence, with 44 more
planned.

Despite the diversity of organizations included under the title of 'CMHC', they share a number of global ideas and an organizing rationale, which seem to fit the ideal type of 'new' mental health provision depicted by Prior above. According to Sayce, one of the motivating forces behind CMHCs is 'a wish to reject a medicalized model of psychiatry' for a more eclectic model of working. This is reflected in the objectives of the current Centres. According to a recent survey, they aim to be local, comprehensive, accessible, non-stigmatizing centres which form the focus for an area's mental health service and encourage coordination between the NHS, social services and other relevant local agencies. Multidisciplinary working and 'key worker' schemes are central, as are holistic methods of working that aim to account for the social and personal, rather than only medical, aspects of a person's problem. Open and self-referral is commonplace and the empowerment of service users and reduction in professional power is also an aim of such centres. Counselling with users is given a high profile, which adds to the role-blurring between mental health professionals.

Despite the growth in the popularity of CMHCs as ideals at a local level (Sayce found that even in localities where there were no centres, policy-makers thought they should have one), they have remained on the margins of community care. They are often established in the face of opposition from conservative forces within the psychiatric profession (Goldie et al. 1989) and are not included in official government plans for replacing asylum beds, as they were, for example, in Italy. As new services they have been subjected to greater scrutiny and evaluations than hospital-based services.

New day places to replace hospital beds were not only slow in coming (between 1975 and 1985 only 9000 new places were made available (Audit Commission 1986)) they were overwhelmingly placed on hospital sites. Similarly, although there was a decrease in the number of in-patients, as outpatients they still attended hospital premises for their appointments. Domiciliary services – the visiting of people in their own homes by mental health professionals – today constitutes only a tiny proportion of this total.

To what extent does this process of 'reinstitutionalization' fulfil a central intention of community care policy, that care environments should reflect, as far as possible, ordinary community life? This was the question that Baruch and Treacher (1978) addressed in their book *Psychiatry Observed*, which examined the policy shift towards providing psychiatric beds in general hospitals. Baruch and Treacher argued that rather than providing for the desegregation of psychiatric patients, such moves merely permitted the desegregation of the psychiatric profession.

An examination of professional literature showed a consensus for the establishment of DGHUs, based on the need for medical students and trainee psychiatrists to be located in teaching hospitals and for psychiatry to be fully integrated into medicine. The latter is particularly relevant given the marginal position and low prestige that psychiatrists have enjoyed vis-à-vis their medical colleagues. The tenuousness of their medical status was exacerbated by their geographical marginalization in the old asylums. Moving to the centre ground of medical practice has allowed for innovations aimed at securing or advancing the professional position of psychiatry. An example here is liaison psychiatry, which takes as its focus of interest the mental health needs of physically ill patients. This points to the adaptive ability of psychiatry as a dominant profession. When psychiatric interests are faced with inevitable social change, as in the closure of the large Victorian asylums, they react by seeking new sites on which to practise.

With regard to organizational structure and therapeutic milieu, a further question posed was, to what extent do DGHUs differ from the isolated mental hospital? The case example Baruch and Treacher (1978: 223) used as the basis of their study suggested that varying the therapeutic location did not appear to lead to major changes in the way in which patients were treated. For instance, there continued to be weak links between the unit and the community:

> . . . staff members were effectively 'institutionalized' – they rarely made domiciliary visits to their patients and they were not involved in the communities from which their patients came, so they could never develop an understanding of the patients' way of life or devise methods for using community resources to help the patients.

Patient management and the division of labour remained under medical control, and a discrepancy between decisions taken at ward level and practice with patients was evident. The therapeutic regime was similar to that provided in the mental hospital, with little in-depth counselling or work with patients and their families. However, there are purported advantages for patients of DGHUs. Raphael (1974) suggested that they preferred the modern building to the isolated and remote mental hospital. None the less, there are added disadvantages. These can be understood with reference to Perrow's analysis of the hospital. Brown (1973) cautioned 25 years ago against reinstitutionalization, on the basis that ordinary hospitals are not designed with the needs of mental patients in mind. DGHs are fashioned to the needs of those who are physically ill. Hence the open 'nightingale' wards and few areas for recreation or privacy. The need for the smooth functioning of the rest of the hospital, for example, operating theatres, may mean extra pressure to constrain patients on psychiatric wards. Moreover, the focus on acute physical conditions may, in turn, lead to the dominance of physical treatments, such as ECT, in psychiatry. The introduction of other therapies (e.g. psychotherapy) into hospital settings were, according to Baruch and Treacher, likely to be perceived as 'alien' and therefore difficult to establish as a mainstream intervention.

A final consideration about the problem of reinstitutionalisation and the inertia of hospital-oriented State funding is the interaction of political interests which have impeded shifts to ordinary living and fuller citizenship for people with mental health problems. The old asylums were a total solution for the social problems associated with mental abnormality. In particular, they provided three main functions:

- semi-permanent or permanent accommodation
- treatment
- social control

All of these functions occurred concurrently in one institution. Whatever disadvantages the old asylum system had for their inmates (by creating a form of disabling apartheid) as well as advantages (see comments from

Gittins earlier), the socio-political benefit for others was that a group of non-conformist, troublesome, worrisome and economically inefficient people were segregated. Mental abnormality was swept away or 'warehoused', out of the sight and mind of the majority of free citizens. The consequences of demolishing these warehouses are thus obvious. The three functions would still be required by society for both economic efficiency and the maintenance of a moral order but now they would have to be reconfigured or reconstructed.

This political challenge has tempted cautious politicians to hold on to revised forms of institutional care. In addition, the latter provided the psychiatric profession with an opportunity to retain its traditional preferred link between power and beds. Moreover, the shift to DGH in-patient units was also an opportunity to increase the professional standing of a low status medical specialty. Families troubled by patients in their midst would also look to new forms of safe residential disposal. Thus, a confluence of interests emerged in the final quarter of the twentieth century to retain a hospital focus to mental health work, despite the run down of the asylum system. However, this has placed unrealistic expectations upon DGH units.

The interest groups just described have become immediately aggrieved about the inefficiency of the units compared to the old asylums, as the shift in scale means that the new units cannot replicate all the functions of the old hospitals. This has led to diverse demands in response. Some of these have centred on requests for more beds (from psychiatrists and patient-relative pressure groups) or calls for a halt to the run down of the old asylums. Others have demanded greater community support to reduce the need for admission (user groups). Also, because the newer units are very small compared to the old local asylum, they have prioritized those patients who are the most 'ill' (i.e. threatening to social order). As a result, the units have become more control orientated. They focus increasingly upon acute psychosis and parasuicidal behaviour and they have re-introduced locked wards. The aggregate overspill from this local trend has been the greater demand for more secure facilities on a regional basis (in Britain, the Regional Secure Unit system). Residential facilities like these are expensive to build and maintain and have high labour costs. Moreover, their small size means that they must fail as semi-permanent residential facilities compared to the asylums.

It can be seen then that the prioritizing of control, professional preferences to treat in in-patient settings and the continued need for people with mental health problems to be accommodated together place pressure upon smaller scale hospital facilities. This pressure has created such political anxiety that in Britain ministers have opted to slow asylum run down and keep high investment levels in beds (Department of Health 1997). In response, critics have argued that the three functions noted above should be dealt with as separate policy questions: accommodation implies social housing not hospitalization; treatment needs to be cost-effective and its appropriate siting clarified; and risk management should be dealt with rationally not prejudicially (Pilgrim and Rogers 1997). The macro policy context together with the micro behaviour of professionals making and dealing with mental health referrals determine the pace and success of community care. A comparison of community-based care for those patients with a diagnosis of schizophrenia in Verona and South Manchester indicated that the organization of services in the former resulted in shorter hospital stays as a result of better integration between hospital and community services (Gater *et al.* 1995).

The current organizational arrangements of psychiatric services are operating within an increasingly loose set of structures and systems. Old asylums, DGH units and community mental health centres are examples of physical structures which largely housed and shaped procedures of care. What has happened in recent years is that although this bricks and mortar style of services has not disappeared, increasingly mechanisms, procedures and forms of care delivery have emerged which are not necessarily tied to structures. An example of this is the emergence of community mental health *teams* (rather than centres). These may be based in a variety of settings and team members may work across a number of sites, including the homes of patients. Another example would be the series of service procedures and legal mechanisms which implicate a number of staff in a variety of settings. Currently in Britain these would include the case management arrangements (Onyett 1994), the care programme approach and supervision registers, which apply to patients living in the community. (These points about changes in acute psychiatry and systems of community mental health care are picked up again in the next chapter.)

Public health, primary care and the new technology revolution

With the fragmentation of old structures like the asylums there has been greater attention paid to considering the cause and solution of mental health problems within a public health context. Previously, psychiatric epidemiology and the treatment of mental disorders were separated conceptually. With the rise of a 'new' public health, which integrates lay with traditional epidemiology, and the emergence of a strong primary health care agenda, epidemiology and treatment are coming closer together as the hospital disappears as the symbolic focus of treatment. Attention shifts instead to inequalities in mental health (discussed in Chapter 2), prevention and the notion of 'positive mental health' (discussed at the end of the last chapter). Alongside this within mental health policy, problem management stretches beyond the structural and organizational arrangements of traditional health services. A multi-sectoral approach to mental health is outlined in the Governments' Green Paper 'Our Healthier Nation'. The policy response to mental health problems here implicates local and central players, community resources, the environment and individual action. Thus, the focus has moved to incorporate aspects of employment, social, community and voluntary organizations in the prevention and management of mental health problems. Within this schema where service contact is needed, primary care is privileged over specialist mental health services. That is, the optimal service response is cast in settings which are as close as possible to the place where the genesis of mental health problems originate and are expressed.

A final and further change is related to the way in which new technologies and information systems have changed the organization of psychiatry. The widespread availability of technology, together with the community location of the overwhelming majority of patients, have changed the face of how mental health services are organized and delivered. This change, in turn, is likely to dramatically alter the power relationships between providers and recipients of mental health services. The proliferation of the use of new forms of mental health services are likely to be reinforced by the cultural shift towards the acceptance of evidenced-based health care discussed in Chapter 7. For example, telephone counselling for patients with 'minor depression' from a primary care base has been found to be both efficient and effective (Lynch *et al.* 1997) as has undertaking a psychiatric assessment and diagnosis over the telephone (Kobak 1997). The ambiguous legitimacy that mental health care professionals hold in the eyes of users is reinforced by research which evaluates the outcomes of services organized along different lines. A randomized controlled trial compared face to face meetings with professionals and another group who used an electronic self-help computer programme in the form of a 'voice bulletin board'. Clients were found to be eight times more likely to participate in the computerised programme and were more satisfied than the group receiving face to face contact (Alemi *et al.* 1996).

The internet and computer-based programmes, by simplifying communication and being readily accessible directly to people has the potential to 'cut out' professionals altogether. It also overcomes the problems caused by geographical location and variable personal quality (mechanical responses can be standardized). It is likely that the use of the internet directly empowers users of mental health services by allowing them to feel in control of their treatment and everyday life more generally. (The issue of users as providers of care is returned to in Chapter 10.) Equally, if not more, importantly is the rapid increase in mutual non-professional support. The social isolation and 'poverty' of social networks have been a recurrent theme in the literature on people with long-term health problems. One of the most important consequences of the technologies is the rapid increase it allows in mutual non-professional support. The anonymous helper in an electronic conference or the support group on the Web provides the bases of a revolution in mental health support that has emerged as an unpredicted and major force in the global organization of mental health care.

Discussion

The old mental asylum system can be thought of as representing part of the modernist project, although other forms of total institution, like the monastery, stretch back to feudal times. But whilst the monastery was guided by theological considerations, the asylum was peculiarly modern because rationality was its guiding organizational principle. Reason, not faith, now permeated the total institution. The pursuit of rational scientific knowledge about lunacy became the aim of modern psychiatry, even when such an aim was rhetorical rather than real. Accordingly, the elimination of mental disease was seen as a possibility, through its systematic organization and treatment in purpose-built institutions designed to segregate embodied irrationality from everyday life. There was no longer what Foucault called a 'dialogue between reason and unreason', rather the latter was trapped and codified by the former.

This Victorian project is now largely over. The crisis of the asylum emerged not only because of considerations of cost but also because of changes in the discourse about mental abnormality and its treatment, in both the lay and professional areas. In Chapter 6 we summarized the expansion of the ambit of psychiatry after the First World War, and Prior (1991), above, argues for a more recent flux in psychiatric theory and practice. The asylum could not adapt to these changes and so its therapeutic legitimacy edged more and more towards crisis. But what of the replacements of the asylums? We have discussed two main British responses – CMHCs and DGHUs. This divided response suggests that there is both a continuity with Victorian modernism and a postmodern break taking place, as far as the organization of mental health work is concerned. The CMHC is consistent with a definition here by Clegg (1990: 53) of postmodern organizations, which are: 'forms of emerging organization that bear little or no relation to modernist variations on the theme of bureaucracy. These organizations are "de-differentiated" . . . flexible, niche marketed and have a multi-skilled workforce held together by information technology, networks and subcontracting.'

The emergence of the CMHC seems to confirm the notion that mental health care delivery is moving into a different era. In this organizational context, role-blurring removes the strict division of labour typical of the hospital. The key worker system and multidisciplinary working brings with it genericism and an increased individual responsibility for practitioners. Outreach work with clients decentralizes or diffuses the locus of power away from the professionals' organizational base. Even that base has lost its architectural salience compared with the hospital: the more successfully 'normalized' it is the more it looks like an ordinary house. The knowledge base used by the professionals is eclectic (incorporating biological, psychological and social notions). Moreover, no two CMHCs are exactly the same. Sayce provided evidence of an emerging diversity of functions offered by the centres – treatment, information, self-help, etc. This picture of diversity and eclecticism in the CMHC no longer squares with Perrow's model of the hospital outlined at the start of the chapter.

However, what does square with such a model is the DGH psychiatric unit. This seems to represent a continuity with the modernist project of Victorian psychiatry. Its power is clearly focused and centralized. There is the retention of a division of labour within the clinical team, and between clinicians and managers. Consultants continue to lead a pyramid of clinical power – they head up 'firms'. However, their power has been subordinated to some extent now to the rules of general management (a bureaucratic process) and the modern hospital has been subjected to the non-bureaucratic principle of marketization. So, whilst the contemporary DGH units represent a strong continuity with the nineteenth-century asylum, the psychiatric profession is enduring peculiar new stresses within its confines.

Another difference between the two centuries is literally visible. The architectural form of the DGHU is actually more clear-cut than the old Victorian hospital, especially when it occurs in the post-war, high rise, concrete block. In the Victorian asylum the expansive grounds might be mistaken for a public park, whereas the modern hospital block containing cramped wards with low ceilings, and no internal or external exercise space, has become a caricature of an impersonal, modern, urban building.

As Samson (1992) notes about the US experience, new hospitals for old marks reinstitutionalization (or it could be dubbed 'trans-hospitalization') not community care. Consequently, if the Victorian asylums were found lacking as therapeutic institutions, then it is likely that this will also be the case for the DGH psychiatric units. With a much smaller physical capacity for beds than the old asylums, these new units are increasingly becoming a focus for the expert coercive regulation of suicidal and psychotic patients. Locked wards have returned ('Special Care Units') and risk assessment and risk management have become the anxious daily pre-occupation of staff. Despite their recent title of acute 'mental health services', these units, more than the Victorian hospitals, closed or closing, function to restrain and segregate, albeit for shorter periods, those deemed to be a risk to themselves or others. They are not about mental health but very much about mental pathology.

A further fragment of the postmodern condition of psychiatry lies with the rise of new technologies in managing mental disorder, where organizational arrangements are largely irrelevant. Directly accessible information to users via the internet and to professionals via telemedicine signals the beginning of a new revolution in the organization and delivery of mental health services.

In conclusion

This chapter has focused on the rise and fall of the asylum and the ambiguities which attend our current post-asylum world. A variety of factors have contributed to the demise of the old large mental hospitals, some of which have been economic and others ideological in influence. What the current social policy controversies surrounding care in the community highlight is that the old hospitals contained the three interweaving functions of care, control and accommodation. Any new arrangement about the organization of mental health work will also involve these functions. Controversies have tended to emerge for the very reason that critics (serving a variety of interests) have complained that government has still not delivered the correct blend of care, control and accommodation.

Questions

1 Why were the large mental hospitals closed down?

2 Why were the large mental hospitals not closed sooner?

3 Do new arrangements about mental health care reflect our postmodern condition?

4 'The pharmacological revolution is a myth' – discuss.

5 'Scull's fiscal crisis of the State thesis was 20 years out of time' – discuss.

6 How might new technology shape community mental health work?

For discussion

If you, or a friend or relative, had a long-term mental health problem how would you like services to be organized in response? When discussing this question, think about the points raised in the chapter about care, control and accommodation.

Further reading

Audit Commission (1994) *Finding A Place: A Review of Mental Health Services For Adults.* London: HMSO.

Baruch, G. and Treacher, A. (1978) *Psychiatry Observed.* London: Routledge.

Martin, J.P. (1985) *Hospitals in Trouble.* Oxford: Blackwell.

Rogers, A. and Pilgrim, D. (1997) *Mental Health Policy in Britain: A Critical Introduction.* Basingstoke: Macmillan.

Chapter 9

Psychiatry and legal control

Chapter overview

This chapter will examine the role of mental health legislation, which is a central feature in the relationship between the State and service delivery. The chapter will cover the following topics:

- Legal versus medical control of madness
- Mentally disordered offenders
- Compulsory and voluntary psychiatric admissions
- Legal aspects of compulsion
- Dangerousness

Legal versus medical control of madness

Since the nineteenth century, legalism has been a central component of social reform in the area of mental health. In England and Wales, the Lunacy Act 1890 prescribed that admissions to hospitals and treatment would be governed by statute. It also ensured that the control and supervision of inmates would be overseen by government bodies. In the twentieth century such safeguards and powers have increasingly involved the legal profession. This contrasts with medical control, which entails mental disorder and its management being under the control of doctors. Diagnosis and admission are seen primarily as the concern of the medical profession. This is the viewpoint underlying both the Mental Health Act 1959 and, in a softened form, the current British legislation, the Mental Health Act 1983.

Historically, legalism has been used to counter what have been viewed as the deficits of medical management. Similarly, the assertion of a medical view of mental disorder has been resorted to at times when legalism was considered to have failed. The tension between legalism and medical control permeates the implementation of mental health legislation. This is true of both civil compulsory admissions of non-offender patients and mentally disordered offenders.

It is not only the psychiatric profession that has resisted the intrusion of law into its work. The use of the law in the mental health area has also been criticized by some social scientists. For example, Jones (1960) a prominent social policy analyst, has argued that there are severe limits to what the law can achieve in mental health services. Jones argues that good practice is likely to be fostered through adequate resource allocation and the development of professional norms and values. She believes that the latter would enhance the appropriate attitudes, skills and treatments needed for the compassionate management of mentally disordered people and interprofessional cooperation. A strict legal framework might inhibit this process. Thus, the use of the law in her view should only be as a last resort.

From a different standpoint, Rose (1986) has argued that legalism is just another form of control that does not ultimately benefit the patient. Instead, he argues that not only does legalism not constrain psychiatric discretion but it also disguises the wider political context of the delivery of mental health services and thereby depoliticizes the debate over how psychiatry is organized and operates: 'legality is merely one mode of regulation and body of professional expertise amongst others, neither conceptually more rigorous, nor necessarily more effective in bringing power to account' (Rose 1986: 209). Rose's criticism centres on the tendency of legal measures to individualize problems. This and Jones' viewpoint have a certain merit. Legalism has had a chequered history with regard to fostering positive values about mental abnormality. The Lunacy Act 1890, for example, led to wide-scale stigma around madness and 'certification', because it allowed only for the forced admission of people to mental asylums via the courts. The Mental Treatment Act 1930 attempted to rectify this by introducing the possibility of voluntary admission to hospital, which, it is argued, fostered a more sympathetic attitude to emotional deviance. Yet, as we have seen in Chapter 8, the appeal to medical means and humanitarianism has not been enough to prevent abuse and neglect in mental hospitals. Nor has it protected the individual rights of patients. Bean (1980) found that, under the Mental Health Act 1959, which represented a swing back from a legal to a medical control, there was an absence of adequate checks and control mechanisms. Over-zealous psychiatrists sometimes placed patients in a vulnerable position by permitting them to be deprived of their liberty for considerable periods of time. Bean related this to the nature of therapeutic law with its open-ended clauses and standards, which leads to a tendency towards *ad hoc* rule enforcement and the playing down of the importance of general rules. In other words, where there is a clash between the views of medicine and legal requirements, medical demands tend to be privileged.

Over the last two decades there has been a global trend towards balancing the medical dominance of therapeutic law with a greater legal presence with a view to giving greater weight to the individual rights of patients. A recent ethnographic study carried out in Sweden examining such arrangements seems to suggest that nothing much changes when the legal role is formally extended. Psychiatric norms and values still dominate patient-professional interaction and the outcome of assessments. Even in a legally-dominated context those with mental health problems are treated as patients rather than adverse parties and there is an inbuilt bias to the proceedings – it is assumed from the beginning that they are mentally ill. There is a tendency for their credibility to be viewed as suspect and expressions of 'sane' behaviour are seen as a temporary effort at self-composure. Where mental health is concerned, an informal atmosphere is often adopted which is atypical of other legal proceedings. This further militates against a view of the patient as a valid legal party (Sjostrom 1997).

Mentally disordered offenders

Issues relating to secure provision have already been touched on in Chapter 1 (lay perceptions of badness and madness) and in Chapter 7 (the scandals associated with the isolation of special hospitals). Here, we will focus on forensic psychiatry and its relation to law.

Forensic psychiatry is concerned with the management of those who are 'doubly deviant' – those who are considered to have committed a criminal act and who are deemed to be mentally abnormal. Forensic psychiatry is charged with the management of lawbreakers and others who come before the courts. Thus, its area of jurisdiction is principally in relation to referrals from the criminal justice system and those patients who are detained in hospitals subject to restriction orders. In England and Wales, recent statistics indicate that the latter comprises a small proportion of mental patients overall. There are about 1800 patients detained in hospitals under restriction orders and most (two-thirds) of these are detained in special hospitals. The rest are residents in Regional Secure Units, which between them have 500–600 beds, and mainstream psychiatric provision. Some forensic psychiatrists consider that up to one-third of the prison population would benefit from psychiatric treatment (Gunn 1978). By contrast, mainstream psychiatry operates alongside other medical specialisms in the National Health Service, concerning itself mainly with voluntary patients or civil compulsory detention.

The view of control discussed at the start of this chapter locates power in the hand of State organizations and agencies and their professional employees (psychiatrists and lawyers). Foucault provides an alternative view of the emergent relationship between psychiatry and the law. Psychiatry's involvement with penal law in the eighteenth and nineteenth centuries came about with the shift from a criminology that focused on the offence and penalty, to one concerned with the crime, the criminal and means of repression. The shift from crime to the criminal meant that the focus changed from what must be punished and how, to who must be punished: 'It is not enough for the accused to say in reply to that question "I am the author of the crimes before you, period. Judge since you must, condemn if you will". Much more is expected of him. Beyond admission, there must be confession, self examination, explanation of oneself, revelations of what one is' (Foucault 1978: 2).

For Foucault, psychiatry took its place in the legal machinery through the concept of 'homicidal mania' (a killing that took place in a domestic setting in the absence of any apparent motive) in the latter half of the eighteenth century. From this moment, crime and insanity became the same thing. He illustrates this type of crime/insanity with reference to notorious cases: a mother who kills her child; a man who breaks into a house kills an elderly woman and departs without stealing and fails to hide himself; a son who kills his mother with whom he has always got on well. Psychiatry justified its involvement in order to make the unintelligibility of this type of crime intelligible. By claiming that insanity manifested itself in crime and vice versa, forensic psychiatry adopted a different focus of interest from the rest of the profession.

Foucault links forensic psychiatry to a type of public hygiene where the focus is on the 'societal body' and social danger rather than the 'individual soul'. Homicidal mania represents insanity in its most harmful form – minimum warning, maximum consequences – which only a specialist eye can detect. According to Foucault, forensic psychiatry's claim to monomania did not include a desire to take over criminality and was not a form of psychiatric imperialism. Rather, it was a means of justifying its function, namely the control of danger emanating from the human condition.

Although Foucault was not concerned with providing an account of specific developments within the psychiatric profession, his account does hint at the possibility of divergent interests between forensic psychiatry and that of mainstream psychiatry. The differing interests of the two branches of the profession are illustrated by their involvement with psychopathy. Psychopathy is usually regarded as a condition which involves seriously irresponsible behaviour:

> The moral principles of the mind are strongly perverted or depraved; the power of self government is lost or greatly impaired and the individual is found to be incapable not of talking or reasoning upon any subject proposed to him, but of conducting himself with decency and propriety in the business of life.
>
> (Prichard 1835, quoted in Ramon 1986: 215)

The definition of psychopathy has not altered greatly since Prichard's medical description. The legal definition of psychopathy appears under the Mental Health Act 1983 as: 'A persistent disorder or disability of mind (whether or not including significant impairment of intelligence) which results in abnormally aggressive or seriously irresponsible conduct on the part of the person concerned.'

Whilst the British concept has changed little (most countries have abandoned it on the grounds that it is beyond definition (Bean 1986)), there has been a shift in the interest of the psychiatric profession.

Mainstream psychiatry shows evidence of wanting to reject psychopaths as patients worthy of their attention. In mainstream psychiatric discourse, psychopaths have come to be regarded as unresponsive to treatment, hence the inclusion under the Mental Health Act 1983 of a treatability clause. The procedures for admission under section 3 of the Mental Health Act (a six-month detention order for the purposes of treatment) includes a clause which states that if a patient is suffering from psychopathic disorder, treatment must be likely to 'alleviate or prevent a deterioration' of the person's condition. Recently, there has also been a marked downward trend in the numbers of in-patients receiving the diagnosis of psychopathic or personality disorder in mainstream psychiatric services. Yet, more than half the residents of special hospitals are still classified as suffering from psychopathic personality disorder (Ramon 1986). This suggests that whilst mainstream psychiatry is busy trying to minimize their management of what are seen as disruptive and undesirable patients, for forensic psychiatry it remains a large part of their 'bread and butter' work.

Why is psychiatry divided in this way about psychopathy? The answer may lie in the lack of responsiveness to treatment of this group of patients. However, this could well apply to other psychiatric diagnoses. For example, the limited success of treating 'schizophrenics' with major tranquillizers has not led to mainstream psychiatry wishing to diminish its contact with this group. A more plausible explanation is connected to changes in segregative control.

Ramon (1986) traces the change in the psychiatric stance towards psychopathy to developments in psychological approaches just after the Second World War. Then, soldier patients showing evidence of psychopathic disorder began to be treated in therapeutic communities. The move away from segregative control in mainstream psychiatry meant that the method to control antisocial behaviour (which is the *sui generis* of the condition) became less feasible. Forensic psychiatry in contrast still had the segregative means to effectively manage such deviance.

Indeed, it seems to be that the precondition of the psychiatric detention of this group is governed by the demands of security and public threat, rather than mental state. As patients who have committed offences, they are likely to be detained for a period at least commensurate with the gravity of their offences (Norris 1984; Peay 1989). This is true also for those who have committed minor offences. A recent American study, using a large random sample of misdemeanour defendants, found that those with a psychiatric history were 'criminally sanctioned more severely than defendants without psychiatric records, and defendants with relatively extensive psychiatric records were even more severely sanctioned' (Hochstedler-Steury 1991: 358).

The importance of the psychopath to forensic psychiatry (in both numerical and therapeutic terms) illustrates the two systems which it tries to bridge. By definition, the mentally disordered offender qualifies for entry into both the criminal justice and mental health systems. This raises particular dilemmas and questions which arise out of a merging of two types of deviance, criminality and mental disorder. Explicitly stated, should individuals be dealt with in the system designed to deal with the criminal aspects of their behaviour (i.e. in prison) or should they be treated for their mental disorder in hospital? This can been framed in terms of the psychiatrization versus criminalization of deviance.

The arguments for psychiatrization are made on the grounds that hospitalization of mentally disordered offenders is less stigmatizing and hospital treatment benefits patients more than do prisons. Prisons are unable to provide the environment or range of treatments that a health care regime can (Abramson 1972). A policy initiative stemming from this reasoning is the diversion of mentally disordered offenders from custody projects, which are also informed by the prevailing ethos of community care. Others (Monahan 1973; Fennell 1991) see psychiatrization as resting on dubious grounds. They point out that mental hospitals are not stigma free. Arguably, in Britain the association of the Special Hospitals with notorious serial killers and gangsters means that they are far more stigmatizing than prisons.

There are also doubts over whether medical treatment regimens are superior. As discussed above, those labelled as psychopathic make up a significant proportion of those in the Special Hospital system, yet there is little evidence to suggest there is an effective treatment for antisocial behaviour. There is evidence that the 'recidivism' rate is lower for those coming out of hospital, i.e. discharged forensic patients are less likely to reoffend than mentally disordered offenders discharged from prison (Fennell 1991). But this may be attributed to the conservative discharge policies of Special Hospitals, which are driven as much by 'security' considerations, as it is to changes in the mental state of patients. Psychopaths in Special Hospitals receive longer periods of detention, on average, than their counterparts in mainstream prison provision, as judged by equivalent index offences (Peay 1989).

There are two main arguments underlying a criminalization position. The first relates to a moral and philosophical argument, that both those who are designated mentally ill and those who are not should be treated as humanely as possible. That is, poor and 'brutalizing' conditions should not exist in either the prison or mental health systems (Monahan 1973). Reforming the prison system has also been argued for on pragmatic grounds. Fennell (1991) suggests that there will always be situations which do not permit the rapid transfer of mentally disordered offenders out of the prison system. Prisoners may not meet the legal criteria for transfer or transfer cannot be arranged quickly enough. Additionally, transfer may not always be the fairest option for prisoners. Sentences are often suspended for prisoners who spend time in Special Hospitals and recommenced if a person is transferred back to prison. (That is, there is no remission for the period that they have been treated as patients, and so their detention is extended beyond their sentence.)

Moreover, increased diversion into psychiatric facilitates is unrealistic, given the burden on existing facilities and the failure to rapidly develop more regional secure facilitates. Fennell argues for a proper legal framework for psychiatric treatment in prisons to be established as a means of improving the standard of care that is currently provided. One recent policy option which tries to bridge the gap between these two positions was proposed by the Tumin Report (Woolfe and Tumin 1990). This suggested that adequately staffed psychiatric intensive care wards in the NHS be provided inside prisons.

Compulsory and voluntary psychiatric admissions

The Mental Treatment Act 1930 first made provision for those wanting to enter hospital without certification. A voluntary patient could be admitted on making 'a written application to the person in charge' which was the medical superintendent in the instance of the public mental hospital. The trend towards voluntary admission was slow to establish itself. Immediately after the 1930 Act, 90 per cent of patients were still admitted compulsorily. By the 1980s about 92 per cent of in-patients were recorded on DHSS statistics as entering hospital on a voluntary basis (DHSS 1987). However, opinion is divided over whether the most recent mental health legislation improved matters for voluntary patients. Informal patients are considered hardly at all in the 1983 Act. Ramon (1983) has argued that, as a result, the individual rights of these patients have been neglected. On the other hand, Bean (1986) points out that certain rights were strengthened, such as the removal of the power to withhold a patient's mail and the right of informal patients to vote whilst in hospital.

A common view from the psychiatric profession is that the large number of informal admissions is an indicator that mental illness is now being treated like any other illness. However, others have pointed to the conditional nature of being a voluntary mental patient. Szasz has argued that whilst there is legislation authorizing compulsory detention there can be no genuine voluntary admission. The latter status is vulnerable to threats of invoking the former. Bean has used the term 'coactus voluit' ('at his will although coerced') (Bean 1986: 5) to describe voluntary admission. In his research into compulsory admissions to hospital Bean found that assessing psychiatrists sometimes gave patients a Hobson's choice. Patients were informed in a non-negotiable way of their impending admission or told that if they did not come into hospital voluntarily they would be compelled to do so (Bean 1980). A recent study also suggested that a substantial minority of patients who are admitted to hospital as voluntary patients regard themselves to be there under coercion (Rogers 1993a).

After admission, the voluntary status of the patient is always precarious. Under the Mental Treatment Act 1930, patients had to give 72 hours' notice in writing of the wish to leave, and those incapable or unwilling to receive treatment could be dealt with under section 5 (compulsory admission) as 'a person of unsound mind'. Similar clauses exist under the 1983 legislation. Section 5 of the Mental Health Act allows for an application for compulsory admission to be made for patients already in hospital on an informal basis. Estimates in the late 1980s suggested that over 8000 detentions per annum involved the subsequent detention of patients admitted voluntarily – approximately one-third of all recorded compulsory detentions (Barnes et al. 1990).

Sections 2 and 3 under Part II of the Mental Health Act 1983 are the main sections authorizing civil compulsory admission. Section 2 is a short-term admission order for the purposes of assessment. Section 3 is for a longer period and allows detention for the purposes of treatment for up to 6 months. Briefly put, the grounds for detention are that the person must be suffering from a mental disorder, and detention is warranted in the interest of the patient's health and safety and/or the safety of other people. This involves the notion of *parens patriae*, that is 'the State as father and protector of the people and the protection of others'. Although, in theory, there is a distinction between the patient's psychiatric condition and his or her need for protection, in practice the grounds for admission are reducible to one another. There is a tendency for a psychiatric condition to be defined as an urgent need for protection and vice versa (Bean 1985).

Legal aspects of compulsion

Variations on the legal theme of civil detention are traceable to cultural differences, to the balance of power over time of professional lobbies and to the resources available in particular societies at particular times. Let us now look at these sources of variation in relation to:

1 Compulsory admission to hospital.
2 Compulsory treatment.
3 Compulsory community control.

Compulsory admission to hospital

Mental health legislation provides the framework and sets out the conditions under which people can be detained, coerced, and given treatment against their will. Bean (1986: 3) views legislation as being concerned with two questions: 'How should patients and staff (that is medical and allied workers) be regulated in the manner in which patients make contact with psychiatric services; second, how should patients and staff be regulated in the manner in which psychiatric treatment is provided.' The way in which the questions are answered reflects both culturally accepted norms on the part of State and society about the limits of acceptable behaviour and the appropriate means used to deal with transgressions. The percentage of the population involved, and the mode of confinement or restriction varies over time and place.

Differences in contemporary compulsory admission/detention legislation also varies from country to country. This reflects a variable relationship between State, society and the use of mental health powers, as illustrated by the following examples.

Cross-national differences in mental health services

Italy

In Italy compulsory admission procedures are partly a civil matter, signified by the involvement of the mayor in compulsory admission proceedings. This may be linked to the Italian tradition of participatory involvement of people in civil, legal and health provision. Unlike in Britain, 'dangerousness' is not a ground for compulsory detention *per se*. Detention for non-offender patients can only take place on grounds of mental illness (Ramon 1988).

Commonwealth of Independent States (CIS)

The former Soviet Union had additional clauses to British legislation. It was not unusual for people to be detained on political grounds. Under a law passed in 1988, mental disorders which 'infringe the rules of the socialist community' were grounds for a compulsory assessment for admission to hospital by a psychiatrist. The inclusion of such a clause may be a legacy of the centralized collective and authoritarian nature of Soviet civil society (Cohen 1989).

Japan

Japan incarcerates many more patients on an involuntary basis than western countries; 80 per cent of in-patients are there under compulsion. This high rate of compulsion perhaps reflects the gravity with which transgressions of societal norms are held in Japanese society. The culturally prescribed codes of behaviour for each rank in society tends to play down individual differences. The behaviour of those experiencing psychological distress are likely to offend traditional values of self-control and modesty (Dingwall *et al.* 1991).

United States of America

Each state in the US passes its own mental health legislation covering mental health detention. This results in a diversity of commitment systems and the heterogenous application of therapeutic law. Overall, about three-quarters of admissions are voluntary and one-quarter compulsory. However, in Connecticut and Alaska, compulsory admissions outnumber voluntary admissions by 3 to 1 (Brakel *et al.* 1985).

As well as these international variations, there are signs of convergence occurring in relation to mental health law (Curran 1979). These include a change from the use of terminology such as 'insane' and 'lunatic' to 'mental illness', reflecting a worldwide trend towards medicalization.

Professional interests and legislation

The professional interests of mental health workers are discernible in recent legislation. This is signified by the clear demarcation of roles and responsibilities outlined in compulsory admission procedures. In England and Wales, the 1959 Act established the medical profession as the key party involved in making applications for compulsory admissions. This was based on the view that mental illnesses require medical treatment (see above). This principle remains unchanged in current mental health legislation. Thus, although another profession is involved (social workers) they participate in Freidson's (1970) terms as a 'subordinate' profession to the dominant medical profession.

Compulsory admission requires two medical recommendations, one of which must be made by a psychiatrist. The other medical practitioner is usually a general practitioner. The rationale for this is linked to the opinion that the different medical practitioners act as a check and balance on the other. General practitioners are assumed to be knowledgeable about the patient at a personal level whilst psychiatrists are supposed to have an expert knowledge of mental illness. In practice, professional power and status mean that the psychiatrist as the specialist acts as the key decision-maker. The general practitioner rubber-stamps the psychiatrist's conclusion rather than making an independent judgement (Bean 1986).

Social workers

Social workers perform a subsidiary and facilitative role. They are the personnel charged with bringing the patient to the attention of the psychiatrist and are thus subordinate to medicine. Bean (1986) views the social worker's role in compulsory detention as due to a historical accident. Certainly, as a predominantly female occupation, social work did not have access to the structures and territory that the male medical profession had when capturing jurisdiction over the control and management of mental disorder (Witz 1990). This is evident in the position that social workers have been ascribed in mental health legislation.

Intraprofessional, as well as interprofessional power and status are also implicated. 'Approved Social Workers' (ASWs) are expected to have 'expertise' in mental health, which their peers do not. They are charged with interviewing patients in 'a suitable manner' and seeking alternatives to admission wherever possible. These roles and responsibilities set ASWs apart from generic social workers. However, unlike the professional politics of nursing in relation to the 1983 Act described below, social workers did not seek or aspire to this enhanced status. It was imposed from outside. There were concerns over the competence and commitment of social workers to carry out their expected responsibilities from those informing and drawing up the new legislation. The reluctant imposition of external professionalization on social workers led to disputes between the social workers' trade union NALGO and their employing authorities. Extra payments were demanded for what were viewed as new responsibilities, and these demands were accompanied by a boycott of ASW training programmes. This response from social workers can be viewed as an example of 'proletarianization' (see Chapter 6). Social workers did not see their interests in competing with the knowledge and skills of other mental health professionals by increasing their own expertise in mental health, preferring instead to adopt an industrialization strategy (Oppenheimer 1975).

Psychiatric nurses

Psychiatric nursing, along with other branches of the profession, has, for the last decade, been engaged in strategies to move from being a semi-profession to a fully autonomous profession. This can be seen in attempts to develop a unique body of knowledge (e.g. nursing theory) and engaging in research. Recognition by the State of the responsibilities and authorization of certain duties is also a prerequisite for the professionalization of an occupation.

The 1983 Act gave psychiatric nurses 'holding powers' to detain voluntary patients who wish to leave hospital (section 5 (4)). During the six-hour period that registered nurses are authorized to prevent a person from leaving, a medical practitioner must consider whether a 'full' holding power should be used. According to Bean (1986) this new power was not really necessary. Existing medical powers and common law provides for the physical restraint of patients. The power granted to nurses thus represented a capitulation to demands for greater recognition of their role, in the context of one of the nursing unions resisting the acceptance of a patient from a special hospital: 'Threats of industrial action, even from members of one union, can seriously disrupt and place patients in a vulnerable position. The holding power under the 1983 Act was an obvious attempt to placate trade union demands' (Bean 1986: 51). Thus, nurses used trade union tactics to gain increased State recognition of their professional status and role. This presents something of a contradiction within the professional ideology of psychiatric nursing. On the one hand, claims to an original body of knowledge rests on nursing's unique skills of 'caring' (as opposed to the curative claims of medicine); on the other, increased professional power was sought via their coercive role in relation to psychiatric patients. The supervisory role of new legally-backed community control have also fallen to mental health nurses outside of a hospital context. This has provided nurses with greater voice and weight in mental health matters nationally but has had unforeseen negative consequences for nurse–patient relationships (Wells 1998).

Discharge from hospital

The conditions for the detention and release of patients are defined legally. The limits to legalism are illustrated by the effect that the availability of resources have on decision-making about patients' destinies. This is illustrated by two studies, one on the discharge of patients from hospital and the other on arrest by police officers under section 136 of the Mental Health Act.

The principal means by which patients are discharged from hospital is through the expiry of their detention orders or at the discretion of the Responsible Medical Officer. Another means of discharge is via Mental Health Review Tribunals (MHRTs). These independent bodies charged with hearing appeals by patients compulsorily detained in hospital, or subject to Guardianship Orders, were set up under the 1959 Act and strengthened under the 1983 Act. MHRTs have the power to order either immediate discharge, or delayed discharged (that is until suitable arrangements have been made for after care). Tribunal panels are drawn from three groups: (1) lawyers; (2) medical practitioners; and (3) lay people with experience of administration or social services.

The power of professionals determines the outcome of tribunals. Far from being independent bodies, they are unduly influenced by the views and recommendations of the Responsible Medical Officers. This conclusion was drawn in a study of decision-making about Special Hospital patients. Over and above professional power, material resources were also found to be influential. Legally, the determinants of whether a Tribunal hearing should discharge a patient centre on the patient's condition (and whether they show remorse in the case of those detained by the Home Secretary). In practice, the lack of appropriate resources and alternatives to Special Hospitals influence a tribunal's decision-making.

> Tribunals also found themselves constrained by their view that there was a lack of suitable alternative placements for patients . . . There were examples where no hostel could be found to accept a patient. But few tribunals were prepared to take the step, seemingly logically demanded by the legal criteria, that if a patient could not be discharged to a hostel place, he should be discharged regardless. Rather they took a step back in their reasoning and merely redefined the patient as not yet ready for discharge.
>
> (Peay 1989: 213)

Similar findings can be found in other studies, which suggest the importance of resources in areas which should be governed solely by prescribed legal criteria. For example, under section 136 of the Mental Health Act 1983, which authorizes police officers to make psychiatric referrals, apprehension in law should be on the basis of a judgement about a person's mental disorder, and the threat they pose to themselves and others. However, in practice, a police officer's discretion is often influenced by the availability of other alternatives, such as accommodation and informal means of support (Rogers 1990).

Compulsory treatment

The three sets of factors discussed above are also implicated in matters relating to Part IV of the Mental Health Act 1983, which sets out the rights of formal patients to refuse treatment. First, the principle that these patients have the right to refuse treatment in the same way as informal patients can be related to prevailing cultural norms, where voluntarism is viewed as desirable even within the limitations of a coercive relationship. This principle often clashes with the second group of factors – the professional norms – about the benefits of treatment and the assumed interests of patients.

Professional processes, in particular the dominance and maintenance of medical values, can be seen in both the conditional nature of consent and in the system of deciding whether a person should receive treatment without their consent. With regard to the former, medication (the most commonly prescribed psychiatric treatment) can be given without the patient's consent for three months before a patient can request a review. The confirmation of whether a patient should be given treatment against their will for ECT and medication is decided by a system of peer review. A member of the same profession judges the decision of their colleague, according to the norms, values and beliefs of their common profession. In the case of consent to psychiatric treatment, another medical practitioner (appointed by the Mental

Health Act Commission) decides whether the patient should receive the unwanted intervention. In this process, other mental health professionals play a subordinate role to the 'second opinion doctor'. They are consulted, but it is the medical practitioner alone who is charged with making the decision.

Thus, it is predominantly medical norms and values which determine whether or not a patient's wishes should be overturned. The notion of an 'independent' second opinion is restricted, in this case, to someone with the same training and socialization as the treating psychiatrist. Not surprisingly, there is a high degree of agreement between the Responsible Medical Officer wanting to impose the treatment and the second opinion doctor (MHAC Biennial Report 1991). Consequently, appeals for a second opinion are often unsatisfactory, as far as the patient's wishes are concerned.

The third group of factors – the range of resources available – may influence the number of patients who receive treatments on a forced basis. Early intervention and prevention may avoid the necessity of compulsory admission and treatment. Resources made available for after-care may prevent the need for re-admission as revolving-door patients. Similarly, the absence of resources may make people more vulnerable to admission and non-consented treatment. In Britain, few crisis intervention teams operate on the basis of providing emergency support in non-hospital settings. This type of service has been a central demand of the mental health service users' movement in providing alternatives to hospitalization (Rogers and Pilgrim 1991).

The need for after-care for patients who have been detained for some time (six months or longer under section 3) was recognized by the statutory duty to provide after-care, under the Mental Health Act 1983 (section 117). However, as successive Mental Health Act Commission (MHAC) reports have noted, the provision of support has been variable because new resources have not been made available or resources have not been diverted from existing hospital-centred interventions (MHAC 1987; 1989; 1991). Thus, the seemingly individual choice over the acceptance or rejection of treatment, and the attendant negotiations between doctors and patients involved in the 'consent to treatment' decisions, are influenced by wider considerations about the funding and prioritizing of mental health services.

Compulsory community control

The control of patients in the community raises questions of who should be controlled and when. Also, who should do the controlling and how much should be spent on this form of intervention? A further issue with which social scientists have been concerned is the nature of community control.

The notion of disciplinary power, the self-surveillance of bodies and 'souls' which has informed a Foucauldian approach to mental health, has been discussed in earlier chapters. The move from institutional to community care has been viewed in terms of new discourses on the mind and madness. Certainly this new community gaze is also evident in the definition and assessment of psychiatric illnesses. For example, recent rating scales used to assess whether patients have 'schizophrenia' are concerned with the way in which people behave in a domestic, not hospital, context (Rogers 1993b).

Undoubtedly, the demise of the asylum in Britain has led to a reduction in the scale of segregation overall. Although it is interesting to note that after the introduction of the Mental Health Act 1983 there was a 6 per cent increase in the number of compulsory admissions to hospital (DHSS 1987). This apparent contradiction is accounted for by the number of revolving-door admissions of the same group of patients. As has been seen, the provision of psychiatric treatment in small units in community settings is a reversal of the policy where emotional deviance was geographically and symbolically separated from the rest of the population in remote institutions. As a result of smaller units now operating, the *proportion* of their residents which are detained compulsorily has increased compared to the populations of the old asylums immediately prior to their run down. A shift towards community care and revolving-door admissions means that these small units are increasingly being used for coercive control and treatment. A manifest example of this is the return of locked wards on these units (euphemistically called 'Special Care' wards).

Despite the shift of psychiatric populations out of in-patient settings, 'repressive power' is still a concept which is applicable to the use of coercion in the community. Leaving aside the question of whether or not repressive power is effective in terms of its intended outcome, examples of it in the area of mental health can be found cross-nationally. These are justified on the same grounds as compulsory admission, i.e. the need to protect the patient's health and well-being and in the interests of other people.

The CIS provides an explicit example of the use of repressive power in the community. Psychiatric dispensaries are to be found in every small town. These are similar to the Community Mental Health Centres set up in the US in the 1960s. These dispensaries keep two types of 'registers' of psychiatric patients. One is for ordinary patients, the other for those whose behaviour is specifically aggressive. The explicit purpose of the registers is to check on patients living in the community. Dispensaries phone family, friends and workplace to monitor patients. Being on the register also means that a patient is not permitted to travel abroad or take up certain types of employment. They are obliged to accept treatment regularly from the dispensary. In 1987 there were 5.5 million people on this register, all of whom were liable to hospital detention. Conditions for a name being removed from the register are that a person remains symptom-free for a minimum of five years.

The measures just described appear Draconian and one could, until recently, have argued that they could be accounted for by the peculiarly authoritarian nature of the State in the Soviet Union. However, there is evidence of a degree of international convergence over the necessity to restrict the movement and freedom of patients living in the community. That is, different countries with seemingly different political, ideological and economic bases are following similar paths. The United States and Britain provide two examples of different coercive community control measures.

In the United States 'involuntary outpatient civil commitment' (IOC) is now widely accepted as a principle in mental health services. Although the use of such powers are still relatively rare, over the last 20 years most States have passed legislation that permits involuntary outpatient intervention on the basis of a need for treatment. Some patients have been placed on IOC indefinitely and the penalty for non-compliance has varied from no action to automatic re-admission, depending on the State involved (Maloy 1992).

In Britain, in 1987, the Royal College of Psychiatrists advocated the need for a 'Community Treatment Order' (CTO). This could have entailed the forced medication by injection with psychotropic drugs of people in their own homes. Advocates for the introduction of legislation permitting this forced treatment argued that a small number of patients were prone to 'relapse' and could not be relied on to take medication. This gave rise to a number of philosophical, ethical and practical difficulties. Who would administer the medication? Although psychiatrists would prescribe it, community psychiatric nurses were reluctant to take on the responsibility for administering drugs, which they viewed as potentially damaging to their relationship with patients. There were also problems related to who would receive compulsory treatment, given the limited effectiveness of major tranquillizers in treating certain patient groups (see Chapter 6), and the strong opposition to the idea on the part of patient advocacy groups (see Chapter 10). These and other problems about implementing CTOs are discussed at length by Bean and Mounser (1993).

Because of these problems, both the Mental Health Act Commission and the Government failed to endorse the bid for a CTO. Consequently, enabling legislation for compulsory treatment in the community was not passed by Parliament. Instead there was an endorsement of an extended use of guardianship for providing community control. Under the 1983 Act a guardian (appointed by the local authority) has three powers: s/he can (1) compel a person to live at a specified place; (2) require a patient to attend at designated times 'for medical treatment education or training' (but cannot compel patients to accept medication); and (3) gain access to the patient for medical practitioners, social workers or any other person specified by the guardian. Until recently, guardianship has been little used. Barnes *et al.* (1990) estimate that there are about 200 orders made each year. This may be linked to the less-developed community care policies of Britain compared with other countries. Hospital-oriented services make compulsory detention in hospital the first choice of control; there may be other reasons. Here, the Mental Health Act Commission has recently attributed the minimal use of guardianship to the lack of sanctions for 'non-compliance' and a legal loophole impeding the implementation of orders: 'The lack of powers to convey patients has widely been cited as the major constraint on the effectiveness of Guardianship and in one county the number of patients fell from 40 to 20 when staff learned that this power did not exist' (MHAC 1991: 50).

Despite these difficulties, official bodies, such as the MHAC, see the extension of the use of such powers as an essential component of future mental health care delivery. In addition to the powers enshrined in legislation, other measures which involve more subtle forms of control are also increasingly being used in relation to voluntary patients. These include the use of 'case registers' and 'case management', which involve close surveillance by key workers of the daily behaviour and activities of patients. There are those who see the control of patients in the community as an appropriate response to managing severe 'mental illness' – essentially liberating patients from the control imposed upon them by hospitalization. Others are more sceptical. There are fears that community control could lead to severe restrictions on patients' civil liberties, without any attendant improvements in service provision. In other words, such mechanisms could lead to a reduction in admissions and length of in-patient stays, but not actually improve the support for patients living in the community (Maloy 1992).

Although formal attempts by psychiatrists in Britain to negotiate powers of compulsory community treatment failed in the late 1980s, the issue was revisited by politicians in the mid-1990s when a series of embarrassing incidents occurred in public involving psychiatric patients. As a result, new legislation was introduced to ensure active follow-up in the community with powers to recall non-compliant patients to hospital (the Supervised Discharge Act 1995 modified the 1983 Act). This legal adaptation of the 1983 Act was reinforced by a raft of procedures including a register of 'at risk' patients and the Care Programme Approach. These administrative mechanisms were a governmental attempt to systematize risk management in the community. The impact of the British legislation still awaits the outcomes of formal evaluation research.

Huxley (1990), for example, describes case management as a system in which care is provided through individually planned combinations of different sources of support. In contrast, research which places the issue of coercion centre stage simultaneously places the issue of ethics high on the agenda. The term 'aggressive outreach' (used in the US) as opposed to the British notions of 'Care Programme Approach', 'care management' or 'assertive outreach' suggest tenacity and surveillance on the part of mental health professionals, which goes beyond paternalistic benevolence. In both types of research positive outcomes include measures of the extent of contact that people with mental health problems have with their worker and a reduction in hospital admission rates. However, the issue of control is more explicit when some terms are used compared to others. In 1998 the British government began a process of reviewing the 1983 Mental Health Act. At that time it made clear its intention to implement new powers of compulsory conveyancing to hospital to ensure treatment compliance.

Dangerousness

In Chapter 1 it was noted that there is a tendency for some lay people to equate mental disorder with violence. Legalism has attempted to separate considerations of the health and interests of the patient from the risk posed to society. In practice the two have become blurred. But is there actually a link between mental disorder and violence? And how accurate is the perception of the lay public (often reflected and reinforced in the media) of people diagnosed as mentally ill being violent? Also what is the link between mental disorder and self-harm?

Violence and mental disorder

Until recently research evidence has not given clear answers to the questions above. However, this research picture has now changed – although, as we note below, public and clinical attitudes to dangerousness may lag behind. Since the early 1990s findings from the US suggests that people experiencing active psychotic symptoms may have a slightly greater tendency towards violence than ordinary community populations. However, generally having been a psychiatric patient in the past apparently bears no relationship to a propensity for violence in the present. The very weak population correlation between psychiatric disorder and violence is accounted for by a subgroup of recurringly dangerous psychotic patients (discussed later) or by those with a diagnosis of psychopathy. The latter category is defined in a circular way in relation to aggressive or antisocial acts, as we noted in Chapter 1, so it is inevitable that psychopathic disorder (in the US called 'sociopathic disorder') is predictive of violence.

This point was made here by an American researcher who conceded a weak relationship between psychiatric diagnosis and violence:

> None of the data give any support to the sensationalized caricature of the mentally disordered served up by the media . . . Compared with the magnitude of risk associated with the combination of male gender, young age, and lower socioeconomic status for example, the risk of violence presented by mental disorder is modest. Compared with the magnitude of risk associated with alcoholism and other drug abuse, the risk associated with major mental disorders such as schizophrenia and affective disorder is modest indeed. Clearly, mental health status makes at best a trivial contribution to the overall level of violence in society.
>
> (Monahan 1992: 510)

The most recent research from the MacArthur Foundation's multimillion dollar investigation of this issue provides a strong empirical base on which to dispel previous assumptions and stereotypes. It also counters or supersedes findings of research based on poor construct validity and small samples. Commentary on the MacArthur research in the *Archives of General Psychiatry* by Link and Stueve (1998) note:

> Steadman and colleagues reassessed former psychiatric patients every 10 weeks for a year following hospital discharge. While they found a modest elevation in rates of violence shortly after hospitalisation, the elevation diminished rapidly and became indistinguishable from rates reported by residents in the communities to which patients were discharged. Second, Steadman *et al.* asked about the targets of violence and found that the vast majority (86%) of violent acts committed by former patients occurred within the context of family and friendship networks. Indeed members of the Pittsburgh public who were violent were slightly (but not significantly) more likely to target strangers (22%) than were Pittsburgh patients (11%).
>
> (Link and Stueve 1998: 1)

The study by Steadman *et al.* (1998) alluded to by Link and Stueve found that psychiatric patients who did not abuse drugs or alcohol had the same rates of violence as their (non-patient) neighbours. In sociological terms there is a strong boundary between the world of research and the public sphere. Despite indications from research that the link between violence and mental disorder has at best been tenuous, and research showing the ways in which images of mental illness and violence have become conflated in the mass media, clinical, political and public opinion remain stubbornly impervious to research findings such as those from Steadman *et al*.

An associated issue is the extent to which one can predict or assess the potential for violence amongst mentally disordered people. There are those that view it as impossible to assess the risk of prospective violent acts. Monahan (1981) summarized three sources of doubts about predicting violence amongst mental patients.

1 The empirical attack. This is a body of research evidence which suggests that accurate prediction is impossible: 'It now seems beyond dispute that mental health professionals have no expertise in predicting future dangerous behaviour either to self or others. In fact predictions of dangerous behaviour are wrong about 90 per cent of the time' (Ennis and Emery 1978: 28).
2 The political attack. From a libertarian position, Szasz has argued that prediction violates patients' civil rights:

> Drunken drivers are dangerous both to themselves and to others. They injure and kill many more people than, for example persons with paranoid delusions of persecution. Yet, people labelled 'paranoid' are readily committable, while drunken drivers are not ... Some types of dangerous behaviour are even rewarded. Racecar drivers, trapeze artists, and astronauts receive admiration and applause ... Thus, it is not dangerousness in general that is at issue here, but rather the manner in which one is dangerous.
>
> (Szasz 1963: 46)

3 Professional dissent. The third source of attack emanates from a minority professional lobby. Because predicting dangerousness is tied to social control, some professionals worry that it is incompatible with a caring and therapeutic role. They resent and resist becoming society's police officers for informal rule rather than law infringement.

Yet, it seems that, within limits, it is possible to predict violent behaviour, and this does not always work against the interests of the majority of psychiatric patients. Some have argued for standardizing the criteria for predicting the likelihood of violent behaviour, because of the *ad hoc* nature of clinical judgements. According to Monahan (1981: 67) clinical judgement in this area is: 'prone to several types of systematic error, including vagueness as to what is being predicted, lack of attention to base rates of violent behaviour, reliance upon erroneous predictor items, and a failure to take into account information regarding the environment in which the individual is to function'. Monahan argues instead for judgements made on statistical predictions (i.e. based on mathematical rules) of known variables associated with dangerousness, such as past history of violence, alcohol/opiate abuse, age, gender and IQ. He does, however, admit that even standardized predictions cannot be devoid of implications for people's civil liberties. However, in other respects it could improve the liberties for patients. More accurate prediction for a minority of patients would lead to a less restrictive regime for

Table 9.1 Mental health and dangerousness

	Sick				Well			
	Law breaker		*Law abiding*		*Law breaker*		*Law abiding*	
	Detained	*Free*	*Detained*	*Free*	*Detained*	*Free*	*Detained*	*Free*
Dangerous	1	2	3	4	5	6	7	8
Non-dangerous	9	10	11	12	13	14	15	16

Cell 1: Mentally disordered offenders.
Cell 2: Mentally disordered offenders prior to detection.
Cell 3: Civil compulsory admissions to psychiatric hospitals.
Cell 4: People who are HIV+ who indulge in unprotected sexual intercourse.
Cell 5: Convicted prisoners.
Cell 6: Drunken/speeding car drivers.
Cell 7: Prisoners of war.
Cell 8: Members of the SAS.
Cell 9: Petty criminal prisoners who are psychologically disturbed.
Cell 10: Petty criminals on probation.
Cell 11: Old people forcibly hospitalized under the 1948 National Assistance Act because they live in insanitary conditions.
Cell 12: People in the community who are depressed.
Cell 13: Prisoners guilty of 'white collar' crimes like fraud.
Cell 14: Unapprehended shop lifters.
Cell 15: Victims of child abuse who are taken into care.
Cell 16: The assumed societal norm.

the majority. It might also lead to the more rational targeting of secure facilitates for those legitimately predicted to have dangerous propensities.

One of the problems, at the moment, is that such a rational targeting runs against the current of a confused mixture of opinion on the part of lay people and professionals about the whole question of dangerousness and responsibility. In Chapter 1, we discussed how both of these groups of people make decisions about the 'disposal' of those committing violent acts, at the interface between psychiatry and the criminal justice system. They do so inconsistently and often in disagreement. As the lay people we discussed in Chapter 1 and many professionals focus on the relationship between mental disorder and dangerousness, albeit inconsistently, it is worth finishing our analysis of the topic here with a table of contingencies (Table 9.1).

These various examples demonstrate that psychiatric patients are only one of many groups that we might consider when thinking about degrees of dangerousness and socio-legal sanction. The question is whether or not psychiatric patients are offered the same rights as others in the table. For instance, currently in Britain people of known dangerousness (like those in cells 4 and 6) are morally condemned but not legally restrained. By contrast, many psychiatric patients who are no proven threat to others are compulsorily detained under the Mental Health Act.

The empirical critique has softened recently as those involved in long-term studies of mental disorder and violence discovered that *some* patients are predictably dangerous (Monahan and Steadman 1994). Whilst diagnosis of mental illness *per se* does not predict violence, rendering categories like 'schizophrenia' redundant for this purpose (see Steadman *et al.* (1998) discussed above), some specific symptoms are predictive. For example, aggressive command hallucinations (voices telling people to act in a hostile way) and delusions with hostile content *are* linked to violent action.

Suicide

The social control of psychiatric patients, both in hospital and community settings, is not limited to the question of violence to others. Mental health services are also concerned with reducing the incidence of self-harm and self-neglect. Rates of suicide amongst psychiatric patients are high for a number of reasons. Their labour market disadvantage places them in a demoralized and devalued position. Their primary disability may include profound feelings of anomie, aimlessness, worthlessness, low mood and low self-esteem, as well as angry feelings which can be trapped and turned inwards. The secondary disability created by psychiatric treatment may be both demoralizing (when coping with drug side-effects and stigma) and an opportunity to act suicidally (the option to self-poison with prescribed psychiatric drugs).

The differential way in which psychiatric patients are treated when violent or potentially violent is also true of self-harm. In Britain suicide is *not* illegal. Despite this, suicidal patients, when identified, are treated in a peculiar way – coercion is applied. The question of suicide in psychiatric populations is thus more contradictory in a legal sense than that of violence to others. The latter in any population, general or psychiatric, is judged to be both immoral and illegal. By contrast, suicide is not illegal and its moral status is contested. Another example of the differential rule application to psychiatric patients in relation to suicide is more subtle and implicit.

When psychiatric patients are suicidal, it is assumed that their intentions are governed singularly by their mental abnormality. However, suicides in non-psychiatric populations are evaluated in a range of ways, which might include a notion of a temporary imbalance of mind, but other motives can be ascribed as well. These include a notion of rational intelligibility, when for various reasons, it is obvious why a person has little or nothing to live for (e.g. severe pain or physical disability or traumatic loss of significant others). Similarly, for reasons noted above, psychiatric patients might for very good reason feel devalued and disabled. And yet, suicidal intent or action on their part tends only to be interpreted as irrational. Thus, whilst the *post hoc* attribution of mental abnormality may be applied to any person committing suicide, there is a greater tendency for this to occur with people who are already psychiatric patients.

Psychiatric diagnosis is a weak predictor of suicide. For example, those with a diagnosis of depression have 15 per cent lifetime risk of suicide and for those with a diagnosis of schizophrenia it is 10 per cent (Morgan 1994). This means that the overwhelming majority of those with a psychiatric diagnosis do *not* commit suicide, although more do so than in the general population. When specific personal and social factors are taken into account, rather than diagnosis, then predictive validity increases. These factors include: drug and alcohol abuse; single or separated status; male gender; low social class; unemployment; poverty; previous parasuicide; age (variable according to diagnosis); and recent violence (received or given) (Platt 1984; Jenkins *et al.* 1994).

When suicide is re-framed as a social, rather than individual, phenomenon then a range of public policy factors can be identified in relation to primary prevention. For example, in the US suicide rates are lower in States with tight gun control than those with lax control. An Australian study revealed that 85 per cent of gunshot deaths were linked to distress rather than criminal action (Dudley, Cantor and Demoore 1996). Suicide has increased with motor car use over the past 20 years (via carbon monoxide self-poisoning) but it decreased when North Sea (non-toxic) gas was introduced in Britain in the 1970s. Given that self-poisoning is a common means of suicide, then lax prescribing of psychiatric drugs by the medical profession increases suicide rates, as does the widespread availability of some over-the-counter drugs like paracetamol.

Impact on patients of their risky image

The legal and empirical debate about dangerousness and mental illness and how to assess risk does include considerations of moral and ethical issues. However, notwithstanding the importance of the latter, sociologically there is a much wider agenda than assessing the points at which it may be considered legitimate or illegitimate to use coercive control. The conflation of violence with mental illness and its expression in language, its importance as a cultural construct, and its impact on the everyday lives of people with psychiatric diagnoses are also worthy of our attention. There is evidence, for example, that psychiatric patients internalize the stigma of dangerousness in a way which comes to impact negatively on their self-image. This has been illustrated in a recent study of the meaning and management of neuroleptic medication in its recipients (Rogers *et al.* forthcoming). This is illustrated by this patient who was interviewed in the study who had no personal history of violent acts or intentions. He reports his reaction to having been told that he had a diagnosis of 'schizophrenia':

> ... the word frightened me to death because books I've read and programmes on telly like, when I heard the word like 'schizophrenic', the word 'schizophrenic' at that time meant to me, I'm not bloody safe. I'm not safe. I'm a dangerous person and that sort of thing, and I'm likely to, be talking nice and calm to someone and the next minute I'm going to be getting a knife or something like that to them you know and I said no, I'm not accepting this ... that word does frighten people, if you were to tell somebody that I was a schizophrenic oh my God you know the first thing they'd say you know is 'I think you'd better keep away from him'.

In the final chapter we explore the way in which media constructs impact on and reinforce 'stereotypes' about users of mental health services.

In this chapter we have been mainly concerned with the way in which psychiatric patients have been contained and confined within psychiatric facilities or in the community by the provisions of therapeutic law. The shift towards community settings have none the less brought to the fore the issue of the rights of psychiatric patients to be involved in the mainstream of society and to participate in the planning and delivery of the mental health services they receive. British legislation, most notably the NHS and Community Care Act 1990, has encouraged the direct participation of service users in the planning and management of care services. However, legislation which encourages and promotes the notion of consumerism in mental and community services does not, in itself, ensure change. The meaning and purpose of user involvement and how service users can best be represented and power shared cannot be legislated for but requires more fundamental changes to take place outside a strict legal framework (Bowl 1996). However, with the rise of the users' movement there has been growing attention placed on the need for a set of positive rights linked to the notion of citizenship. This perspective has stressed the need for equal opportunities about, and rights of access to, employment and housing for all psychiatric patients (Rooke-Matthews and Lindow 1997).

Discussion

Psychiatric patients are singled out and treated in a separate way by legislation. First, involuntary patients admitted to hospital under civil sections of mental health legislation have no one to act as their advocate to retain their freedom at the time of admission. They have only the right to argue for their freedom after their detention. Second, they can be singled out in terms of their potential rather than their actual behaviour. Thus, therapeutic law is used for purposes of preventive detention. Whereas criminals have a prescribed period of detention, mental patients do not, in the sense that legal powers allow their periods of detention to be renewed. Criminals lose their liberty as a consequence of a proven transgression of the law. Mental patients can lose their liberty even if there has been no such transgression – to offend public or family rules of decorum is all that is required. And even when a patient has committed an offence, they are not prescribed a defined period of detention if they are sent to a secure psychiatric facility.

Thus, Szasz is correct to point out that psychiatric patients are treated in a particularly discriminatory way in modern society. Moreover, some people who are not labelled as mentally disordered are manifestly dangerous (like those in cells 4 and 6 of Table 9.1 above) yet they suffer none of the infringements of liberty imposed on non-offending psychiatric patients. This discrimination against psychiatric patients is not implicit or covert, as is the case in so much of sexual and racial discrimination, but is explicit and legally legitimized.

Although British mental health legislation seemingly exists to protect the rights of patients, it actually helps facilitate this discrimination, rather than alleviating it, since it frequently fails to adequately protect or enhance patients' civil liberties or their quality of life. Instead, the law legitimizes 'the institutionalization of society's unfounded prejudice and fear regarding madness'. The latter phrase is used by Campbell and Heginbotham (1991) when arguing that there is little justification for maintaining a separate legislative framework for those considered to be mentally disordered. Rather, the law should provide for the protection of victims and control of perpetrators on the basis of those who are proved to be dangerous, whatever its assumed causes (i.e. independent of mental health status). Campbell and Heginbotham argue that the only legislation that might be warranted on the basis of psychiatric history is anti-discriminatory legislation, similar to equal opportunities legislation. Such legislation might attempt to reverse the discrimination which has led to an inequitable access to social and material resources, for people who have received a diagnosis of mental illness.

Having reviewed the interplay between legal and medical control, it seems that their conceptual separation, and assumed antagonism, does not always translate neatly into practice. Currently, the two feed off one another or form complementary contributions to the constraint of mental abnormality. In Britain, for instance, both lawyers and doctors sit on Mental Health Review Tribunals. The Mental Health Act Commission, which arose out of legislation (the 1983 Act), contains both doctors and lawyers. Moreover, although the Commission is a manifestation of legalism, it enshrines the collegial loyalties enjoyed by doctors. For instance, it appoints and pays second opinion doctors to review the appropriateness of the treatment of detained patients at the hands of other doctors. Disagreements with the 'treating psychiatrist' are uncommon. Thus, arguably, in the field of mental health, lawyers and psychiatrists are bedfellows, not adversaries.

A wider approach to understanding mental health care and coercion from within the social sciences and health services research is likely to add to analysis provided from within the existing legal framework. A greater focus on social and contextual aspects of violence and mental health suggests a response at a different level (for example, a public health agenda about mental health). Additionally, the adoption of a patient-centred approach to the framing of questions of care and control in coercion research is likely to balance the dominance of disciplinary approaches from within psychiatry and the law. The social construction of violence and mental illness at a socio-political level, the wider role played by services and professionals and the risks faced by patients living in the community should arguably be at the centre, rather than at the periphery, of research and analysis on coercion.

In conclusion

Legalism has played an important role in the field of mental health. It has set certain limits on medical power and discretion. It has also codified two separate social processes which are at odds with one another: the rights of patients to exercise choice; and the rights of professionals to impose their actions against the wishes of patients. Psychiatric patients have also had special legal provision when they commit criminal offences. The legal rules applied to them have been different to those of other offenders, highlighting the special (arguably discriminatory) way in which people with mental health problems are treated. This special treatment also applies to self-injurious behaviour. Although suicide itself is not illegal, suicidal intent detected in people with mental health problems can trigger peculiar forms of lawful control.

Questions

1 Should dangerous psychiatric patients be treated differently to other dangerous people?

2 Discuss the evidence about mental health status and dangerousness.

3 What contradictions exist in mental health law?

4 In which respects did mental health law in Britain change during the twentieth century?

5 Can consumerism operate whilst we have coercive mental health law?

6 Should mental health legislation be abandoned?

For discussion

Consider the different ways in which psychiatric patients might be denied informed consent and examine legal options to improve their lot in this regard.

Further reading

Aldridge, D. (1997) *Suicide: The Tragedy of Hopelessness*. London: Jessica Kingsley.

Bean, P. (1986) *Mental Disorder and Legal Control*. Cambridge: Cambridge University Press.

Monahan, J. and Steadman, H.J. (eds) (1994) *Violence and Mental Disorder*. Chicago: Chicago University Press.

Sjostrom, S. (1997) *Party or Patient?: Discursive Practices Relating to Coercion in Psychiatric and Legal Settings*. Borea: Spinettstraket.

Chapter 10

Users of mental health services

Chapter overview

This chapter will explore the different ways in which those who use mental health services can be understood sociologically. These are not merely different perspectives. They reflect the changing role of psychiatric patients in mental health services. A shift over a 30-year period in which they started only as patients but latterly have become providers of mental health services themselves highlights this point. The following topics will be discussed:

- The diffuse concept of service use

- The relatives of psychiatric patients

- The user as patient

- The user as consumer

- The user as survivor

- The user as provider

- The mass media and psychiatric patients

The diffuse concept of service use

In the British context, the term 'user' of mental health services has generally been common in recent years. The term is eschewed in the US because of its narrow connotation of drug misuse. There, patient groups tend to prefer the term 'patient' or 'survivor'. These discourses will be examined later in this chapter but for now we are simply noting a semantic caution. There is a second problem, not related to terminology, about the concept of service use. Psychiatric services provide, amongst other things, one form of social control in society (see Chapters 8 and 9). As a consequence, social groups other than designated patients benefit from the existence of mental health services. Moreover, some of these groups have regular service contact. The legal framework in Britain recognizes this. The Mental Health Act 1983 (which at the time of writing is about to be reviewed and probably revised) is split into two broad parts – one about civil sections and the other about mentally disordered offenders. This separation implies, and at times spells out, that mental health services will interface with, or be accessed by, a range of statutory and civil groups of wider society: the criminal justice system, social services, the immigration service, primary health care and relatives of people entering the psychiatric patient role. These legal administrative arrangements indicate that groups within this list are in regular contact with, and effectively constitute users of, mental health services. Some of these relationships have been discussed in earlier chapters. Here we will focus on the relatives of psychiatric patients before considering patients themselves in the next section.

The relatives of psychiatric patients

Whether or not psychiatric patients enter the role voluntarily or involuntarily, it is not unusual for their relatives (or 'significant others') to be interested parties about service contact. Not only might they be involved in formal decision-making about hospital admission, they might have previously been involved in engendering, coping with, and eventually informally labelling the incipient patient's mental abnormality. Also, once the patient role is then formally established by diagnostic and treatment action from professionals, relatives may have service contact as visitors. Sometimes they act as advocates for patients (demanding improved services). Sometimes they might express concern that services are not being coercive enough in ensuring treatment compliance or in prematurely discharging patients. Within some treatment rationales relatives are framed by professionals as implicit or adjunct service clients in order to engender change in the patient or minimize the chances of relapse in their condition. Because of wide-ranging powers of professional discretion within services, this imputed role is variegated and relatives may not always be informed of the assumptions operating about them in a particular service setting. A number of examples of this point can be given.

- *Family role in aetiology* In the controversial model of 'schizophrenia' being intelligible within mystifying and dysfunctional family communication patterns, some professionals sought to engage with relatives to render the patient's behaviour and experience intelligible or to trace causal anteced-ents (Lidz, Laing and his colleagues, Bowen and Jackson). A critical review of this strand of therapeutic work is provided by Howells and Guirguis (1985).
- *Family role in relapse* A less controversial model relates to relapse. Here, professionals do not necessarily question either the validity of psychiatric diagnosis or the role of genetic factors in causality. Instead they argue that relatives who are intrusive and emotionally labile (high on 'expressed emo-tion') place stress upon mentally ill people which increases the probability of relapse in those diagnosed as depressed or schizophrenic. Within this model, relatives may be contacted in a process of 'psycho-education' in order to reduce levels of 'expressed emotion' during their contact with the identified patient. This work is summarized by Jenkins and Karno (1992). It has been critiqued by Johnstone (1993).
- *Relatives as risk assessors* A paradoxical effect of the above two therapeutic approaches is that they may have changed professional norms about the credibility and involvement of family members. However, involving fam-ilies by asking their views about risk in their relative-patient increases the accuracy of risk assessment and efficiency of risk management (Klassen and O'Connor 1987).
- *Relatives as perpetrators and victims of abuse* Leaving aside the particular controversy noted above about family aetiology in 'schizophrenia', the families of people with a psychiatric diagnosis, may be sites of victimiza-tion. In Chapter 5 we discussed the raised levels of diagnosis in survivors of childhood sexual abuse. The 'schizophrenia' literature may be contested about causal antecedents, but the long-term post-traumatic effects of child-hood abuse are clear. In the other direction, some relatives may at times become the victims of violence at the hands of children who are psychi-atric patients (Estroff and Zimmer 1994).

Over and above these variable professional assumptions operating about the antecedent and current role of relatives for psychiatric patients, family mem-bers have also become an important self-organizing lobby. In Britain, groups such as SANE (Schizophrenia A National Emergency) Concern (see Chapter 2) and the National Schizophrenia Fellowship are dominated by relatives, as is the National Alliance for the Mentally Ill in the US (Manthorpe 1994). These groups focus on lobbying politicians and professional organizations nationally and locally. Sometimes they also set up direct support services in localities. The lobbying power of relative-dominated groups has been evident in recent years in Britain. It has been commonplace for the NSF and SANE to seek and gain more publicity about mental health issues like community care and violence and mental disorder than patient lobby groups like MIND.

The current mental health service managerial discourse in Britain often entails a recurring amalgam phrase of 'users and carers'. Up to now we have deliberately avoided the notion of 'carer' in this section for a number of reasons. First, relatives may or may not subjectively care for their patient relative; the notion of 'care-as-emotion' cannot be taken for granted in a family relationship. Second, they may or may not offer practical care – shelter, tangible support and domestic tending. Third, patients themselves may, when not in hospital, be the carer of their non-mentally ill relatives (e.g. their children and elderly parents). Fourth, sometimes those offering a caring role to someone who is mentally distressed are not family members.

For these reasons, caution needs to be exercised, purely on logical grounds, about conflating the term 'carer' and 'relative'. Despite our caution, there is a growing literature which uses the term 'carer' simplistically to mean family relative. For example, there is the review book of *Family Caregiving in Mental Illness* (Lefley 1996). The extensive literature it contains depicts relatives as victims of care burden created by (genetically caused) mental illness. Another conceptual problem with this 'burden' focused literature is the tendency to see mental illness as creating similar political demands for relatives and patients alike. As a consequence, the self-advocacy movements (NB plural) of patients and their relatives are not properly separated for academic analysis and are assumed to arise for similar reasons and to have the same interests (for example, see Watkins and Callicutt 1997). We return to this point in the next section.

Elsewhere (Rogers and Pilgrim 1996) we have argued that social scientists should avoid stereotypical assumptions about the role of family members. Sociologically we can see two dominant currents of professional discourse – one which tends to blame relatives for their aetiological role and the other which tends to sympathize with the martyrdom created by 'care burden'. It may be that relatives can be both victims of circumstance when, for example, struggling to cope with a disruptive and distressing son or daughter, and a causal source of distress when, for example, they abused an incipient patient in childhood. A whole range of other contingent styles of relating can exist between prospective and current patients and their relatives.

The stress of living with people who have severe mental health problems can itself lead to distress in relatives. For this reason, it is not unusual for relatives to seek professional help for their own emotional difficulties and thus become patients themselves (Perring *et al.* 1990). It is little surprising that relatives, when asked, will express the need for services to support them as well as the primary identified patient (Goldberg *et al.* 1993).

Having discussed the wider notion of service use and looked at patients' relatives, we will now discuss the specific question of what services might describe as the 'identified patients' – people who formally enter the sick role voluntarily or against their will. We will examine the different ways in which the psychiatric patient's voice has been portrayed or conceptualized. We concentrate on four views of mental health service users, which reflect different discourses and interests:

1 The user as patient.
2 The user as consumer.
3 The user as survivor.
4 The user as provider.

The user as patient

The main way in which users of psychiatric services have been portrayed is as objects of the clinical gaze of mental health professionals. This is clearly seen in the academic literature which forms the basis of most psychiatric and psychological knowledge. Clinical research in the area of mental health has tended either to exclude the views of patients or to portray them as the passive objects of study. Their individual characteristics and feelings are mostly variables to be 'controlled out' in order to ensure valid results. For example, if one looks at the Medical Research Council's (1989) priorities for the funding of schizophrenia research, the emphasis is on promoting genetic and biological studies. Evaluation of services to patients is number eight out of the ten priorities, and user evaluation of services and treatment is not mentioned at all. Explicitly or implicitly, 'mental patients' are portrayed in a way which emphasizes their pathology. A review of the literature provides a number of interesting examples of this claim. Here we mention four forms in which patients are denied a valid viewpoint.

1 The disregarding by researchers of those users' views that do not coincide with the views of mental health professionals

In an early attempt at providing a genuine user perspective, Mills (1962) found some interesting results. The study, which mainly used the accounts of patients and their relatives, found that users of services preferred contact with non-professionals to contact with social and health services personnel. When the latter were 'from a different social class [they] were often received with hostility'. The greatest forms of support were regarded as coming from people such as the local publican, the secretary of the local darts club and homehelps, who were seen to provide 'down to earth common sense'. However, a reviewer of this work appeared to dismiss this errant view of services on the grounds that it could not be cross-validated.

> It is hard to believe that there were no sympathetic and sensible social workers in the area . . . The material is taken very largely from patients and their relatives and no attempt at validation appears to have been made. Since some of the patients were suffering from paranoia, and others from depression, it would have been a basic precaution to check the objective value of statements with the medical records or the responsible psychiatrist.
>
> (Jones 1962: 343)

This criticism insists that patients' views are to be treated with inevitable suspicion and that a professional view inevitably carries a greater claim to validity or truth.

2 The notion that psychiatric patients are continually irrational and so incapable of giving a valid view

Discussions around informed consent, which are relevant to the administration of treatments and participation in research programmes, also tend to invalidate the views of users. 'Schizophrenics' are a particular group thought inherently incapable of giving genuine informed consent. This is not infrequently linked to the high rate of 'non-compliance' to prescribed medication: 'Since the majority of clients with schizophrenia deny their illness, special difficulties are encountered in the criteria for understanding the nature of the psychiatric condition . . . Denial is a major psychopathological mechanism which can impair appreciation . . .' (Davidhazar and Wehlage 1984: 385).

Why those labelled as schizophrenic should 'deny' their 'illness' is left unexplored. There is an assumption that this is due to a lack of 'insight'. That is, patients fail to agree with the opinion of their treating psychiatrist, which in itself is viewed as a symptom of mental illness (see Chapter 7). In the example given, the diagnostic label of schizophrenia is taken as a neutral one, that can only be of benefit to patients.

Assumptions about the inability of patients to hold valid opinions are held by therapists of all kinds. This is summarized in a literature review of consumer satisfaction with mental health treatment by Lebow (1982: 254), who notes that therapists often suggest that the consumer cannot adequately judge the treatments they are given:

> Distortion is seen as inherent in consumer evaluation because of the client's intensity of involvement in treatment and impaired mental status, and the client is viewed as lacking the requisite experience to assess treatment adequately. Consumer satisfaction is regarded as principally determined by transference projections, cognitive dissonance, unconscious processes, folie a deux, client character, and a naïvety about treatment, rather than an informed decision process reflecting the adequacy of treatment.

So the second form of patient invalidation to be found in the literature emphasizes the inevitable inadequacy of views which are expressed by people who are mentally ill.

3 Patients and relatives are assumed to share the same perspective, and where they do not, the views of the former are disregarded by researchers

Another tendency in clinical work, that superficially gives credence to the consumer voice, is the conflation of the patient's view with that of their relatives. This is evident in a study which set out to examine the impact of the Mental Health Act 1959 (Hoenig and Hamilton 1969). The authors of the study conclude that: 'On the whole, [therefore] the general picture given here is of a large degree of satisfaction on the part of patients and their relatives' (Hoenig and Hamilton 1969: 130).

However, if one scrutinizes their results in detail, there are some important discrepancies found between relatives' and patients' views. Whereas 84 per cent of the relatives' group were favourably disposed to the admission of the patient, only 47 per cent of the patients were content to be admitted, with 43 per cent being reluctant. Yet, the implication of these findings, which seem to suggest on close reading that the interests of these two groups may at times be divergent, was not noted by the researchers. Moreover, disquieting results were glossed over and excused by referring to patient pathology. For instance, complaints made by patients about services were dismissed thus: 'Their complaints referred to rough handling by nursing staff. It must be remembered that they were rather sick patients, and it was also not within our brief to verify individual complaints' (Hoenig and Hamilton 1969: 126).

4 Framing patient views in terms which suit professionals

Often, lay conceptions of mental health problems are researched in such a way that there is little room for people to express their own view about the subject in hand. One example, from a psychologist's perspective (Furnham 1984) involved a research design aimed at examining lay people's conceptions of 'neuroticism'. Leaving aside the problem of representativeness (the experimental group was 'a fairly homogeneous young, well-educated sample'), such questionnaires leave little room for self-expression, since all the items are predetermined as standardized items by the researcher, with no open-ended questions.

Even where credence is given to the freely expressed views of patients, there is a tendency on the part of some researchers, who are also mental health practitioners, to adopt a 'victim blaming' approach. This approach tends to leave practitioners' own role and that of their service unquestioned. One example of this is a study which found that clients attending a psychiatric day unit found it stigmatizing (Teasdale 1987). Patients preferred to 'hide' the reasons for attendance, because a label of 'mental illness' was experienced to be unhelpful. The analysis focused on the need for clients to be helped, 'to arrive at unambiguous personal interpretations and management of the stigmatising reaction of the local community' (Teasdale 1987: 345). It is suggested that this might be achieved 'if they [the patients] are supported in their attempts to understand and manage the resulting stigma, then the social and therapeutic effectiveness of the service should increase'. The professional's signal's role in alleviating stigma was outlined as the 'need to encourage clients to be open about their fears, and to help them demystify the idea of psychiatric care'.

Another example is that of a study reported in the *British Medical Journal* (McIntyre *et al.* 1989), the aim of which was to obtain the views of psychiatric in-patients. The most important finding of the study appeared to be that the 'thing psychiatric in-patients value most about being in hospital is their ability to leave'. The use of drugs was not rated highly and 'talking' to a care giver was seen as the most valuable aspect of being an in-patient. The authors conclude that 'talking therapy' should be given a higher priority in psychiatric training. However, the authors did not take the customer's view about leaving hospital to its logical conclusion. If they had, they would have had to question the value, in principle, of becoming an in-patient in a District General Hospital psychiatric unit.

The user as consumer

An alternative way of conceptualizing psychiatric patients is not as the objects of clinical interventions but as consumers of services. The term 'consumerism' implies the existence of choice between products, and an active insistence on value for money. Consumerism is a relatively new ideology, which has informed health policy-making in Britain since the beginning of the 1980s. It is linked to the introduction of general management principles in the NHS, which has tended to modify the clinical view of services. The administration of the health services by consensus decision-making amongst different clinical groups was replaced by the concentration of responsibility for services and management in the general manager. Part of this trend towards general management has involved what Offe (1984) has referred to as the 'commodification' of welfare services. This has introduced the logic of the wider economic system into the health service. An example of this is the tendering-out of health service catering and laundry services. Another example can be seen in the previous Conservative government's attempt to introduce an internal market for services by creating 'purchasers' and 'providers' of services under the NHS and Community Care Act 1990.

One of the effects of this philosophy has been a growing acknowledgement of the importance of consumer satisfaction. The Griffith's Report (Community Care: Agenda for Action (1988)), for example, emphasized the importance of the health service being accountable to the patient. The importance of consumer choice has also been stressed in recent government consultative documents on primary care. Thus, there is now a clear acceptance within health policy circles that more credence and authority should be given to a user perspective. Attention given to psychiatric views and levels of satisfaction with services has, until recently, tended to lag behind other client groups using health service facilities. This may be a result of the assumption that the accounts of psychiatric patients lack credibility (see Chapter 7).

There are a number of difficulties associated with viewing patients as consumers. Although general management has encouraged in the NHS a market-influenced system permitting consumer choice, the extent to which the health service has actually achieved this has been restricted by the 'clinical autonomy' exercised by the medical profession in treating patients. Britten (1991) showed that consultants who adhered to a biomedical rather than psychosocial model of illness were less likely to agree with a proposed policy of patient access to their own records. Professionals sometimes claim that patients do not wish to know that they are ill.

There are also doubts about whether users of health services are currently in a position to make informed choices. Customers of health care do not have the same access to clinical knowledge as health care professionals, who have many years of training and experience on which to base their choices. Informed consent, in which the benefits and negative effects of treatment are made available to patients, has only recently been acknowledged as an area which needs attention. As we noted in Chapter 7, patients do not have access to information about their treatment whereas professionals do. In particular, there is the bias set up by professionals selectively withholding information which might alarm or demoralize the patient.

Market forces		Professional power
−	+	
Psychiatric patient	Private patient	+
Acute medical/surgical NHS patient	Complementary medicine user	−

Figure 10.1   Typology of health consumers.

There are also objections to the notion of consumer being used specifically in relation to psychiatric patients. 'Consumer' tends to denote a positive choice from a range of alternatives. As one user representative put it:

> Consumer tends to be rejected because of its connotations with Tory consumerism but also because consumer implies you are getting something of value. The majority of people in the users' movement do not feel that they have consumed anything of value and many say quite clearly that the real consumers of mental health services are relatives, the police and the state.
>
> (cited in Rogers and Pilgrim 1991: 136)

Clearly, then, being a 'consumer' of health services is a complex affair. In order to understand the health care consumer's position, and in particular that of the psychiatric patient, we also require an analysis in terms of their relationship to market forces on the one hand, and professional power on the other. Figure 10.1 provides a way of conceptualizing these variables, putting psychiatric patients in a context of other medical service users. It can be seen that there are some areas of health care to which the term 'consumer' seems more applicable than others.

Complementary medicine (bottom right) provides a service predominantly in the private sector where market forces operate most freely. (There is little provision for alternative medicine within the NHS.) This allows for free competition between individual practitioners who compete for patients. Prices charged for therapies take place in a competitive environment. The necessity for social control on the part of professionals is also minimized. The typical person who chooses alternative medicine is middle class, articulate, and consults for non-life-threatening illness, under a voluntary contract which involves regular but limited service contact. Here the term 'consumer' seems to be highly appropriate.

The private patient using conventional medicine (top right) can choose health care according to the range of private hospitals available. However, professional control is greater than in the case of the complementary medicine user. General practitioners control access to specialist medical services, so the patient is not totally free of professional constraints. Moreover, in terms of professional power, in the private sector the internal constraints (such as complaints procedures and health authority policies) which govern clinical practice in the NHS are absent. Here the term 'consumer' is plausible, but the power of professionals to impede or dictate consumer choice renders it problematic.

Professional power is still influential in relation to NHS acute patients. However, this is arguably not as strong as in the private sector given the constraints placed on professional dominance through policy-making and fiscal arrangements determined by the State. For example, as well as the gate-keeping function of GPs, the NHS acute medical patients' free choice is constrained by the rationing of health services made available by health authority funds (see Figure 10.1, bottom left). If demand outstrips supply (clinical resources of manpower and technology), access to public health care is usually rationed according to the notion of a waiting list. In other instances, such as kidney dialysis, other selection criteria may also apply. In the case of fertility treatment for example, sexual orientation, marital status, socio-economic status, and number of existing children are factors which may be taken into consideration in permitting the uptake of services. Thus, the term 'consumer' becomes more dubious in this group of service recipients, given limited resources and mechanisms to filter out 'unworthy' cases.

Users of psychiatric services (top left) experience professional power even more acutely, whilst being denied the freedom to choose their therapist or service (compare this with the consumer of alternative medicine). Psychiatric patients can be forced into the sick role by means of compulsory admission. Even though this relates to only a small minority of patients, the fact that a person may be forced to enter hospital or receive treatment makes any notion of free positive choice tenuous (see Chapter 9). Being excluded from employment in the main, psychiatric patients are also a group with very little 'buying power' and so they penetrate little into either of the boxes on the right of the figure. By the time we reach the top left box, the term 'consumer' hardly appears to be apposite at all.

In measuring satisfaction in the area of mental health, there appear to be a number of other differences between patients who use services for acute physical problems and those who receive psychiatric services:

1 Contact with services for those with mental health problems is far more extensive than for most others who use the health and social services. (Although they have this in common with some groups of physically disabled people.) Those who enter hospital for acute physical problems, such as appendicitis, are patients for a short time only, whether or not they experience their hospitalization as positive or negative. Thus, the quality of service and treatment does not have as many long-term consequences as for those who are psychiatric patients. The latter often spend many years of their lives in contact with the services and professionals.

2 The consequences of being labelled 'ill' are often greater for a person who is given a psychiatric diagnosis. For the majority of those with physical problems, the diagnosis itself is often only temporary and is often not stigmatizing. Since the diagnosis of a person as 'mentally ill' is done primarily on the basis of a judgement about a person's conduct, there is always a risk of invalidating their whole identity or sense of self. Again, certain physical disabilities (such as epilepsy) may carry with them stigma, and so the mental patient is not unique.

3 There are social and economic consequences of contact with psychiatric services which apply much less often when acute medical services are used. Those labelled as mentally ill are discriminated against by present

and prospective employers and, as a result, are often subjected to a life of poverty. Educational opportunities are curtailed, family and intimate relationships affected and making social contact with people is fraught with difficulties. Again, some of these impediments to citizenship often apply to people with long-term physical disabilities.

Despite these differences between psychiatric and acute medical patients, let us look briefly at the literature which has included mental health service users within a discourse of being 'consumers' or 'clients', particularly in relation to 'quality assurance'.

Literature on psychiatric patient satisfaction and dissatisfaction

The emerging body of satisfaction research about mental health services has commonly adopted a needs assessment approach. This has usually assessed patient satisfaction according to 'normative need'; that is need defined by an acknowledged expert (Bradshaw 1972; Prior 1989) and typically ascertained by means of standardized assessment tools. These approaches have been linked to the emphasis on 'quality assurance', which is a type of evaluation research which is concerned with patient satisfaction. According to the WHO (1979), the aim of quality assurance is: '. . . to assure that each patient receives such a mix of diagnostic and therapeutic health services as is most likely to produce the optimal achievable health care outcome for that patient.' This form of evaluation of 'client need' focuses on the narrow measurement of the behaviour of the mental health client. Unlike the view of patients defined by psychopathology, this approach treats people as complete individuals in the sense that understanding is based on the everyday actions and language of individuals. However, this approach is still defined professionally, as this account of the observations of one quality assurance programme suggests:

> Once out of the client's hearing, however, the results of these interactions are often reanalysed in terms of a specific (and professionalised) linguistic framework. Thus, a game of ten-pin bowling is reanalysed in terms of 'motor skills'. A discussion about food is reanalysed in terms of coping skills. A lapse of memory is discussed in terms of a syndrome and a leisure time activity is analysed in terms of affective disorder. In fact client 'problems' are in many respects newly created through the application of behaviourist discourse to what are called 'activities of daily living'.
> (Prior 1991: 141–2)

In addition to this behaviourist approach, there is a small amount of research conducted from within statutory services which does not presume that mental health services are only there to do people good. Rather than 'normative need' this research has focused on 'felt need' (Bradshaw 1972). An early example of this was Mayer and Timms' (1970) work in which social workers were encouraged to take seriously the views expressed by clients. The work of Beresford and Croft (1986) also highlights the views of users of social services and emphasizes the need for genuine participation by users in research about services.

Whilst professionally defined needs tend to focus on behaviour and the effectiveness of prescribed treatments, the 'felt need' evaluations tend to emphasize the material and social aspects of people's everyday lives. Kay and Legg (1986) found that the need to have a job was a high priority for those recently discharged from hospital. An example is a survey which examined the expressed needs of patients *vis-à-vis* their living arrangements and material and social support (Hatfield *et al.* 1992). A sizeable minority of patients expressed dissatisfaction with their living arrangements. Those living in staffed accommodation were particularly critical and did not view their living situations as a result of their own positive choice. The survey also identified a 'substantial level of felt need for work'.

A more recent survey of discharged patients revealed a number of aspects about their quality of life in the community. These included their sense of vulnerability, the benefits of community care, an appreciation of the support of others, an awareness of the impact of scarce resources and disappointment about poor co-ordination between health and social services (MacDonald and Sheldon 1997).

Two other examples are illustrative of an acceptance of the users' perspective as it is actually expressed. The Community Psychiatric Nurses Association (1988) produced a booklet in which verbatim quotes on a range of issues affecting their lives were recorded from patients discharged from hospital. These included stigma, finances, 'what's needed in hospital', living alone and moving out of hospital, attitudes towards services, treatments and accommodation and ways of coping. Similarly, a publication produced by Islington Mental Health Forum examined a group of users' views regarding the effects of diagnosis and medication and suggestions about alternatives. Both of these publications, based on gathering information from local groups of patients, are a marked departure from the dominant way in which psychiatric patients' views are depicted.

The user as survivor

There has been some analysis of the users' views of services from those who do not work directly with people in service settings either as clinicians or as managers. The position of psychiatric users in a wider social context is the object of these analyses. Two perspectives can be identified in this regard. The first has adopted a phenomenological approach to understanding the social position of the mental patient. The second has tried to analyse the structural position of users as a social group within wider society. In particular there is an interest in users campaigning collectively as a 'new social movement'.

The phenomenology of surviving the psychiatric system

An example of the expansion of the felt need approach to users described above is provided by a phenomenological study. This is concerned with understanding the subjective meaning that people give to their experience of the social world. An example of this is the work of Barham and Hayward (1991), who made use of personal accounts of mental patients to explore their experiences of trying to live outside of hospital. The aim of this study was:

> To attempt to bring people with mental illness under the concept of personhood, required of us will be what Bernard Williams terms an 'effort at identification', in which the person 'should not be regarded as the surface to which a certain label can be applied, but one should try to see the world (including the label) from his point of view'.
>
> (Barham and Hayward 1991)

In adopting this approach, their work takes us beyond the measuring of consumer satisfaction. Rather, the concern is with the mental patient's identity and social position in everyday life. The themes identified from the subjects themselves were:

1 Exclusion from participation in social life.
2 Burden, which 'refers to the cultural freight which agents are obliged to carry'
3 Reorientation, which refers to 'coping' with their vulnerabilities.

Everyday encounters reported by subjects suggested the continuing marginalization of people labelled as schizophrenic, as illustrated by this quote from one respondent who struck up a conversation in a pub: 'I said I was schizophrenic and he said "You don't want to tell people things like that, they might take you out and beat you up outside". Anyway, I just got up and left because I didn't want any trouble' (Barham and Hayward 1991: 16). Participants in the study were also reluctant to enter or re-enter patienthood. Most wanted to establish their credibility as ordinary people with rights of citizenship, such as adequate employment and housing. The participants were only marginally more willing to be incorporated into community services than the old custodial regime. This suggests a fundamental questioning of the utility of services from the perspective of users themselves. Such a questioning is not acknowledged by the other two views (of patient and consumer) discussed above. Phenomenological analysis gives primacy to the individual experience of the patient in relation to the mental hospital or community. The wider collective role of mental health consumers, as a group within civil society, is also an aspect which is important in understanding the contemporary position of mental patients.

Survivors as a new social movement

The growing collective activities of mental health users over the last two decades has been noted by a number of commentators (Haafkens *et al.* 1986; Burstow and Weitz 1988; Chamberlin 1988; Rogers and Pilgrim 1991). During the 1970s, the Dutch and US survivors' movements gained national and state recognition. By 1977, 35 organizations were represented in the Netherlands. Organized mental patient pressure in the US has recently resulted in funding both for research and for mental health services to be run exclusively by patients (Campbell and Schraiber 1989). More recently, similar developments have been taking place in Britain.

Three examples from the British survivors' movement give a flavour of the type of activism that has emerged in the area of user participation and mental health services. In 1988, a campaign was launched by users in London to oppose changes being advocated by the Royal College of Psychiatrists to the Mental Health Act 1983. The proposed Community Treatment Order (CTOs) would have allowed doctors to treat patients in the community on a compulsory basis. This hostility to CTOs culminated in over a hundred users and their allies marching from Hyde Park to Belgrave Square. There, a wreath was laid at the steps of the Royal College of Psychiatrists, in honour of the deceased recipients of ECT and major tranquillizers. Speeches were made (including one from a Labour MP) and patients read poems critical of psychiatric treatment.

A second example of the activity during this period was the organized opposition to the poster campaign, in the south of England, of SANE (Schizophrenia a National Emergency). This advertising campaign enjoyed the patronage of Prince Charles and the pop singer Sting. It was heavily financed by, amongst others, Rupert Murdoch and P&O ferries. The posters depicted psychiatric patients as frenziedly dangerous and called for a halt to the hospital closure programme. In response, London-based users' groups lobbied the Advertising Standards Authority about the offending posters.

A third example was the lobby of the then opposition (Labour Party) spokespeople in Parliament by a national network of 56 different users' groups. This network is dispersed throughout the country. The MPs agreed to meet the groups, to hear their complaints about existing services and their recommendations for changes in mental health policy.

Thus, user dissatisfaction has now reached such a point that, in terms of numbers and organizations, it constitutes a nascent 'new social movement'. Social movements can be defined as certain groups engaged in informal efforts in order to promote their interests in opposition to dominant forms of power and organization preferred by the State (Toch 1965). 'New' social movements can be distinguished conceptually from 'old' social movements in that they are further removed from the arena of production than the latter. Additionally, rather than seeking to defend existing social and property rights from erosion by the State, they seek to establish new agendas and conquer new territory (Habermas 1981).

Scott (1990) contrasts new social movements with the Labour (or workers') movement (the focus of the Marxian tradition in sociology). This movement has become a part of the political process through organized industrial action and negotiation (e.g. the TUC and the Labour Party). Its organization has become formalized or bureaucratized and its aims have been economic and political. By contrast, the new social movements (feminism, ecology, black and gay liberation, etc.) have mainly had social and cultural aims and have emphasized direct action and non-hierarchical forms of organization. Some social scientists have gone as far as arguing that the absorption of the Labour movement into the established political process, in capitalist society, leaves the new social movements as the only remaining radical challenge to the status quo (Marcuse 1964). The mental health service survivors' movement would seem to fit conceptually into this new political pattern of radicalism.

Whilst the rise of survivors' groups suggests that there is a groundswell of dissatisfaction, which health and social services have, overall, failed to contain, this new social movement is not homogenous. Rogers and Pilgrim (1991) found disparities in ideology between the British users' groups over attitudes to conceptualizing mental health problems, professionals and treatment. Some groups uncritically accepted the paradigm of mental illness, whilst others were wholly rejecting of the medical model and its attendant treatments.

In the US, where the movement is more developed, user groups have been classified according to two models – 'structural' and 'clinical'. The first is concerned with offering self-help services and is oriented towards social change through legal advocacy, public education and providing information. The second model is concerned with individual change through group support meetings, drop-in centres and alternative therapies. The analysis of the relationship between these groups and professionals shows that the former are more likely to develop partnerships than the latter. However, there was a tendency on the part of both types of group to reject alliances with mental health professionals who had a narrow clinical conception of mental illness (Emerick 1990).

Sang (1989) has pointed out that the term 'advocacy' has been co-opted by professionals and is used loosely by them to include 'meeting clinical needs'. He distinguishes this professional discourse from two separate notions from service users themselves: citizen advocacy and self-advocacy. In the first of these, ordinary citizens (i.e. not professionals) form a relationship with a psychiatric patient to represent their interests as if they were their own. In the second case, psychiatric patients work together to represent their individual and collective interests independently of non-patients.

A final point about survivors' groups is that they have shared several concerns which were first highlighted by critical professionals during the 1960s (the so-called 'antipsychiatry' movement). Whereas that critique was highly intellectual and came from professionals themselves, the more recent critique has come from service users directly and is less theoretically oriented. Instead, practical direct action characterizes its form. However, the 'clinical' group described in the US clearly draws upon the therapeutic alternatives, which the 'antipsychiatrists' themselves developed and advocated at an earlier point.

The user as provider

One development of the users' movement, which has converged with the interests of health service managers, is the development of user-led service innovations. For example, user-led services can be found in the voluntary sector in Britain and occasionally they are supported by statutory authorities. The large range of user-controlled facilities available in the US is reviewed by Mowbray et al. (1997) This activity varies from the latent role of patients being self-caring and mutually supportive in professionally-led services (Rogers et al. 1993; Mental Health Foundation 1996) and self-help groups, right through to funded projects which are managed and staffed by users themselves

(Chamberlin 1988; Lindow 1994; Wallcraft 1996). The type of service the latter provide (such as safe houses and drop-in day centres) reflect the users' movement's priorities of voluntary relationships, alternatives to hospital admission, crisis intervention and personal support.

Between the diffuse self-care strategies and mutual support occurring spontaneously between patients in statutory services and funded user-led services, there is another layer of user involvement. In recent years, service providers have, to various degrees in different localities, sought the collaboration of users to support service developments. Minimally this has entailed surveys or consultation exercises about local need identification (an extension of the role of user-as-consumer). It has also included: the formal acceptance by professional providers of innovations such as patients' councils; users being paid to train mental health staff (Crepaz-Keay *et al.* 1998) and users' and carers' groups being called upon to improve services in collaborative experiments in service development (Carpenter and Sbaraini 1997; Pilgrim and Waldron 1998).

User-led services have also introduced an alternative philosophical base to the management and treatment of mental health problems. At times this has had a feedback impact on traditional services. The Hearing Voices Network, informed by the work of Romme, works positively with people's experiences of hearing voices. Rather than attempting to obliterate the voices, as a traditional symptom-based approach might do, this user-led initiative attributes meaning to voice hearing. This offers alternative means of coping with voices that may at times cause their recipients distress.

The limits of the user-as-provider are essentially set by the willingness (or lack of it) to encroach upon the coercive social control role which professionals have traditionally taken. Professional norms have included State delegated powers to detain and forcibly intervene in the lives of people who are socially deviant or incompetent (under the paternalistic guise of the 'treatment' of illness). Not only do user-led projects not include this function currently, because of the absence of legal powers, it is unlikely that they would want to accrue this traditional psychiatric professional service role, given that the main stimulus for the development of the service users' movement internationally was the civil libertarian objection to the coercive role of psychiatry in society. This point is made in a critical way by an academic psychiatric nurse: 'What matters here is that such services can show that they can provide safe and effective care to a high standard. The fact that all [*sic*] such services so far have had to institute rules that enable difficult people to be excluded indicates that such services are developing in a way that is supplementary rather than alternative to psychiatry' (Bowers 1998: 138).

Whilst it is an open empirical question whether or not the vast array of user-led service experiments have *all* excluded 'difficult people', rather than a presumed 'fact', Bowers is probably correct in highlighting the tendency of user projects to eschew a coercive role and embrace voluntary relationships. However, what user-led projects do provide is an alternative to the readiness of psychiatry to coercively control those who are not 'difficult' (in the sense of being dangerous rule-breakers) but who are harmlessly unintelligible to their fellows (e.g. voice hearers and those with inoffensive delusions). Currently, psychiatrists regularly use their legal powers to remove the liberty of these types of patients – to be deemed to be mentally ill and without insight is sufficient for a forced psychiatric admission. User-led projects offer more benign alternatives to this group of people and in so doing provide a redefinition of who is difficult, by showing how this latter group can be helped where traditional services have failed.

A second criticism we would make of Bowers' position is that the lack of capacity (or willingness) of user projects to fully replace psychiatry's societal function also clarifies it. In other words, at times some extreme rule-breaking, such as sexual assault, violence or incorrigible madness, is simply beyond the capability of ordinary people to cope with and respond to safely, whether in domestic or public settings. In such circumstances, State delegated social control is understandably invoked – 'something has to be done'. The police or psychiatry are called in then as part of a repressive State apparatus which is requested, respected and gratefully received by ordinary people who are *not* (or not deemed to be) the rule-breakers in particular social crises (Coulter 1973). By stopping short of this role, user-led services clarify the embodied constitution of repressive social control, i.e. some psychiatric, some social work and most police action.

The mass media and psychiatric patients

The mass media operate in a highly ambiguous and ambivalent way about mental health matters and they are a powerful factor in the construction of images about mental abnormality, and thus on how mental health users are seen in the public eye. In order to unpack this ambiguity and ambivalence we will address the role of the mass media under three subheadings:

1 The interest mediation role of the mass media.
2 Negative image portrayal.
3 Public psychological exploration.

The interest mediation role of the mass media

The mass media can act as conduits for interest groups. Several examples of this can be given in recent years in Britain. In the 1980s, MIND, in conjunction with Esther Rantzen's *That's Life* television programme, stimulated a national campaign about the need to reduce the prescription of benzodiazepines. Also in the 1980s the Channel Four series *Mind's Eye* offered a range of opportunities for both professionals and service users to express their views about a number of topics. For example, one programme, *We're Not Mad We're Angry* allowed users to express their anger about the way in which psychiatry treated them. More recently, in 1997 a BBC *Panorama* programme took a lengthy account from a psychiatrist operating in an inner city mental health unit to highlight his professional concerns about resources.

These examples highlight how the mass media pass on and publicize the values and goals of interest groups. These allow such groups to argue, persuade and special plead in the presence of a wide audience which might normally be excluded from the fine grain of mental health debates.

Negative image portrayal

Whilst the above points highlight that a variety of perspectives are at times represented by the mass media, viewpoints are not put forward randomly or even-handedly. This bias is generated by the tendency of the mass media to sell their wares on the back of sensation, untoward events, crises and the anticipated audience desire for the shock and intrigue these create. Complex arguments are often boring and negative images create a stronger audience reaction than positive images. Stories are constructed by the media in a series of themes, each with a connecting moral panic. This process usually has at its centre a clear alien and hostile target, with an identifiable social group being demonized, criticized or feared at particular times (e.g. homosexuals, social security scroungers, single mothers, HIV carriers, psychiatric patients). In relation to mental health, occasionally this critical attention can be about services or staff. Examples of this include the two television programmes which preceded and triggered official inquiries about mistreatment at the Special Hospitals of Rampton and Ashworth (DHSS 1980; HMSO 1992b). However, this negative media portrayal of psychiatric personnel is much less common than are sinister images of psychiatric *patients*. This was made clear in the content analysis of British media output about mental health during April 1993 (Philo *et al.* 1994). Of 562 images analysed, the overwhelming majority (66 per cent) referred to patient violence to others. Other categories described were: sympathetic coverage (18 per cent); harm to self (13 per cent); comic images (2 per cent); and criticism of accepted definitions of mental illness (1 per cent).

Public psychological exploration

The mass media are not only driven in their focus by untoward events, moral panics and negative images of psychiatric patients. Other anticipated audience motives shape programme or story production. In particular, the 'human interest' aspect of a report appeals to a broad public audience. Rose (1990) following Foucault, argues that the confessional is now at the heart of many operations of modernity, including the mass media. In recent years, the exploration of personal problems and distress in the mass media has been evident in a number of ways. Popular magazines for both women and men carry 'problem pages' authored by psychiatric experts and 'Agony Aunts'. Radio stations have phone-in periods in which people confess their difficulties and seek advice. The glossiest version of this type of public exploration is celebrated in programmes such as the American Oprah Winfrey and Ricki Lake shows which are also broadcast in Britain. These programmes are a source of reference for people about their own mental health and their daily coping with stress (Rogers and Pilgrim 1997).

These media outlets also at times allow mental health issues to be explored in programmes about treatments, such as ECT and major tranquillizers, and their iatrogenic problems. These may furnish information to users of services to allow them to critically evaluate the treatments they receive. The Philo *et al.* study noted above would suggest that these media events are less frequent though than stories projecting psychiatric patients as a menacing social problem.

Discussion

The four ways of viewing service users described in the second part of this chapter illustrate the construction of the mental patient from different vantage points. The first has a narrow clinical conception of the user of services – as an extension or carrier of the mental illness he or she is deemed to be suffering. The conceptualization of the user as consumer defines the user of services as a whole person, who has needs over and above those defined from a diagnostic viewpoint. This approach tends still to be professionally defined and is limited to the parameters of the provision and delivery of existing or achievable services. The third approach takes the expressed view of users as the main reference point of analysis, along with the collective structural position of mental patients within a wider social context. The fourth and most recent view of users is that they can be providers of care for other people with mental health problems.

The implications that stem from these conceptualizations are consequently different. The first accepts that professionally-led services are most appropriate, given the paternalism that mental illness is deemed to necessitate. The second modifies this by recognizing the notion of the positive choice that the ideology of consumerism implies. The third position marks a departure from a professionally defined discourse because by giving a voice to user demands, professionally delivered services are brought into question or are rendered problematic. The fourth position opens up even more ambiguity by shifting care from the professional domain to that of the mutual care of patients.

The clinical conception points to a traditional therapist/patient relationship. Consumerism envisages a larger role for mental health users in health care. There is an implicit assumption that views and participation should be in relation to existing services, whether some of these are expanded or diminished as a result of feedback on the basis of 'felt need'. The survivor and provider views in eschewing or distrusting professional interventions emphasizes that the fundamental needs of patients are for rights rather than specialized services. This would imply an increase in material and social resources, for example, improved access to housing and employment opportunities. A further requirement might be legislation aimed at ensuring that people with a psychiatric label are not discriminated against in civil society, along the lines of that already existing for race and sex.

These divergent implications of the four conceptions of the mental patient outlined above suggest that rather than being neutral or value free, each is imbued with, or reflects, a set of competing interests and ideologies related to the three groups central to contemporary mental health services: clinicians, managers and users. The power of each of these interest groups interact to determine the types of priorities that come to prevail in the organization, distribution and delivery of services and resources to those with mental health problems in society. The interaction is also affected by media portrayals of psychiatric patients and by the influence of groups of their relatives. Thus, any social understanding of the role, status and credibility of people who use mental health services needs to be reached after an appraisal of the relative salience of a number of dynamic processes and disparate actors which surround and inscribe a set of identities upon them.

In conclusion

This chapter has highlighted some basic problems about defining who exactly is a user of mental health services. Although the term 'user' (in Britain) has become a new shorthand for 'psychiatric patient', we drew attention to the other parties being served and thus arguably 'using' these services. If a variety of parties use services then it is inevitable that they are a source of disappointment as the different interest groups often seek different ends. Both the relatives of psychiatric patients and patients themselves have become important social movements which have shaped the character of mental health services. The emergence of user-led mental health provision has also highlighted the shortcomings of professional work (from a patient perspective) and defined the social control role of psychiatry more clearly.

Questions

1 Describe the reasons for the rise of the mental health service users' movement.

2 Compare and contrast the expectations which patients and their relatives are likely to have about mental health services.

3 How does the mass media shape our views of psychiatric patients?

4 What have 'survivors' of the psychiatric system 'survived'?

5 What do user-led services tell us about mainstream mental health provision?

6 Why is the term 'carer' problematic in the field of mental health?

For discussion

If you were the relative of a person who became psychotic what would you want from services? Think about this question again but now as the patient. Compare and contrast both parts of the exercise.

Further reading

Crepaz-Keay, D., Binns, C. and Wilson, E. (1998) *Dancing With Angels: Involving Survivors in Mental Health Training*. London: CCETSW.

Crossley, N. (1998) Transforming the mental health field: the early history of the National Association of Mental Health. *Sociology of Health and Illness*, 20(4): 458–88.

Mowbray, C.T., Moxley, D.P., Jasper, C.A. and Howell, L.L. (eds) (1997) *Consumers As Providers in Psychiatric Rehabilitation*. Columbia: International Association of Psychosocial Rehabilitation Services.

Pilgrim, D. and Waldron, L. (1998) User involvement in mental health service development: how far it can it go? *Journal of Mental Health* 7, 1: 95–104.

Rogers, A., Pilgrim, D. and Lacey, R. (1993) *Experiencing Psychiatry: Users' Views of Services*. Basingstoke: Macmillan.

References

Abbott, P. and Wallace, C. (eds) (1990) *The Sociology of the Caring Professions*. London: Falmer Press.

Abel, B. (1988) *The British Legal Profession*. Oxford: Blackwell.

Abel, G., Becker, J., Mittleman, M. *et al*. (1987) Self-reported sex crimes of non-incarcerated paraphiliacs. *Journal of Interpersonal Violence*, 2(1): 3–25.

Abraham, J. and Sheppard, J. (1998) International comparative analysis and explanation in medical sociology: demystifying the Halcion anomaly. *Sociology*, 32(1): 141–62.

Abramson, M. (1972) The criminalisation of mentally disordered behaviour: possible side effects of a new mental health law. *Hospital and Community Psychiatry*, 23(3): 101–5.

Adorno, T.W., Frenkel-Briunswik, E., Levinson, D.J. and Sanford, R.N. (1950) *The Authoritarian Personality*. New York: Harper and Brothers.

Al-Issa, I. (1977) Social and cultural aspects of hallucinations. *Psychological Bulletin*, 84: 570–87.

Al-Issa, I. (1987) Gender roles, in L. Diamant (ed.) *Male and Female Homosexuality: Psychological Approaches*. New York: Hemisphere.

Alemi, F., Mosavel, M., Stephens, R. *et al*. (1996) Electronic self-help and support groups. *Medical Care*, 34(10): 32–44.

Allen, H. (1986) Psychiatry and the feminine, in P. Miller and N. Rose (eds) *The Power of Psychiatry*. Cambridge: Polity Press.

Althusser, L. (1971) *Lenin and Philosophy and Other Essays*. London: New Left Books.

Alzheimer's Disease Report (1992). London: Alzheimer's Disease Society.

Anthias, F. (1992) Connecting race and ethnic phenomena. *Sociology*, 26(3): 421–38.

Arber, S. and Gilbert, N. (1989) Men: the forgotten carers. *Sociology*, 23(1): 111–18.

Arber, S. and Ginn, J. (1991) *Gender and Later Life*. London: Sage.

Armstrong, D. (1980) Madness and coping. *Sociology of Health and Illness*, 2(3): 393–413.

Atkinson, P. (1983) The reproduction of the professional community, in R. Dingwall and P. Lewis (eds) *The Sociology of the Professions*. London: Macmillan.

Audit Commission (1986) *Making a Reality of Community Care*. London: HMSO.

Audit Commission (1994) *Finding A Place: A Review of Mental Health Services For Adults*. London: HMSO.

Backett, K. and Davison, C. (1995) Lifecourses and life style – the social and cultural location of health behaviour. *Social Science and Medicine*, 40(5): 629–38.

Baker, A.W. and Duncan, S.P. (1985) Child sexual abuse: a study of prevalence in Great Britain. *Child Abuse and Neglect*, 9: 457–67.

Baker, D. and Taylor, H. (1997) Inequality in health and health service use for mothers of young children. *Journal of Epidemiology and Community Health*, 51: 74–9.

Bakker, C.B. (1975) Why people don't change. *Psychotherapy: Theory, Research and Practice*, 12: 164–72.

Bannister, D. (1968) The logical requirements of research into schizophrenia. *British Journal of Psychiatry*, 114: 1088–97.

Bannister, D. and Fransella, F. (1970) *Inquiring Man*. Harmondsworth: Penguin.

Barham, P. and Hayward, R. (1991) *From the Mental Patient to the Person*. London: Routledge.

Barnes, M. and Maple, N. (1992) *Women and Mental Health: Challenging the Stereotypes*. Birmingham: Venture Press.

Barnes, M., Bowl, R. and Fisher, M. (1990) *Sectioned: Social Services and the 1983 Mental Health Act*. London: Routledge.

Barrett, M. and Roberts, H. (1978) Doctors and their patients, in H. Smart and B. Smart (eds) *Women, Sexuality and Social Control*. London: Routledge and Kegan Paul.

Bartley, M., Blane, D. and Davey-Smith, G. (1998) Beyond the Black Report. *Sociology of Health and Illness*, 20(5): 563–77.

Bartley, M., Davey-Smith, G. and Blane, D. (1997) Vital comparisons: the social construction of mortality measurement, in M.A. Elston (ed.) *The Sociology of Medical Science and Technology*. Oxford: Blackwell.

Barton, W.R. (1959) *Institutional Neurosis*. Bristol: Wright and Sons.

Baruch, G. and Treacher, A. (1978) *Psychiatry Observed*. London: Routledge and Kegan Paul.

Bassuk, E., Rubin, L. and Lauriat, A. (1984) Is homelessness a mental health problem? *American Journal of Psychiatry*, 141: 1546–50.

Bean, P. (1979) Psychiatrists' assessments of mental illness: a comparison of Thomas Scheff's approach to labelling theory. *British Journal of Psychiatry*, 135: 122–8.

Bean, P. (1980) *Compulsory Admissions to Mental Hospital*. Chichester: Wiley.

Bean, P. (1985) Social control and social theory in secure accommodation, in L. Gostin (ed.) *Secure Provision*. London: Tavistock.

Bean, P. (1986) *Mental Disorder and Legal Control*. Cambridge: Cambridge University Press.

Bean, P. and Mounser, P. (1993) *Discharged from Mental Hospitals*. London: Macmillan.

Bean, P., Bingley, W., Bynoe, I. et al. (1991) *Out of Harm's Way: MIND's research into police and psychiatric action under Section 136 of the Mental Health Act*. London: MIND.

Bebbington, P.E., Hurry, J. and Tennant, C. (1981) Psychiatric disorders in selected immigrant groups in Camberwell. *Social Psychiatry*, 16: 43–51.

Beck, A.T. (1970) Cognitive therapy: nature and relation to behaviour therapy. *Behaviour Therapy*, 1: 184–200.

Beck, U. and Beck-Gersheim, E. (1995) *The Normal Chaos of Love*. Oxford: Polity Press.

Beck-Sander, A. (1998) Is insight into psychosis meaningful? *Journal of Mental Health*, 7(1): 25–34.

Becker, J.V. (1988) The effects of child sexual abuse on adolescent sexual offenders, in G.E. Wyatt and G.J. Powell (eds) *Lasting Effects of Child Sexual Abuse*. New York: Sage.

Beliappa, J. (1991) *Illness or Distress? Alternative Models of Mental Health*. London: Confederation of Indian Organisations.

Bendalow, G. and Williams, S. (1998) *Emotions in Social Life: Critical Themes and Contemporary Issues*. London: Routledge.

Bentall, R.P. (ed.) (1990) *Reconstructing Schizophrenia*. London: Routledge.

Bentall, R.P. and Pilgrim, D. (1993) Thomas Szasz, crazy talk and the myth of mental illness. *British Journal of Medical Psychology*, 66: 69–76.

Bentall, R.P. and Slade, P. (1985) Reality testing and auditory hallucinations: a signal detection analysis. *British Journal of Clinical Psychology*, 24: 159–69.

Bentall, R.P., Jackson, H. and Pilgrim, D. (1988) Abandoning the concept of schizo-phrenia: some implications of validity arguments for psychological research into psychotic phenomena. *British Journal of Clinical Psychology*, 27: 303–24.

Beresford, P. and Croft, S. (1986) *Whose Welfare? Private Care or Public Service*. London: Lewis Cohen Urban Studies.

Bergin, A.E. (1971) The evaluation of therapeutic outcomes, in A.E. Bergin and S. Garfield (eds) *Handbook of Psychotherapy and Behaviour Change*. New York: Wiley.

Bergin, A. and Lambert, M. (1978) The evaluation of therapeutic outcomes, in S. Garfield and A. Bergin (eds) *Handbook of Psychotherapy and Behaviour Change*, 2nd edn. Chichester: Wiley.

Bhaskar, R. (1978) *A Realist Theory of Science*. New Jersey: Hassocks.

Bhaskar, R. (1989) *Reclaiming Reality*. London: Verso.

Bhui, K., Christie, Y. and Bhugra, D. (1995) The essential elements of culturally sensitive psychiatric services. *International Journal of Social Psychiatry*, 41(4): 242–56.

Biafora, F. (1995) Cross cultural perspectives on illness and wellness – implications for depression. *Journal of Social Distress and the Homeless*, 4(2): 105–29.

Bifulco, A., Harris, T.O. and Brown, G.W. (1992) Mourning or inadequate care? Re-examining the relationship of maternal loss in childhood with adult depression and anxiety. *Development and Psychopathology*, 4: 119–28.

Bifulco, A. and Moran, A. (1998) *Wednesday's Child: Research into Women's Experience of Neglect and Abuse in Childhood and Adult Depression*. London: Routledge.

Bion, W.R. (1959) *Experiences in Groups*. New York: Basic Books.

Blaxter, M. (1990) *Health and Lifestyles*. London: Routledge.

Blaxter, M. (1998) Class time and biography, in S.J. Williams, J. Gabe and M. Calnan (eds) *Theorising Health Medicine and Society*. London: Sage.

Bolton, P. (1984) Management of compulsorily admitted patients to a high security unit. *International Journal of Social Psychiatry*, 30: 77–84.

Bowers, L. (1998) *The Social Nature of Mental Illness*. London: Routledge.

Bowl, R. (1996) Legislating for user involvement in the United Kingdom mental health services and the NHS and Community Care Act. *International Journal of Social Psychiatry*, 42(3): 165–80.

Bowlby, J. (1951) *Maternal Care and Mental Health*. Geneva: World Health Organisation.

Boyle, M. (1991) *Schizophrenia: A Scientific Delusion*. London: Routledge.

Bracken, P.J., Greenslade, L., Griffen, B. and Smyth, M. (1998) Mental health and ethnicity: an Irish dimension. *British Journal of Psychiatry*, 172: 103–5.

Bracken, P. and Thomas, P. (1998) A new debate in mental health. *Open Mind*, 89 (February): 17.

Bradshaw, J. (1972) The concept of social need. *New Society*, 640–3.

Brady, M. (1995) Culture in treatment, culture as treatment: a critical appraisal of developments in addiction programmes for indigenous North Americans and Aus-tralians. *Social Science and Medicine*, 41: 1487–98.

Braginsky, B.M., Braginsky, D.D. and Ring, K. (1973) *Methods of Madness: The Mental Hospital as a Last Resort*. New York: Holt, Rinehart and Winston.

Brakel, J., Parry, J. and Weiner, B. (1985) *The Mentally Disabled and the Law*. Chicago: American Bar Foundation.

Brayne, C. and Ames, D. (1988) The epidemiology of mental disorders in old age, in B. Gearing, M. Johnson and T. Heller (eds) *Mental Health Problems in Old Age*. London: Wiley.

Breggin, P. (1993) *Toxic Psychiatry*. London: HarperCollins.

Briere, J. and Runtz, M. (1987) Post-sexual abuse trauma: data implications for clinical practice. *Journal of Interpersonal Violence*, 2: 367–79.

Briere, J. and Runtz, M. (1988) Post-sexual abuse trauma, in G.E. Wyatt and G.J. Powell (eds) *Lasting Effects of Child Sexual Abuse*. New York: Sage.

Britten, N. (1991) Hospital consultants' views of their patients. *Sociology of Health and Illness*, 13(1): 83–97.

Brodsky, A. and Holdroyd, J. (1975) Report of the task force on sex bias and sex role stereotyping in psychotherapeutic practice. *American Psychologist*, 30: 1169–75.

Broverman, D., Clarkson, F., Rosenkratz, P. *et al.* (1970) Sex role stereotypes and clinical judgements of mental health. *Journal of Consulting and Clinical Psychology*, 34: 1–7.

Brown, G.W. (1959) Experiences of discharged chronic schizophrenic patients in various types of living group. *Millbank Memorial Fund Quarterly*, 37: 105.

Brown, G.W. (1973) The mental hospital as an institution. *Social Science and Medicine*, 7: 407–21.

Brown, G.W. (1996) Onset and course of depressive disorders: summary of a research programme, in C. Mundt, M. Goldstein, K. Hahlweg and P. Fiedler (eds) *Interpersonal Factors in the Origin and Course of Affective Disorders*. London: Gaskell.

Brown, G.W. and Harris, T.O. (1978) *The Social Origins of Depression*. London: Tavistock.

Brown, G.W. and Wing, J.K. (1962) A comparative clinical and social survey of three mental hospitals. *The Sociological Review Monograph*, 5: 145–71.

Brown, G.W., Harris, T.O. and Bifulco, A. (1986) Long term effects of early loss of parent, in M. Rutter, C. Izard and P. Read (eds) *Depression In Childhood: Developmental Perspectives*. New York: Guilford Press.

Brown, G.W., Harris, T.O. and Hepworth, C. (1995) Loss, humiliation and entrapment among women developing depression: a patient and non-patient comparison. *Psychological Medicine*, 25: 7–21.

Brown, P. (1995) Naming and framing: the social construction of diagnosis and illness. *Journal of Health and Social Behaviour*, Extra Issue: 34–52.

Brown, P. and Funk, S.C. (1986) Tardive dyskinesia: barriers to the professional recognition of iatrogenic disease. *Journal of Health and Social Behaviour*, 27: 116–32.

Browne, A. and Finklehor, D. (1986) Impact of child sexual abuse: a review of the research. *Psychological Bulletin*, 99: 66–77.

Browne, D. (1990) *Black People, Mental Health and the Courts*. London: NACRO.

Bullough, V.L. (1987) The first clinicians, in L. Diamant (ed.) *Male and Female Homosexuality: Psychological Approaches*. New York: Hemisphere.

Burrows, R., Bunton, R. and Nettleton, S. (1995) *The Sociology of Health Promotion: Critical Analyses of Consumption, Lifestyle and Risk*. London: Routledge.

Burstow, B. and Weitz, D. (eds) (1988) *Shrink Resistant: The Struggle Against Psychiatry in Canada*. Vancouver: New Star.

Bury, M. (1986) Social constructionism and the development of medical sociology. *Sociology of Health and Illness*, 8: 137–69.

Bury, M. and Gabe, J. (1990) Hooked? Media responses to tranquillizer dependence, in P. Abbott and G. Payne (eds) *New Directions in the Sociology of Health*. London: Falmer Press.

Busfield, J. (1982) Gender and mental illness. *International Journal of Mental Health*, 11(12): 46–66.

Busfield, J. (1986) *Managing Madness*. London: Hutchinson.

Busfield, J. (1988) Mental illness as a social product or social construct: a contradiction in feminists' arguments? *Sociology of Health and Illness*, 10: 521–42.

Busfield, J. (1991) A female malady? Men, women and madness in nineteenth century Britain. Paper given to the British Sociological Association Medical Sociology Conference: York.

Busfield, J. (1996) *Men, Women and Madness: Understanding Gender and Mental Disorder*. London: Macmillan.

Buss, A.H. (1966) *Psychopathology*. New York: Wiley.

Cahill, C., Llewelyn, S.P. and Pearson, C. (1991) Long term aspects of sexual abuse which occurred in childhood: a review. *British Journal of Clinical Psychology*, 30: 117–30.

Cameron, E. and Bernardes, J. (1998) Gender and disadvantage in health: men's health for a change. *Sociology of Health and Illness*, 20(5): 673–93.

Campbell, J. and Schraiber, R. (1989) *In Pursuit of Wellness: The Well-being Project*. Sacramento: the California Department of Mental Health.

Campbell, T. and Heginbotham, C. (1991) *Mental Illness, Prejudice Discrimination and the Law*. Dartmouth: Aldershot.

Carchedi, G. (1975) On the economic identification of the new middle class. *Economy and Society*, 4(1): 1–85.

Carpenter, L. and Brockington, I. (1980) A study of mental illness in Asians, West Indians and Africans living in Manchester. *British Journal of Psychiatry*, 137: 201–5.

Carpenter, J. and Sbaraini, S. (1997) *Choice, Information and Dignity: Involving Users and Carers in Care Management in Mental Health*. London: Policy Press.

Carpenter, M. (1980) Asylum nursing before 1914: a chapter in the history of nursing, in C. Davies (ed.) *Re-writing Nursing History*. London: Croom Helm.

Carstairs, G.M. and Kapur, R.C. (1976) *The Great Universe of Kota: Stress, Change and Mental Disorder in an Indian Village*. London: Hogarth Press.

Castel, F., Castel, R. and Lovell, A. (1979) *The Psychiatric Society*. New York: Columbia Free Press.

Castel, R. (1983) Moral treatment: mental therapy and social control in the nineteenth century, in S. Cohen and A. Scull (eds) *Social Control and the State*. Oxford: Basil Blackwell.

Chamberlin, J. (1988) *On Our Own*. London: MIND.

Chen, E., Harrison, G. and Standen, P. (1991) Management of first episode psychotic illness in Afro-Caribbean patients. *British Journal of Psychiatry*, 158: 517–22.

Chesler, P. (1972) *Women and Madness*. New York: Doubleday.

Ciompi, L. (1984) Is there really a schizophrenia? The long term course of psychotic phenomena. *British Journal of Psychiatry*, 145: 636–40.

Clare, A. (1974) Mental illness in the Irish emigrant. *Journal of the Irish Medical Association*, 67: 20–4.

Clare, A. (1976) *Psychiatry In Dissent*. London: Tavistock.

Clausen, J.A. and Kohn, M.L. (1959) Relation of schizophrenia to the social structure of a small city, in B. Pasamanick (ed.) *Epidemiology of Mental Disorders*. Washington, DC: American Association for the Advancement of Science.

Clegg, S.R. (1990) *Modern Organisations*. London: Sage.

Cochrane, R. (1977) Mental illness in immigrants to England and Wales: an analysis of mental hospital admissions 1971. *Social Psychiatry*, 12: 2–35.

Cochrane, R. (1983) *The Social Creation of Mental Illness*. London: Longman.

Cochrane, R. and Bal, S. (1989) Mental hospital admission rates of immigrants to England: a comparison of 1971 and 1981. *Social Psychiatry*, 24: 2–11.

Cohen, D. (1989) *Soviet Psychiatry*. London: Paladin.

Cohen, D. (1997) A critique of the use of neuroleptic drugs in psychiatry, in S. Fisher and R.P. Greenberg (eds) *From Placebo to Panacea*. New York: Wiley.

Cole, M.G. and Bellavance, F. (1997) Depression in elderly inpatients: a meta-analysis of outcomes. *Canadian Medical Association Journal*, Oct. 15, 157: 1055–60.

Community Psychiatric Nurses Association (1988) The Patient's Case. London: CPNA Publications.

Cooper, D. (1968) *Psychiatry and Anti-Psychiatry*. London: Tavistock.

Cooperstock, R. (1978) Sex differences in psychotropic drug use. *Social Science and Medicine*, 12: 179–86.

Cope, R. (1989) The compulsory detention of Afro-Caribbeans under the Mental Health Act. *New Community*, 15(3): 343–56.

Copeland, J., Dewey, M., Wodd, N. *et al.* (1987) Range of mental illness among the elderly in the community. *British Journal of Psychiatry*, 150: 815–23.

Coulter, J. (1973) *Approaches to Insanity*. New York: Wiley.

Craib, I. (1989) *Psychoanalysis and Social Theory: The Limits of Sociology*. Hemel Hempstead: Harvester Wheatsheaf.

Craib, I. (1997) Social constructionism as a social psychosis. *Sociology*, 31(1): 1–15.

Craib, I. (1998) *Experiencing Identity*. London: Sage.

Crawford, D. (1989) The future of clinical psychology; whither or wither? *Clinical Psychology Forum*, 20: 29–31.

Crepaz-Keay, D., Binns, C. and Wilson, E. (1998) *Dancing With Angels: Involving Survivors in Mental Health Training*. London: CCETSW.

Crompton, R. (1987) Gender, status and professionalism. *Sociology*, 21(3): 413–28.

Crossley, N. (1998) Transforming the mental health field: the early history of the National Association of Mental Health. *Sociology of Health and Illness*, 20(4): 458–88.

Crow, T.J., MacMillan, J.F., Johnson, A.L. and Johnstone, E.C. (1986) The Northwick Park study of first episodes of schizophrenia II: a controlled trial of prophylactic neuroleptic treatment. *British Journal of Psychiatry*, 148: 120–7.

Cuffe, S.P., Waller, J.L., Cuccaro, M.L., Pumariega, A.J. and Garrison, C.Z. (1995) Race and gender differences in the treatment of psychiatric disorders in young adolescents. *Journal of the American Academy of Child and Adolescent Psychiatry*, 34(11): 1536–43.

Curran, W. (1979) Comparative analysis of mental health legislation in forty-three countries: a discussion of historical trends. *International Journal of Law and Psychiatry*, 1(1): 79–92.

Currer, C. (1986) Concepts of well- and ill-being: the case of Pathan mothers in Britain, in C. Currer and M. Stacey (eds) *Concepts of Health, Illness and Disease*. Leamington Spa: Berg.

Curtis, S. and Jones, I. (1998) Is there a place for geography in the analysis of health inequality? *Sociology of Health and Illness*, 20(5): 645–72.

Davey Smith, G., Bartley, M. and Blane, D. (1990) The Black Report on socio-economic inequalities in health 10 years on. *British Medical Journal*, 301: 373–7.

Davidhazar, D. and Wehlage, D. (1984) Can the client with chronic schizophrenia consent to nursing research? *Journal of Advanced Nursing*, 9: 381–90.

Davidson, M.J. and Earnshaw, J. (1991) *Vulnerable Workers: Psychosocial and Legal Issues*. London: Wiley.

Davis, A., Llewellyn, S.P. and Parry, G. (1985) Women and mental health: a guide for the approved social worker, in E. Brook and A. Davis (eds) *Women, the Family and Social Work*. London: Tavistock.

Dean, G., Walsh, D., Downing, H. and Shelly, P. (1981) First admission of native-born and immigrants to psychiatric hospitals in South-East England 1976. *British Journal of Psychiatry*, 139: 506–12.

De Boer, F. (1991) Sex differences in the construction of mental health care problems. Paper presented at the British Sociological Association Medical Sociology Conference: York.

de la Cuesta, C. (1993) Fringe work: peripheral work in health visiting. *Sociology of Health and Illness*, 15(5): 665–82.

Denney, D. (1992) *Racism and Anti-Racism in Probation*. London: Routledge.

Department of Health (1997) press release re IRG.

Department of Health (1998) *Our Healthier Nation*. London: Department of Health.

DHSS (1980) *Inequalities in Health: Report of a Working Group* (The Black Report). London: HMSO.

DHSS (1987) Mental illness and Mental Handicap Hospitals and Units in England: Legal Statistics 1982–85. *DHSS Statistical Bulletin* 2/87, London: HMSO.

DHSS (1988) *Community Care: Agenda for Action* (The Griffiths Report). London: HMSO.

DeSwaan, A. (1990) *The Management of Normality*. London: Routledge.

Diamont, L. (1987) *Male and Female Homosexuality: Psychological Approaches*. New York: Hemisphere.

Dimock, P.T. (1988) Adult males sexually abused as children; characteristics and implications for treatment. *Journal of Interpersonal Violence*, 3: 203–21.

Dingwall, R., Tanaka, H. and Minamikata, S. (1991) Images of parenthood in the United Kingdom and Japan. *Sociology*, 25(3): 423–46.

Dohrenwend, B.P., Brice, P., Levar, I. *et al.* (1992) Socioeconomic status and psychiatric disorders: the causation selection issue. *Science*, 255: 946–51.

Dohrenwend, B. and Dohrenwend, B.S. (1977) Sex differences in mental illness: a reply to Gove and Tudor. *American Journal of Sociology*, 82: 1336–41.

Donnelly, M. (1983) *Managing the Mind*. London: Tavistock.

Donzelot, J. (1979) *The Policing of Families*. London: Hutchinson.

Dover, S. and McWilliam, C. (1992) Physical illness associated with depression in the elderly in community based and hospital patients. *Psychiatric Bulletin*, 16: 612–13.

Dowrick, C., May, R., Richardson, M. and Bundred, P. (1996) The biopsychosocial model of general practice: rhetoric or reality? *British Journal of General Practice*, 46: 105–7.

Dreitzel, H.P. (ed.) (1973) *Childhood and Socialization*. London: Macmillan.

Dudley, M., Cantor, C. and Demoore, G. (1996) Jumping the gun – firearms and the mental health of Australians. *Australian and New Zealand Journal of Psychiatry*, 3: 370–81.

Dunham, H. (1957) Methodology of sociological investigations of mental disorders. *Journal of Social Psychiatry*, 3: 7–17.

Dunham, H.W. (1964) Social class and schizophrenia. *American Journal of Orthopsychiatry*, 34: 634–46.

DYG Corporation (1990) *Public Attitudes Toward People with Chronic Mental Illness*. Elmsford, NY: DYG Corporation.

Eastman, M. (1984) *Old Age Abuse*. Portsmouth: Grovesnor Press.

Eichenbaum, L. and Orbach, S. (1982) *Outside In Inside Out*. Harmondsworth: Penguin.

Elias, N. (1978) *The Civilising Process*. Oxford: Blackwell.

Elliot, A. (1992) *Social Theory and Psychoanalysis in Transition*. Oxford: Blackwell.

Ellis, A. (1970) *The Essence of Rational Psychotherapy*. New York: Institute for Rational Living.

Emerick, R.E. (1990) Self help groups for former patients: relations with mental health professionals. *Hospital and Community Psychiatry*, 41(4): 401–7.

Emerson, R.M. and Pollner, M. (1975) Dirty work designations: their features and consequences in a psychiatric setting. *Social Problems*, 3: 243–54.

English, B. and Ehrenreich, D. (1976) *Complaints and Disorders: The Sexual Politics of Sickness*. London: Writers and Readers Publishing Cooperative.

Ennis, B. and Emery, R. (1978) *The Rights of Mental Patients – An American Civil Liberties Union Handbook*. New York: Avon.

Estroff, S. and Zimmer, C. (1994) Social networks, social support and violence among persons with severe and persistent mental illness, in J. Monahan and H. Steadman (eds) *Violence and Mental Disorder: Developments in Risk Assessments*. Chicago: Chicago University Press.

Evans, G. (1992) Is Britain a class divided society? *Sociology*, 26(2): 233–58.

Eysenck, H.J. (1952) The effects of psychotherapy: an evaluation. *Journal of Consulting Psychology*, 16: 319–24.

Eysenck, H.J. (1955) Psychiatric diagnosis as a psychological and statistical problem. *Psychological Reports*, 1: 3–17.

Eysenck, H.J. (1975) *The Future of Psychiatry*. London: Methuen.

Fabrikant, B. (1974) The psychotherapist and the female patient: perceptions and change, in V. Franks and V. Burtle (eds) *Women in Therapy*. New York: Brunner Mazel.

Faris, R.E.L. (1944) Ecological factors in human behaviour, in R.E.L. Farris and H.W. Dunham (eds) *Mental Disorders In Urban Areas: An Ecological Study of Schizophrenia*. Chicago: Chicago University Press.

Faris, R. and Dunham, H. (1939) *Mental Disorders in Urban Areas*. Chicago: University of Chicago Press.

Faulkner, A. (1997) 'Strange bedfellows' in the laboratory of the NHS? An analysis of the new science of health technology assessment in the United Kingdom, in M.A. Elston (ed.) *The Sociology of Medical Science and Technology*. Oxford: Blackwell.

Felton, C., Stansty, P., Shern, D. *et al.* (1995) Consumers as peer specialists on intensive case management teams – impact on client outcomes. *Psychiatric Services*, 46(10): 1037–44.

Fennell, G., Phillipson, C. and Evers, H. (1988) *The Sociology of Old Age*. Milton Keynes: Open University Press.

Fennell, P. (1991) Diversion of mentally disordered offenders from custody. *Criminal Law Review*: 333–48.

Fenton, S. and Sadiq, A. (1991) *Asian Women and Depression*. London: Commission for Racial Equality.

Fenton, S. and Sadiq-Sangster, A. (1996) Culture, relativism and mental distress. *Sociology of Health and Illness*, 18(1): 66–85.

Fernando, S. (1988) *Race and Culture in Psychiatry*. Tavistock: Routledge.

Fernando, S. (1995) *Mental Health in a Multi-Ethnic Society*. London: Routledge.

Fernando, S., Ndegwa, D. and Wilson, M. (1998) *Forensic Psychiatry, Race and Culture*. London: Routledge.

Fevre, R. (1984) *Cheap Labour and Racial Discrimination*. Aldershot: Gower.

Field Institute (1984) *In Pursuit of Wellness: A Survey of California Adults*. Sacramento: California Department of Mental Health.

Finkelhor, D. (1979) *Sexually Victimized Children*. New York: Free Press.

Finkelhor, D. (1984) *Child Sexual Abuse: New Theory and Research*. New York: Free Press.

Finn, S.E., Bailey, M., Schultz, R.T. and Faber, R. (1990) Subjective utility ratings of neuroleptics in treating schizophrenia. *Psychological Medicine*, 20: 843–8.

Fisher, S. and Greenberg, R.P. (eds) (1997) *From Placebo to Panacea: Putting Psychiatric Drugs to the Test*. New York: Wiley.

Ford, G., Ecob, R., Hunt, K., Macintyre, S. and West, P. (1994) Patterns of class inequality in health through the life span. Class gradients at 15, 35, and 55 yrs in the West of Scotland. *Social Science and Medicine*, 39(8): 1037–50.

Forsythe, B. (1990) Mental and social diagnosis and the English Prison Commission 1914–1939. *Social Policy and Administration*, 24(3): 237–53.

Foucault, M. (1961) *Folie et deraison: Histoire de la Folie a l'age classique*. Paris: Plon.

Foucault, M. (1965) *Madness and Civilisation*. New York: Random House.

Foucault, M. (1978) About the concept of the 'dangerous individual' in 19th century legal psychiatry. *International Journal of Law and Psychiatry*, 1: 1–18.

Foucault, M. (1980) *Power/Knowledge*, in C. Gordon (ed.) Brighton: Harvester Press.

Foucault, M. (1981) *The History of Sexuality*. Harmondsworth: Penguin.

Foucault, M. (1988) Technologies of the self, in L. Martin (ed.) *Technologies of the Self*. London: Tavistock.

Francis, E. (1989) Black people, dangerousness and psychiatric compulsion, in A. Brackx and C. Grimshaw (eds) *Mental Health Care in Crisis*. London: Pluto.

Francis, E., Pilgrim, D., Rogers, A. and Sashidaran, S. (1989) Race and 'schizophrenia': a reply to Ineichen. *New Community*, 17: 161–3.

Franks, C.M. (1993) Cognitive-behavioural assessment and therapy with adolescents. *Psychotherapy*, 30(4): 698–9.

Frederick, J. (1991) *Positive Thinking for Mental Health*. London: The Black Mental Health Group.

Freidson, E. (1970) *Profession of Medicine*. New York: Harper and Row.

Freud, S. (1920) Beyond the pleasure principle, in the *Standard Edition of the Complete Psychological Works of Sigmund Freud*, vol. 18. London: Hogarth Press.

Freud, S. (1930) *Civilisation and Its Discontents*. London: Hogarth Press.

Freund, P. (1988) Understanding socialised human nature. *Theory and Society*, 17: 839–64.

Fromm, E. (1942) *Fear of Freedom*. New York: Routledge, Kegan and Paul.

Fromm, E. (1955) *The Sane Society*. New York: Holt, Rinehart and Winston.

Fromm, E. (1970) *The Crisis of Psychoanalysis*. Harmondsworth: Penguin.

Fryer, D. (1995) Labour market disadvantage, deprivation and mental health. *The Psychologist*, 8(6): 265–72.

Furnham, A. (1984) Lay conceptions of neuroticism. *Personality and Individual Difference*, 5(1): 95–103.

Gabe, J. and Bury, M. (1996) Halcion nights: a sociological account. *Sociology*, 30(3): 447–71.

Gabe, J. and Lipshitsz-Phillips, S. (1982) Evil necessity? The meaning of benzodiazepine use for women patients from one general practice. *Sociology of Health and Illness*, 4(2): 201–11.

Gabe, J. and Thorogood, N. (1986) Prescribed drug use and the management of everyday life: the experiences of black and white working class women. *Sociological Review*, 34: 737–72.

Gamarnikow, E. (1978) Sexual division of labour: the case of nursing, in A. Kuhn and A. Wolpe (eds) *Feminism and Materialism: Women and Modes of Production*. London: Routledge and Kegan Paul.

Garfinkel, H. (1956) Conditions of successful degradation ceremonies. *American Journal of Sociology*, 61: 420–4.

Gater, R., Amaddeo, F., Tansella, M., Jackson, G. and Goldberg, D. (1995) A comparison of community based care for schizophrenia in Verona and South Manchester. *British Journal of Psychiatry*, 166: 344–52.

Gelinas, D. (1983) The persisting negative effects of incest. *Psychiatry*, 46: 312–32.

Gerard, D.L. and Houston, L.G. (1953) Family setting and the ecology of schizophrenia. *Psychiatric Quarterly*, 27: 90–101.

Gergen, K. (1985) The social construction movement in modern psychology. *American Psychologist*. 40, 266–75.

Giddens, A. (1984) *The Constitution of Society*. Cambridge: Polity Press.

Giddens, A. (1992) *The Transformation of Intimacy*. Cambridge: Polity Press.

Gilbert, P. (1992) *Depression: The Evolution of Powerlessness*. Hove: Lawrence Erlbaum.

Gilroy, P. (1987) *There Ain't No Black in the Union Jack*. London: Hutchinson.

Ginn, J. and Arber, S. (1995) 'Only connect': gender relations and ageing, in S. Arber and J. Ginn (eds) *Connecting Gender and Ageing: A Sociological Approach*. Buckingham: Open University Press.

Gittens, D. (1998) *Madness in its Place*. London: Routledge.

Godfrey, M. and Wistow, G. (1997) The user perspective on managing for health outcomes: the case of mental health. *Health and Social Care in the Community*, 5(5): 325–32.

Goffman, E. (1961) *Asylums*. Harmondsworth: Penguin.

Goldberg, D. and Huxley, P. (1980) *Mental illness in the Community*. London: Tavistock.

Goldberg, D. and Morrison, S.L. (1963) Schizophrenia and social class. *British Journal of Psychiatry*, 109: 785–802.

Goldberg, D., Sharp, D., Strathdee, G. *et al.* (1993) *Developing a Strategy for a Primary Care Focus for Mental Health Services for the People of Lambeth, Southwark and Lewisham*. London: Institute of Psychiatry.

Goldie, N. (1977) The division of labour among mental health professionals – a negotiated or an imposed order? in M. Stacey and M. Reid (eds) *Health and the Division of Labour*. London: Croom Helm.

Goldie, N., Pilgrim, D. and Rogers, A. (1989) *Community Mental Health Centres: Policy and Practice*. London: Good Practices in Mental Health.

Goldthorpe, J.H. and Marshall, G. (1992) The promising future of class analysis: a response to recent critiques. *Sociology*, 26(3): 381–400.

Goode, W. (1957) Community within a community: the professions. *American Sociological Review*, xx(1), 194–200.

Gorbien, M.J., Bishop, J. and Beers, M.H. (1992) Iatrogenic illness in hospitalised elderly people. *Journal of American Geriatrics Society*, 40: 1031–47.

Gottesman, I.I. and Shields, J. (1972) *Schizophrenia and Genetics*. London: Academic Press.

Gough, I. (1979) *Political Economy of the Welfare State*. London: Macmillan.

Gould, A. (1981) The salaried middle class in the corporist welfare state. *Policy and Politics*, 9(4), 401–8.

Gouldner, A.W. (1979) *The Future of Intellectuals and the Rise of the New Class*. London: Macmillan.

Gove, W. (1970) Societal reaction as an explanation of mental illness: an evaluation. *American Sociological Review*, 35: 873–84.

Gove, W. (1984) Gender differences in mental and physical illness: the effects of fixed roles and nurturant roles. *Social Science and Medicine*, 19(2): 77–91.

Gove, W. and Geerken, M. (1977) Response bias in surveys of mental health: an empirical investigation. *American Journal of Sociology*, 82: 1289–317.

Gove, W.R. (1975) The labelling theory of mental illness: a reply to Scheff. *American Sociological Review*, 40: 242–8.

Greenslade, L. (1992) White skin, white masks: psychological distress among the Irish in Britain, in P. O'Sullivan (ed.) *The Irish in the New Communities*. Leicester: Leicester University Press.

Greenwood, J.D. (1994) *Realism, Identity and Emotion: Reclaiming Social Psychology*. London: Sage.

Guidano, G.F. (1987) *Complexity of the Self*. New York: Guilford Press.

Gunn, J. (1978) *Psychiatric Aspects of Imprisonment*. London: Academic Press.

Haafkens, J., Nijhof, G. and van der Poel, E. (1986) Mental health care and the opposition movement in the Netherlands. *Social Science and Medicine*, 22: 185–92.

Habermas, J. (1972) *Knowledge and Human Interests*. London: Heinemann.

Habermas, J. (1975) *Legitimation Crisis*. Boston: Beacon Press.

Habermas, J. (1981) New social movements. *Telos*, 48: 33–7.

Habermas, J. (1987) *The Philosophical Discourse of Modernity*. Cambridge: Polity Press.

Habermas, J. (1989) The tasks of a critical theory of society, in S.E. Bronner and D.M. Kellner (eds) *Critical Theory and Society: A Reader*. London: Routledge.

Halpern, D. (1993) Minorities and mental health. *Social Science and Medicine*, 36(5): 597–607.

Hamid, W. (1991) Homeless people and community care: an assessment of the needs of homeless people. Unpublished PhD: University of London.

Hammer, M. (1968) Influence of small social networks as factors on mental hospital admission, in S.P. Spitzer and N.K. Denzin (eds) *The Mental Patient*. New York: McGraw-Hill.

Hannay, D. (1979) *The Symptom Iceberg: A Study of Community Health*. London: Routledge.

Hardt, R.H. and Feinhandler, S.J. (1959) Social class and mental hospital prognosis. *American Sociological Review*, 24: 815–21.

Harrison, G., Owens, D., Holton, A. *et al.* (1988) A prospective study of severe mental disorder in Afro-Caribbean patients. *Psychological Medicine*, 11: 289–302.

Harvey, D. (1989) *The Condition of Postmodernity*. Oxford: Basil Blackwell.

Hatfield, B., Huxley, P. and Hadi, M. (1992) Accommodation and employment: a survey into the circumstances and expressed needs of the users of mental health services in a northern town. *British Journal of Social Work*, 22(4): 32–50.

Hayes, J. and Nutman, P. (1981) *Understanding the Unemployed*. London: Tavistock.

Healy, D. (1997) *The Anti-Depressant Era*. London: Harvard University Press.

Hearn, J. (1982) Notes on patriarchy, professionalisation and the semi-professions. *Sociology*, 16(2): 184–202.

Heitman, E. (1996) The public's role in the evaluation of health care technology – the conflict over ECT. *International Journal of Technology Assessment in Health*, 12(4): 657–72.

Hemmenki, E. (1977) Polypharmacy among psychiatric patients. *Acta Psychiatrica Scandinavica*, 56: 347–56.

Hemsi, L. (1967) Psychiatric morbidity of West Indian immigrants. *Social Psychiatry*, 2: 95–100.

Hennelly, R. (1988) Myth making and the major tranquillisers. *Inter-disciplinary Mental Health Worker's Bulletin*, 8: 5–9.

Hensing, G., Alexanderson, K., Allebeck, P. and Bjurulf, P. (1996) Sick leave due to psychiatric disorder. *British Journal of Psychiatry*, 169: 740–6.

Hirsch, S.R. (1986) Clinical treatment of schizophrenia, in P.B. Bradley and S.R. Hirsch (eds) *The Psychopharmacology and Treatment of Schizophrenia*. Oxford: Oxford University Press.

Hirst, P. and Woolley, P. (1982) *Social Relations and Human Attributes*. London: Tavistock.

Hitch, P. (1981) Immigration and mental health: local research and social explanations. *New Community*, 9: 256–62.

Hitch, P. and Clegg, P. (1980) Modes of referral of overseas immigrant and native-born first admissions to psychiatric hospital. *Social Science and Medicine*, 14A: 369–74.

HMSO (1992a) *Health of the Nation*. London: HMSO.

HMSO (1992b) *Report of the Committee of Inquiry into Complaints about Ashworth Hospital*. London: HMSO.

Hochschild, A. (1983) *The Managed Heart: The Commercialisation of Human Feeling*. Berkeley: University of California Press.

Hochstedler-Steury, E. (1991) Specifying 'criminalization' of the mentally disordered misdemeanants. *Journal of Criminal Law and Criminality*, 82 (Summer): 334–59.

Hoenig, J. and Hamilton, M. (1969) *The Desegregation of the Mentally Ill*. London: Routledge and Kegan Paul.

Hoggett, B. (1990) *Mental Health Law*. London: Sweet and Maxwell.

Holland, R. (1978) *Self and Social Context*. London: Macmillan.

Hollander, D. (1991) Homelessness and mental illness in developing countries, in M. Page and R. Powell (eds) *Homelessness and Mental Illness: The Dark Side of Community Care*. London: Concern Publications.

Hollingshead, A. and Redlich, R.C. (1958) *Social Class and Mental Illness*. New York: Wiley.

Horkheimer, M. (1931) Die gegenwartige Lage der Socialphilisophie und die Aufgaben eines Instituts fur sozialforschung. *Frankfurter Universitatsreden*, 37: 13–20.

Horsfall, J. (1997) Psychiatric nursing: epistemological contradictions. *Advances in Nursing Science*, 20(1): 56–65.

Horwitz, A. (1977) The pathways into psychiatric treatment: some differences between men and women. *Journal of Health and Social Behaviour*, 18: 169–78.

Horwitz, A. (1983) *The Social Control of Mental Illness*. New York: Academic Press.

Howells, J.G. and Guirguis, W.R. (1985) *The Family and Schizophrenia*. New York: International Universities Press.

Hughes, E. (1971) *The Sociological Eye: Selected Papers*. Chicago: Aldine Atherton.

Humphrey, M. and Haward, L. (1981) Sex differences in recruitment to clinical psychology. *Bulletin of the British Psychological Society*, 34: 413–14.

Hunt, S. (1990) Emotional distress and bad housing. *Health and Hygiene*, 11: 72–9.

Huxley, P. (1990) *Effective Community Mental Health Services*. Aldershot: Avebury.

Hydle, I. (1993) Abuse and neglect of the elderly – a Nordic perspective. *Scandinavian Journal of Social Medicine*, 2(2): 126–8.

Hyndman, S.J. (1990) Housing, dampness and health among British Bengalis in East London. *Social Science and Medicine*, 30: 131–41.

Illich, I. (1977a) *Limits To Medicine*. Harmondsworth: Penguin.

Illich, I. (1977b) Disabling professions, in I. Illich, I.K. Zola, J. McKnight *et al.* (eds) *Disabling Professions*. London: Marion Boyars.

Illsley, R. (1986) Social class, selection and class differences in relation to stillbirths and infant deaths. *British Medical Journal*, 229: 1520–4.

Ineichen, B. (1987) The mental health of Asians in Britain: a research note. *New Community*, 4: 1–2.

Ingleby, D. (ed.) (1981) *Critical Psychiatry*. Harmondsworth: Penguin.

Ingleby, D. (1983) Mental health and social order, in S. Cohen and A. Scull (eds) *Social Control and the State*. Oxford: Blackwell.

Jacobs, H. (1991) The battle for inpatient care, in M. Page and R. Powell (eds) *Homelessness and Mental Illness: The Dark Side of Community Care*. London: Concern Publications.

Jacoby, R. (1975) *Social Amnesia: A Critique of Contemporary Psychology from Adler to Laing*. Boston: Beacon Press.

Jahoda, M. (1958) *Current Concepts of Positive Mental Health*. New York: Basic Books.

James, A. and Prout, A. (1990) *The Social Construction of Childhood*. London: Routledge.

James, N. (1989) Emotional labour: skill and work in the social regulation of feelings. *Sociological Review*, 37: 15–42.

Jefferys, M. (ed.) (1989) *Growing Old in the Twentieth Century*. London: Routledge.

Jehu, D. (ed.) (1995) *Patients As Victims*. London: Wiley.

Jenkins, J.H. and Karno, M. (1992) The meaning of expressed emotion: theoretical issues raised by cross-national research. *American Journal of Psychiatry*, 149: 9–21.

Jenkins, R., Griffiths, S., Wylie, I. *et al.* (eds) (1994) *The Prevention of Suicide*. London: HMSO.

Jodelet, D. (1991) *Madness and Social Representations*. London: Harvester Wheatsheaf.

Johnson, T. (1977) The professions in the class structure, in R. Scase (ed.) *Industrial Society: Class, Cleavage and Control*. London: George Allen and Unwin.

Johnstone, L. (1993) Family management in 'schizophrenia': its assumptions and contradictions. *Journal of Mental Health*, 2: 255–69.

Jones, A. (1997) High psychiatric morbidity amongst Irish immigrants: an epistemological analysis. Unpublished PhD thesis: Open University.

Jones, G. and Berry, M. (1986) Regional secure units: the emerging picture, in G. Edwards (ed.) *Current Issues in Clinical Psychology*, 4. London: Plenum Press.

Jones, K. (1960) *Mental Health and Social Policy 1845–1959*. London: Routledge and Kegan Paul.

Jones, K. (1962) Review. *Sociological Review*, 8: 343–4.

Jones, L. and Cochrane, R. (1981) Stereotypes of mental illness: a test of the labelling hypothesis, *International Journal of Social Psychiatry*, 27: 99–107.

Jones, R. (1991) *Mental Health Act Manual* (3rd edn). London: Sweet and Maxwell.

Kadushin, C. (1969) *Why Do People Go to Psychiatrists?* New York: Atherton.

Kane, J.M. (1985) Compliance issues in outpatient treatment. *Journal of Clinical Psychopharmacology*, 5: 220–70.

Kaplan, M.S. and Marks, G. (1995) Appraisal of health risks: the roles of masculinity, femininity and sex. *Sociology of Health and Illness*, 17(2): 206–21.

Karon, B.P. and VandenBos, G.R. (1981) *Psychotherapy of Schizophrenia: The Treatment of Choice*. New York: Jason Aronson.

Kay, A. and Legg, C. (1986) *Discharged into the Community*. London: Good Practices in Mental Health.

Kay, D., Beamish, P. and Roth, M. (1964) Old age mental disorders in Newcastle upon Tyne, part 1, a study of prevalence. *British Journal of Psychiatry*, 110: 146–8.

Kaye, C. and Franey, A. (1998) *Managing High Security Psychiatric Care*. London: Jessica Kingsley.

Kazdin, A.E., Stolar, M.J. and Marciano, P.L. (1995) Risk factors for dropping out of treatment among white and black families. *Journal of Family Psychology*, 9(4): 402–17.

Kellam, A.M.P. (1987) The neuroleptic syndrome, so called: a survey of the world literature. *British Journal of Psychiatry*, 150: 752–9.

Kenny, V. (1985) The post-colonial personality. *Crane Bag*, 9: 70–8.

Kitwood, T. (1988) The contribution of psychology to the understanding of senile dementia, in B. Gearing, M. Johnson and T. Heller (eds) *Mental Health Problems in Old Age*. London: Wiley.

Kitwood, T. and Bredin, K. (1992) Towards a theory of dementia care: personhood and well-being. *Ageing and Society*, 10: 177–96.

Klass, A. (1975) *There's Gold in Them Thar Pills*. Harmondsworth: Penguin.

Klassen, D. and O'Connor, W. (1987) Predicting violence in mental patients: cross-validation of an actuarial scale. Paper presented at the annual meeting of the American Public Health Association.

Klatte, E., Liscomb, W., Rozynko, V. and Pught, L. (1969) Changing the legal status of mental hospital patients. *Hospital and Community Psychiatry*, 20: 199–202.

Kleinman, A. (1986) Some uses and misuses of the social sciences in medicine, in D.W. Fiske and R.A. Shweder (eds) *Metatheory and Social Science*. Chicago: Chicago University Press.

Kleinman, A. (1988) *Rethinking Psychiatry*. New York: Free Press.

Kobak, J. (1997) A computer-administered telephone interview to identify mental disorders. *Journal of the American Medical Association*, 278(11): 905–10.

Koffman, J., Fulop, N.J., Pashley, D. and Coleman, K. (1997) Ethnicity and the use of psychiatric beds: a one day survey in North and South Thames regions. *British Journal of Psychiatry*, 171: 238–41.

Kovel, J. (1988) *The Radical Spirit: Essays on Psychoanalysis and Society*. London: Free Association Press.

Krause, I.B. (1989) Sinking heart: a Punjabi communication of distress. *Social Science and Medicine*, 29(4): 563–7.

Kubie, S. (1954) The fundamental nature of the distinction between normality and neurosis. *Psychoanalytical Quarterly*, 23: 167–204.

Lacey, R. (1991) *The MIND Complete Guide to Psychiatric Drugs*. London: Ebury Press.

Laing, R.D. (1959) *The Divided Self*. London: Tavistock.

Laing, R.D. (1967) *The Politics of Experience and the Bird of Paradise*. Harmondsworth: Penguin.

Laing, R.D. and Esterson, A. (1964) *Sanity, Madness and the Family*. Harmondsworth: Penguin.

Langer, T.S. and Michael, S.T. (1963) *Life Stress and Mental Health*. Glencoe: Free Press.

Lapouse, R., Monk, M. and Terris, W. (1956) The drift hypothesis and socioeconomic differentials in schizophrenia. *American Journal of Public Health*, 46: 968–86.

Lasch, C. (1978) *The Culture of Narcissism*. New York: Norton.

Lashmar, P. (1995) Feel bad factor. *New Statesman and Society*, 9 June: 55–7.

Latour, B. (1987) *Science in Action: How to Follow Scientists and Engineers Through Society*. Cambridge MA: Harvard University Press.

Learoyd, B. (1980) Psychotropic drugs and the elderly patient. *Medical Journal of Australia*, 2: 1131–3.

Lebow, J. (1982) Consumer satisfaction with mental health treatment. *Psychological Bulletin*, 91(2): 244–59.

Lees, S. (1997) How lay is lay? Chinese students' perceptions of anorexia nervosa in Hong Kong. *Social Science and Medicine*, 44(4): 491–502.

Lefley, H.P. (ed.) (1996) *Family Caregiving in Mental Illness*. London: Sage.

Lemert, E. (1951) *Social Pathology*. New York: McGraw-Hill.

Lemert, E. (1967) *Human Deviance, Social Problems and Social Control*. Englewood Cliffs: Prentice-Hall.

Lemert, E. (1974) Beyond reach: the social reaction to deviance. *Social Problems*, 21: 457–67.

Lepine, J.P. and Lellouch, J. (1995) Diagnosis and epidemiology of agoraphobia and social phobia. *Clinical Neuropharmacology*, 18(2): 15–26.

Lidz, C., Meisel, A., Zerubavel, E. *et al.* (1984) *Informed Consent: A Study of Decision Making in Psychiatry*. London: Guilford.

Lindow, V. (1994) *Self-help Alternatives to Mental Health Services*. London: MIND Publications.

Link, B. and Phelan, J. (1995) Social conditions as fundamental causes of disease. *Journal of Health and Social Behaviour*, No SISI: 80–94.

Link, B. and Stueve, A. (1998) Editorial. *Archives of General Psychiatry*, 55: 1–3.

Littlewood, R. and Cross, S. (1980) Ethnic minorities and psychiatric services. *Sociology of Health and Illness*, 2: 194–201.

Littlewood, R. and Lipsedge, M. (1982) *Aliens and Alienists*. Harmondsworth: Penguin.

Longo, R. (1982) Sexual learning and experiences among adolescent sexual offenders. *International Journal of Offender Therapy and Comparative Criminology*, 26: 235–41.

Lowenthal, M. (1965) Antecedents of isolation and mental illness in old age. *Archives of General Psychiatry*, 12: 245–54.

Lupton, D. (1998) *The Emotional Self.* London: Sage.

Lynch, D., Tamburrino, M. and Nagel, R. (1997) Telephone counselling for patients with minor depression: preliminary findings in a family practice setting. *Journal of Family Practice*, 44(3): 293–8.

MacDonald, G. and Sheldon, B. (1997) Community care services for the mentally ill: consumers' views. *International Journal of Social Psychiatry*, 43(1): 35–55.

McGovern, D. and Cope, R. (1987) The compulsory detention of males of different ethnic groups with special reference to offender patients. *British Journal of Psychiatry*, 150: 505–12.

McIntyre, K., Farrell, M. and David, A. (1989) What do psychiatric inpatients really want? *British Medical Journal*, 298: 159–60.

Macintyre, S., MacIver, S. and Sooman, A. (1993) Area, class and health: should we be focusing on places or people? *Journal of Social Policy*, 22: 213–34.

MacLachlan, M. (1997) *Culture and Health.* London: Wiley.

Main, T. (1946) The hospital as a therapeutic institution. *Bulletin of the Menniger Clinic*, 10: 66–70.

Maloy, K. (1992) *Critiquing the Empirical Evidence: Does Involuntary Outpatient Commitment Work?* Washington, DC, Mental Health Policy Center.

Mann, A.H., Graham, N. and Ashby, D. (1984) Psychiatric illness in residential homes for the elderly: a survey in one London borough. *Age and Ageing*, 113: 257–65.

Manthorpe, J. (1994) The family and informal care, in N. Malin (ed.) *Implementing Community Care.* Buckingham: Open University Press.

Marcuse, H. (1964) *One Dimensional Man.* London: Routledge and Kegan Paul.

Marshall, R. (1990) The genetics of schizophrenia: axiom or hypothesis? in R.P. Bentall (ed.) *Reconstructing Schizophrenia.* London: Routledge.

Martin, J.P. (1985) *Hospitals in Trouble.* Oxford: Blackwell.

Marzillier, J. and Hall, J. (1987) *What Is Clinical Psychology?* Oxford: Oxford Medical Publications.

Masson, J. (1985) *The Assault on Truth: Freud's Suppression of the Seduction Theory.* Harmondsworth: Penguin.

Masson, J. (1988a) *A Dark Science: Women, Sexuality and Psychiatry in the Nineteenth Century.* New York: Noonday Press.

Masson, J. (1988b) *Against Therapy.* London: HarperCollins.

Masson, J. (1990) *Final Analysis.* London: HarperCollins.

Maule, M., Milne, J. and Williamson, J. (1984) Mental illness and physical health in older people. *Age and Ageing*, 13: 349–56.

Mayall, B. (1998) Towards a sociology of child health. *Sociology of Health and Illness*, 20(3): 269–88.

Mayer, J. and Timms, N. (1970) *The Client Speaks.* London: Routledge and Kegan Paul.

Mayer-Gross, W., Slater, E. and Roth, M. (1954) *Clinical Psychiatry.* London: Cassell.

Mazza, D. and Dennerstein, L. (1996) Psychotropic drug use by women: could violence account for the gender difference? *Journal of Psychosomatic Obstetrics and Gynaecology*, 17(4): 229–34.

Medawar, C. (1992) *Power and Dependence.* London: Social Audit.

Medical Research Council (1989) *Research into Schizophrenia: Report of the Schizophrenia and Allied Conditions Committee to the Neurosciences Board.* London: Medical Research Council.

Mental Health Act Commission (1987) *Second Biennial Report.* London: HMSO.

Mental Health Act Commission (1989) *Third Biennial Report.* London: HMSO.

Mental Health Act Commission (1991) *Fourth Biennial Report*, 1989–1991. London: HMSO.

Mental Health Foundation (1996) *Knowing Our Own Minds.* London: Mental Health Foundation.

Mercer, K. (1986) Racism and transcultural psychiatry, in P. Miller and N. Rose (eds) *The Power of Psychiatry.* Cambridge: Polity Press.

Meyer, J.E. (1988) The fate of the mentally ill in Germany during the Third Reich. *Psychological Medicine,* 18: 575–81.

Mheen, H., Stronks, K. and Mackenbach, J. (1998) A life course perspective on socio-economic inequalities in health. *Sociology of Health and Illness,* 20(5): 754–77.

Miller, P. (1986) Critiques of psychiatry and critical sociologies of madness, in P. Miller and N. Rose (eds) *The Power of Psychiatry.* Cambridge: Polity Press.

Miller, P. and Rose, N. (1988) The Tavistock programme: the government of subjectivity and social life. *Sociology,* 22(2): 171–92.

Milliren, J.W. (1977) Some contingencies affecting the utilisation of tranquillisers in the long term care of the elderly. *Journal of Health and Social Behaviour,* 18: 206–11.

Mills, E. (1962) *Living with Mental Illness.* London: Institute of Community Studies/ Routledge and Kegan Paul.

Mitchell, J. (1974) *Psychoanalysis and Feminism.* Harmondsworth: Penguin.

Mohan, D., Murray, K., Taylor, P. and Stead, P. (1997) Developments in the use of regional secure unit beds over a 12-year period. *Journal of Forensic Psychiatry,* 2: 321–35.

Monahan, J. (1973) The psychiatrization of criminal behaviour: a reply. *Hospital and Community Psychiatry,* 24(2): 105–7.

Monahan, J. (1981) *Predicting Violent Behaviour.* Beverly Hills: Sage.

Monahan, J. (1992) Mental disorder and violent behaviour perceptions and evidence. *American Psychologist,* 47(4): 511–21.

Monahan, J. and Steadman, H.J. (eds) (1994) *Violence and Mental Disorder: Developments in Risk Assessment.* Chicago: Chicago University Press.

Morgan, H.G. (1994) *Suicide Prevention: The Assessment and Management of Suicide Risk.* Anglia University.

Morgan, K. and Gilleard, C. (1981) Patterns of hypnotic prescribing and usage in residential homes for the elderly. *Neuropharmacology Journal,* 20: 1355–6.

Morris, R.G., Morris, L.W. and Britton, P.G. (1988) Factors affecting the emotional well-being of the care-givers of dementia sufferers. *British Journal of Psychiatry,* 152: 147–56.

Mowbray, C.T., Moxley, D.P., Jasper, C.A. and Howell, L.L. (eds) (1997) *Consumers As Providers in Psychiatric Rehabilitation.* Columbia: International Association of Psychosocial Rehabilitation Services.

Murphy, E. (1982) Social origins of depression in old age. *British Journal of Psychiatry,* 141: 135–42.

Murphy, E. (1988) Prevention of depression and suicide, in B. Gearing, M. Johnson and T. Heller (eds) *Mental Health Problems in Old Age.* London: Wiley.

Myers, J. (1974) Social class, life events and psychiatric symptoms: a longitudinal study, in B.S. Dohrenwend and B.P. Dohrenwend (eds) *Stressful Life Events: Their Nature and Effects.* New York: Wiley.

Myers, J. (1975) Life events, social integration and psychiatric symptomatology. *Journal of Health and Social Behavior,* 16: 121–7.

Navarro, V. (1979) *Medicine Under Capitalism.* New York: Prodist.

Nazroo, J. (1995) Uncovering gender differences in the use of marital violence: the effect of methodology. *Sociology,* 29(3): 475–9.

Nazroo, J. (1997) *Ethnicity and Mental Health.* London: Policy Studies Institute.

Nazroo, J. (1998) Genetic, cultural or socio-economic vulnerability? Explaining ethnic inequalities in health. *Sociology of Health and Illness,* 20(5): 710–30.

Nazroo, J.Y., Edwards, A.C. and Brown, G.W. (1998) Gender differences in the prevalence of depression: artefact, alternative disorders, biology or roles? *Sociology of Health and Illness,* 20(3): 3112–330.

Nettleton, S. and Burrows, R. (1998) Mortgage debt, insecure home ownership and health: an exploratory study. *Sociology of Health and Illness,* 20(5): 731–53.

Newnes, C. (1995) A counselling scheme for NHS employees. *Clinical Psychology Forum*, 3(2): 4–7.

Newton, J. (1988) *Preventing Mental Illness*. London: Routledge.

Noble, P. and Rodger, S. (1989) Violence by psychiatric in-patients. *British Journal of Psychiatry*, 155: 384–90.

Norris, M. (1984) *Integration of Special Hospital Patients into the Community*. Aldershot: Gower.

Offe, C. (1984) *Contradictions of the Welfare State*. London: Hutchinson.

Ogg, J. and Bennet, C. (1992) Elder abuse – a national survey. *British Medical Journal*, 305: 998–9.

Olfson, M. and Pincus, H.A. (1994) Use of benzodiazepines in the community. *Archives of Internal Medicine*, 154(11): 1235–40.

Olsen, M. and Pincus, H. (1994) Outpatient psychotherapy in the US patterns of utilization. *American Journal of Psychiatry* 1, 51(9): 1289–94.

O'Mahony, P. and Delanty, G. (1998) *Rethinking Irish History: Nationalism, Identity and Ideology*. Basingstoke: Macmillan.

Onyett, S. (1994) *Community Mental Health Teams*. London: Avebury.

OPCS (1977) *Mortality Statistics*. London: HMSO.

Oppenheimer, M. (1975) The proletarianisation of the professional. *Sociological Review Monograph*, 20.

Orbell, S., Hopkins, N. and Gillies, B. (1993) Measuring the impact of informal care. *Journal of Community and Applied Social Psychology*, 3: 149–63.

Ostamo, A. and Lonnqvist, J. (1992) Parasuicide rates by gender in Helsinki, 1988–91. Poster paper at Joint Conference of the British Sociological Association Medical Sociology Group and the European Society of Medical Sociology, Edinburgh.

Padgett, D.K., Patrick, C., Burns, B.J. and Schlesinger, H.J. (1994) Women and out-patient mental health services: use by black, Hispanic and white women in a nationally insured population. *Journal of Mental Health Administration*, 21(4): 347–60.

Page, M. and Powell, R. (eds) (1991) *Homelessness and Mental Illness: The Dark Side of Community Care*. London: Concern Publications.

Page, S. (1993) Gender and support for mental health research. *Canadian Journal of Psychiatry*, 38(10): 665–70.

Pahl, R.E. (1993) Does class analysis without class theory have a promising future? A reply to Goldthorpe and Marshall. *Sociology*, 27(2): 253–8.

Park, R. (1936) Human ecology. *American Journal of Sociology*, 43: 1–15.

Parker, I., Georgaca, E., Harper, D., McLaughlin, T. and Stowell-Smith, M. (1995) *Deconstructing Psychopathology*. London: Sage.

Parkhouse, J. (1991) *Doctors' Careers: Aims and Experiences of Medical Graduates*. London: Routledge.

Parry, N. and Parry, G. (1977) Professionalism and unionism: aspects of class conflicts in the National Health Service. *Sociological Review*, 25(4): 823–40.

Parsons, T. (1939) The professions and the social structure. *Social Forces*, 17: 457–67.

Parsons, T. (1951) *The Social System*. Glencoe, IL: Free Press.

Paveza, G.J., Cohen, J.G., Eisdorfer, C. *et al.* (1992) Severe family violence and Alzheimer's Disease: prevalence and risk factors. *Gerontologist*, 32(4): 493–7.

Pearson, V. (1995) Goods on which one loses: women and mental health in China. *Social Science and Medicine*, 41(8): 1159–73.

Peay, J. (1989) *Tribunals on Trial: A Study of Decision-making Under the Mental Health Act 1983*. Oxford: Oxford University Press.

Perring, C., Twigg, J. and Atkin, J. (1990) *Families Caring for People Diagnosed as Mentally Ill: The literature re-examined*. London: Social Policy Research Unit.

Perrow, C. (1965) Hospitals: technology, structure and goals, in J.G. March (ed.) *Handbook of Organisations*. Chicago: Rand McNally.

Phillips, D. (1968) Social class and psychological disturbance: the influence of positive and negative experiences. *Social Psychiatry*, 3: 41–6.

Phillipson, C. (1989) Developing a political economy of drugs and older people. *Ageing and Society*, 9: 431–40.

Philo, G., Secker, J., Platt, S. *et al.* (1994) The impact of the mass media on public images of mental illness. *Health Education Journal*, 53: 271–81.

Philo, G., Secker, J., Platt, S. *et al.* (1996) Media images of mental distress in T. Heller *et al.* (eds) *Mental Health Matters: A Reader.* Basingstoke: Macmillan.

Pilgrim, D. (1988) Psychotherapy in special hospitals: a case of failure to thrive. *Free Associations*, 7: 11–26.

Pilgrim, D. (1992) Psychotherapy and political evasions, in W. Dryden and C. Feltham (eds) *Psychotherapy and Its Discontents.* Milton Keynes: Open University Press.

Pilgrim, D. (1996) From discrete inquiries to collective responsibility: some ideas about reducing sexual abuse in therapy. *Clinical Psychology Forum*, 98: 6–8.

Pilgrim, D. (1997a) *Psychotherapy and Society.* London: Sage.

Pilgrim, D. (1997b) Some reflections on 'quality' and 'mental health'. *Journal of Mental Health*, 6(6): 567–76.

Pilgrim, D. (1998) Medical sociology and psychoanalysis: a rejoinder to Lupton. *Sociology of Health and Illness*, 20(4): 537–44.

Pilgrim, D. and May, C. (1998) Social scientists and the British National Health Service. *Social Sciences in Health*, 4(1): 42–54.

Pilgrim, D. and Rogers, A. (1994) Something old, something new . . . sociology and the organisation of psychiatry. *Sociology*, 28(2): 521–38.

Pilgrim, D. and Rogers, A. (1997) A confined agenda? Guest editorial. *Journal of Mental Health*, 6(6): 539–42.

Pilgrim, D., Rogers, A., Clarke, S. and Clark, W. (1997) Entering psychological treatment: decision-making factors for GPs and service users. *Journal of Interprofessional Care*, 11(3): 313–23.

Pilgrim, D. and Treacher, A. (1992) *Clinical Psychology Observed.* London: Routledge.

Pilgrim, D. and Waldron, L. (1998) User involvement in mental health service development: how far can it go? *Journal of Mental Health*, 7(1): 95–104.

Pillemer, K.A. and Finkelhor, D. (1988) The prevalence of elder abuse: a random sample survey. *Gerontologist*, 28: 51–7.

Pitt, B. (1988) Characteristics of depression in the elderly, in B. Gearing, M. Johnson and T. Heller (eds) *Mental Health Problems in Old Age.* London: Wiley.

Platt, S. (1984) Unemployment and suicidal behaviour: a review of the literature. *Social Science and Medicine*, 39: 93–115.

Post, F. (1969) The relationship to physical health of the affective illnesses in the elderly. *Eighth International Congress of Gerontology Proceedings*, Washington, DC.

Potier, M. (1992) *Evidence recorded by the Report of the Committee of Inquiry About Complaints at Ashworth Hospital.* London: HMSO.

Power, C., Matthews, S. and Manor, O. (1996) Inequalities in self-related health in the 1958 birth cohort – lifetime social circumstances or social mobility? *British Medical Journal*, 313: 449–53.

Prentky, R. (1995) A rationale for the treatment of sex offenders: Pro Bono Publico, in J. McGuire (ed.) *What Works: Reducing Offending.* London: Wiley.

Prior, L. (1989) Evaluation research and quality assurance, in J. Gubrium and D. Silverman (eds) *The Politics of Field Research.* London: Sage.

Prior, L. (1991) Mind, body and behaviour: theorisations of madness and the organisation of therapy. *Sociology*, 25(3): 403–22.

Pritchard, J. (1835) *A Treatise on Insanity and Other Disorders Affecting the Mind.* London: Sherwood, Gilbert and Piper.

Rachman, S. (1971) *The Effects of Psychotherapy.* Oxford: Pergamon Press.

Rack, P. (1982) *Race, Culture and Mental Disorder.* London: Tavistock.

Ramon, S. (1983) The Mental Health (Amendment) Act 1982: reform or cosmetics? *Critical Social Policy*, 3(1): 38–53.

Ramon, S. (1985) *Psychiatry In Britain: Meaning and Policy.* London: Gower.

Ramon, S. (1986) The category of psychopathy: its professional and social context in Britain, in P. Miller and N. Rose (eds) *The Power of Psychiatry*. Cambridge: Polity Press.

Ramon, S. (1988) Introduction, in S. Ramon and M.G. Giannichedda (eds) *Psychiatry in Transition: The British and Italian*. Cambridge: Polity Press.

Ranger, C. (1989) Race, culture and 'cannabis psychosis': the role of social factors in the construction of a disease category. *New Community*, 15(3): 357–69.

Raphael, W. (1974) *Just an Ordinary Patient*. London: King Edward's Fund for London.

Regier, D., Boyd, J., Burke, J. *et al.* (1988) Prevalence of mental disorders in the United States. *Archives of General Psychiatry*, 45: 977–85.

Reich, W. (1942) *The Function of the Orgasm*. New York: Noonday Press.

Reich, W. (1933/1975) *The Mass Psychology of Facism*. London: Pelican.

Reiner, R. (1986) *The Politics of the Police*. London: Harvester Wheatsheaf.

Rhodes, A. and Goering, P. (1994) Gender differences in the use of outpatient mental health services. *Journal of Mental Health Administration*, 21(4): 338–46.

Richards, B. (ed.) (1984) *Capitalism and Infancy*. London: Free Associations.

Richards, B. (ed.) (1985) *Capitalism and Infancy*. London: Free Associations.

Rickwood, D.J. and Braithwaite, V.A. (1994) Social psychological factors affecting help seeking for emotional problems. *Social Science and Medicine*, 39(4): 563–72.

Ritzer, G. (1995) *The McDonaldization of Society*. London: Sage.

Ritzer, G. (1997) *The McDonaldization Thesis*. London: Sage.

Rogers, A. (1988) Psychiatric referrals from the police: an investigation of police officers' actions and interactions with psychiatrists. Unpublished PhD thesis: University of Nottingham.

Rogers, A. (1990) Policing mental disorder: controversies, myths and realities. *Social Policy and Administration*, 24(3): 226–37.

Rogers, A. (1993a) Coercion and voluntary admissions: an examination of psychiatric patients' views. *Behavioural Sciences and the Law* (in press).

Rogers, A. (1993b) Police and psychiatrists: a case of professional dominance. *Social Policy and Administration*, 27(1): 33–45.

Rogers, A. and Pilgrim, D. (1989) Citizenship and mental health. *Critical Social Policy*, 26: 25–32.

Rogers, A. and Pilgrim, D. (1991) 'Pulling down churches': accounting for the British mental health users' movement. *Sociology of Health and Illness*, 13(2): 129–48.

Rogers, A. and Pilgrim, D. (1996) *Mental Health Policy in Britain*. London: Macmillan.

Rogers, A. and Pilgrim, D. (1997) The contribution of lay knowledge to the understanding and promotion of mental health. *Journal of Mental Health*, 6(1): 23–35.

Rogers, A., Day, J., Williams, B. *et al.* (1998) The meaning and management of medication: perspectives of patients with a diagnosis of schizophrenia. *Social Science and Medicine*, 47(9): 1313–23.

Rogers, A., Pilgrim, D. and Lacey, R. (1993) *Experiencing Psychiatry: Users' Views of Services*. London: Macmillan.

Rogers, C.M. and Terry, T. (1984) Clinical interventions with boy victims of sexual abuse, in I. Stuart and J. Greer (eds) *Victims of Sexual Aggression*. New York: Van Nostrand Reinhold.

Romme, M. and Escher, S. (1993) *Accepting Voices*. London: Mind.

Rooke-Mathews, S. and Lindow, V. (1997) *A Survivors' Guide to Working in Mental Health Services*. London: Mind/Joseph Rowntree.

Rose, N. (1986) Law, rights and psychiatry, in P. Miller and N. Rose (eds) *The Power of Psychiatry*. Cambridge: Polity Press.

Rose, N. (1990) *Governing the Soul*. London: Routledge.

Rosen, G. (1968) *Madness In Society*. New York: Harper.

Rosen, G. (1979) The evolution of scientific medicine, in H. Freeman, S. Levine and L. Reeder (eds) *Handbook of Medical Sociology*. Englewood Cliffs: Prentice-Hall.

Rosenhan, D.L. (1973) On being sane in insane places. *Science*, 179: 250–8.

Roth, M. (1973) Psychiatry and its critics. *British Journal of Psychiatry*, 122: 174–6.

Rothblum, E.D. (1994) 'I only read about myself on bathroom walls.' The need for research on the mental health of lesbians and gay men. *Journal of Consulting and Clinical Psychology*, 62(2): 213–20.

Rothman, D. (1983) Social control: the uses and abuses of the concept in the history of incarceration, in S. Cohen and A. Scull (eds) *Social Control and the State*. Oxford: Basil Blackwell.

Royal College of Psychiatrists (Scottish Division) (1973) *The Future of Psychiatric Services in Scotland*. London: Royal College of Psychiatrists.

Royal College of Psychiatrists (1995) *The ECT Handbook (Council Report 39)*. London: Royal College of Psychiatrists.

Runciman, W.G. (1990) How many classes are there in contemporary British society? *Sociology*, 24(3): 377–96.

Russell, D. (1983) The incidence and prevalence of intrafamilial sexual abuse of female children. *Child Abuse and Neglect*, 7: 133–45.

Rwegellera, G.G.C. (1977) Psychiatric morbidity among West Africans and West Indians living in London. *Psychological Medicine*, 7: 317–29.

Ryle, A. (1990) *Cognitive-Analytical Therapy: Active Participation in Change*. Chichester: Wiley.

Saks, M. (1983) Removing the blinkers? A critique of recent contributions to the sociology of the professions. *The Sociological Review*, 33: 1–21.

Saks, M. (ed.) (1992) *Alternative Medicine in Britain*. Oxford: Clarendon Press.

Samson, C. (1992) Confusing symbolic events with realities: the case of Community Mental Health in the USA. Paper presented at the BSA Medical Sociology Group and European Society of Medical Sociology, Edinburgh.

Samson, C. (1995) The fracturing of medical dominance in British psychiatry. *Sociology of Health and Illness*, 17(2): 245–68.

Sang, B. (1989) The independent voice of advocacy, in A. Brackx and C. Grimshaw (eds) *Mental Health Care in Crisis*. London: Pluto Press.

Sartre, J.-P. (1963) *Search for a Method*. New York: Knopf.

Sashidharan, S.P. (1986) Ideology and politics in transcultural psychiatry, in J.L. Cox (ed.) *Transcultural Psychiatry*. London: Croom Helm.

Sashidharan, S.P. (1993) AfroCaribbeans and schizophrenia: the ethnic vulnerability hypothesis re-examined. *International Review of Psychiatry*, 5: 129–44.

Sayce, L. (1989) Community Mental Health Centres – rhetoric or reality? in A. Brackx and C. Grimshaw (eds) *Mental Health Care in Crisis*. London: Pluto.

Scambler, A. (1998) Gender, health and the feminist debate on postmodernism, in G. Scambler and P. Higgs (eds) *Modernity, Medicine and Health*. London: Routledge.

Scambler, A., Scambler, G. and Craig, D. (1981) Kinship and friendship networks and women's demand for primary care. *Journal of the Royal College of General Practitioners*, 26: 746–50.

Scheff, T. (1966) *Being Mentally Ill: A Sociological Theory*. Chicago: Aldine.

Scheper-Hughes, N. (1979) *Saints, Scholars and Schizophrenics*. Berkeley: University of California Press.

Schnitzer, P.K. (1996) 'They don't come in' stories told, lessons taught about poor families and therapy. *American Journal of Orthopsychiatry*, 66(4): 572–82.

Schoener, G.R. and Lupker, E.L. (1996) Boundaries in group settings: ethical and practical issues, in B. DeChant (ed.) *Women and Group Psychotherapy*. New York: Guilford Press.

Scott, A. (1990) *Ideology and The New Social Movements*. London: Unwin Hyman.

Scott, R.D. (1973) The treatment barrier, part 1. *British Journal of Medical Psychology*, 46: 45–53.

Scull, A. (1977) *Decarceration: Community Treatment and the Deviant – A Radical View*. Englewood Cliffs, NJ: Prentice-Hall.

Scull, A. (1979) *Museums of Madness*. Harmondsworth: Penguin.

Sedgwick, P. (1982) *Psychopolitics*. London: Pluto Press.

Sennett, R. and Cobb, J. (1973) *The Hidden Injuries of Class*. New York: Knopf.

Shaikh, S. (1985) Cross-cultural comparison: psychiatric admissions of Asian and indigenous patients in Leicestershire. *International Journal of Social Psychiatry*, 31: 3–11.

Shaw, M., Dorling, D. and Brimblecombe, D. (1998) Changing the map: health in Britain 1951–1991. *Sociology of Health and Illness*, 20(5): 694–709.

Sheppard, M. (1990) Social work and psychiatric nursing, in P. Abbott and C. Wallace (eds) *The Sociology of the Caring Professions*. London: Falmer Press.

Sheppard, M. (1991) General practice, social work and mental health sections: the social control of women. *British Journal of Social Work*, 21: 663–83.

Showalter, E. (1987) *The Female Malady*. London: Virago.

Sjostrom, S. (1997) *Party or Patient? Discursive Practices Relating to Coercion in Psychiatric and Legal Settings*. Borea: Spinettstraket.

Slater, P. (1977) *Origin and Significance of the Frankfurt School*. London: Routledge.

Smail, D. (1987) *Taking Care*. London: Dent.

Smail, D. (1996) *Getting By Without Psychotherapy*. London: HarperCollins.

Smaje, C. (1996) The ethnic patterning of health: new directions for theory and research. *Sociology of Health and Illness*, 18(2): 139–71.

Snow, D., Baker, S., Anderson, L. and Martin, M. (1986) The myth of pervasive mental illness amongst the homeless. *Social Problems*, 33: 407–23.

Snowden, J. and Donnelly, M. (1986) A study of depression in nursing homes. *Journal of Psychiatric Research*, 20: 327–33.

Soskis, D.A. (1978) Schizophrenia and medical inpatients as informed drug consumers. *Archives of General Psychiatry*, 35: 645–7.

Spagnoli, A., Foresti, G., MacDonald, A. and Williams, P. (1986) Dementia and depression in Italian geriatric institutions. *International Journal of Geriatric Psychiatry*, 1: 15–23.

Spector, M. and Kitsuse, J. (1977) *Constructing Social Problems*. Menlo Park: Cummings.

Srole, L., Langer, T.S., Michael, S.T. *et al.* (1962) *Mental Health in the Metropolis: The Midtown Manhattan Study*. New York: McGraw-Hill.

Steadman, H.J., Mulvey, E.P., Monahan, J. *et al.* (1998) Violence by people discharged from acute psychiatric inpatient facilities and by others in the same neighbourhoods. *Archives of General Psychiatry*, 55: 393–401.

Stein, J., Golding, J., Seigel, J. *et al.* (1988) Long term psychological sequelae of child sexual abuse: the Los Angeles epidemiologic catchment area study, in G.E. Wyatt and G.J. Powell (eds) *Lasting Effects of Child Sexual Abuse*. New York: Sage.

Stein, L. (1957) 'Social class' gradient in schizophrenia. *British Journal of Preventative and Social Medicine*, 11: 181–95.

Stevenson, P. (1992) *Evidence cited in Report of the Committee of Inquiry into Complaints about Ashworth Hospital*. London: HMSO.

Stone, M. (1985) Shellshock and the psychologists, in W.F. Bynum, R. Porter and M. Shepherd (eds) *The Anatomy of Madness*, Vol. 2. London: Tavistock.

Sweeting, H. and Gillhooly, M. (1997) Dementia and the phenomenon of social death. *Sociology of Health and Illness*, 19(1): 93–117.

Sweeting, H. and West, B. (1995) Family health in adolescence: a role for culture in the health inequalities debate. *Social Science and Medicine*, 40(2): 163–75.

Szasz, T.S. (1961) The uses of naming and the origin of the myth of mental illness. *American Psychologist*, 16: 59–65.

Szasz, T.S. (1963) *Law, Liberty and Psychiatry*. New York: Macmillan.

Szasz, T.S. (1971) *The Manufacture of Madness*. London: Routledge and Kegan Paul.

Szasz, T.S. (1992) Crazy talk: thought disorder or psychiatric arrogance? *British Journal of Medical Psychology*: 65.

Teasdale, K. (1987) Stigma and psychiatric day care. *Journal of Advanced Nursing*, 12: 339–46.

Tietze, C., Lemkau, P. and Cooper, M. (1941) Schizophrenia, manic depressive psychosis and socio-economic status. *American Journal of Sociology*, 47: 167–75.

Toch, H. (1965) *The Social Psychology of Social Movements.* New York: Bobbs Merrill.

Townsend, P. (1981) The structured dependency of the elderly: a creation of social policy in the twentieth century. *Ageing and Society*, 1: 1–28.

Trent, D.R. and Reed, C.A. (eds) (1997) *Promotion of Mental Health.* London: Ashgate.

Tuckett, D. (1976) The organisation of hospitals, in D. Tuckett (ed.) *An Introduction to Medical Sociology.* London: Tavistock.

Turner, B.S. (1987) *Medical Power and Social Knowledge.* London: Sage.

Turner, B.S. (1990) The interdisciplinary curriculum: from social medicine to post-modernism. *Sociology of Health and Illness*, 12(1): 1–23.

Tyrer, P. (1987) Benefits and risks of benzodiazepines. *Proceedings of the Royal Society of Medicine*, 114: 7–11.

Unger, R. (1984) *Passion: An Essay on Personality.* New York: Free Press.

Ussher, J. (1994) Women and madness – a voice in the dark of women's despair. *Feminism and Psychology*, 4(2): 288–92.

Verbrugge, L. and Wingard, M. (1987) Sex differentials in health and mortality. *Women and Health*, 12(2): 103–43.

Wadsworth, D., Butterfield, W.J. and Blaney, R. (1971) *Health and Sickness: The Choice of Treatment.* London: Tavistock.

Waldron, I. (1977) Increased prescribing of Valium, Librium and other drugs – an example of economic and social factors in the practice of medicine. *International Journal of Health Services*, 7: 41.

Walker, A. (1980) The social creation of poverty and dependency in old age. *Journal of Social Policy*, 9: 49–75.

Wallcraft, J. (1996) Some models of asylum and help in times of crisis, in D. Tomlinson and J. Carrier (eds) *Asylum In the Community.* London: Routledge.

Walters, V. (1993) Stress, anxiety and depression – women's accounts of their health problems. *Social Science and Medicine*, 36(4): 393–402.

Warner, R. (1985) *Recovery from Schizophrenia: Psychiatry and Political Economy.* London: Routledge.

Warr, P. (1987) *Work, Unemployment and Mental Health.* Oxford: Oxford University Press.

Watkins, T.R. and Callicutt, J.W. (1997) Self-help and advocacy groups in mental health, in T.R. Watkins and J.W. Callicutt (eds) *Mental Health Policy and Practice.* London: Sage.

Watters, C. (1996) Representations of Asians' mental health in psychiatry, in C. Samson and N. South (eds) *The Social Construction of Social Policy.* London: Macmillan.

Weinberg, S.K. (1960) Social psychological aspects of schizophrenia, in J. Appleby (ed.) *Chronic Schizophrenia.* Glencoe, IL: Free Press.

Weissman, M. and Klerman, G. (1977) Sex differences and the epidemiology of depression. *Archives of General Psychiatry*, 34: 98–111.

Wells, J. (1998) Severe mental illness, statutory supervision and mental health nursing in the United Kingdom: meeting the challenge. *Journal of Advanced Nursing*, 27(4): 698–706.

Wenger, G.C. (1989) Support networks in old age: constructing a typology, in M. Jeffries (ed.) *Growing Old in the Twentieth Century.* London: Routledge.

Westergaard, J. (1992) About and beyond the underclass: some notes on influence of social climate on British sociology today. BSA Presidential Address. *Sociology*, 26: 575–87.

Westermeyer, J. and Kroll, J. (1978) Violence and mental illness in a peasant society: characteristics of violent behaviours and 'folk' use of restraints. *British Journal of Psychiatry*, 133: 529–41.

White, S. (1996) Regulating mental health and motherhood in contemporary welfare services. *Critical Social Policy*, 16: 67–94.

Whitely, J. (1955) 'Down and Out in London' – mental illness in the lower social groups. *The Lancet*, 1: 529–41.

Whitton, A., Warner, R. and Appleby, L. (1996) The pathway to care in post-natal depression: women's attitudes to post-natal depression and its treatment. *British Journal of General Practice*, 46(408): 427–8.

Wilkinson, R.G. (1996) *Unhealthy Societies: The Afflictions of Inequality*. London: Routledge.

Williams, P., Tarnopolosky, A., Hand, D. and Sheperd, M. (1986) Minor psychiatric morbidity and general practice consultations: the West London Survey. *Psychological Medicine Monograph*, Supplement, 9.

Williams, S.J. (1998) Capitalising on emotions? Rethinking the inequalities in health debate. *Sociology*, 32(1): 121–40.

Wing, J.K. (1962) Institutionalism in mental hospitals. *British Journal of Social and Clinical Psychology*, 1: 38–51.

Wing, J. (1978) *Reasoning about Madness*. Oxford: Oxford University Press.

Wing, J.K. and Freudenberg, R.K. (1961) The response of severely ill chronic schizo-phrenic patients to social stimulation. *American Journal of Psychiatry*, 118, 311.

Winnicott, D.W. (1958) *Collected Works*. London: Hogarth Press.

Witz, A. (1990) *Professions and Patriarchy*. London: Routledge.

Woolfe, J. and Tumin, S. (1990) *Prison Disturbances 1990* (The Tumin Report). London: HMSO, Cmnd 1456.

Woolgar, S. and Pawluch, D. (1985) Ontological gerrymandering: the anatomy of social problems' explanations. *Social Problems*, 32: 214–27.

World Health Organization (1979) *Schizophrenia: An International Follow-Up Study*. Chichester: Wiley.

World Health Organization (1986) *Ottawa Charter for Health Promotion*. Ottawa: WHO.

Wrong, D.H. (1961) The oversocialised conception of man in modern sociology. *American Sociological Review*, 26(2): 183–93.

Wyatt, G.E. and Powell, G.J. (eds) (1988) *Lasting Effects of Child Sexual Abuse*. New York: Sage.

Yarrow, M.J., Schwartz, C., Murphy, H. and Deasy, L. (1955) The psychological mean-ing of mental illness. *Journal of Social Issues*, 11: 12–24.

Yates, A. (1970) *Behaviour Therapy*. New York: Wiley.

Index

RESEARCH METHODS IN HEALTH
INVESTIGATING HEALTH AND HEALTH SERVICES

Ann Bowling

- What research methods are used in the investigation of health and health services?
- What are the principles of the research method that should be followed?
- How do I design a research project to describe the topic of interest and to answer cause and effect questions?

This is the first comprehensive guide to research methods in health. It describes the range of methods that can be used to study and evaluate health and health care. Ann Bowling's impressive range and grasp of research methodology are manifest in the simplicity of her style and in the organization of the book. The text is aimed at students and researchers of health and health services, including those in: demography, economics, epidemiology, health management, health policy, health psychology, health sciences, history, medical sociology, medicine, nursing, pharmaceutics and other health care disciplines. It has also been designed for health professionals and policy makers who have responsibility for applying research findings in practice, and who need to know how to judge the value of the research.

Contents
Preface – Section 1: Investigating health services and health: the scope of research – Evaluating health services: multidisciplinary collaboration – Social research on health: sociological and psychological concepts and approaches – Health needs and their assessment: demography and epidemiology – Costing health services: health economics – Section 2: The philosophy, theory and practice of research – The philosophical framework of measurement – The principles of research – Section 3: Quantitative research: sampling and research methods – Sample size for quantitative research – Quantitative research: surveys – Quantitative research: experiments and other analytic methods of investigation – Sample selection and group assignment methods in experiments and other analytic methods – Section 4: The tools of quantitative research – Data collection methods in quantitative research: questionnaires, interviews and their response rates – Questionnaire design – Techniques of survey interviewing – Preparation of quantitative data for coding and analysis – Section 5: Qualitative and combined research methods, and their analysis – Unstructured and structured observational studies – Unstructured interviewing and focus groups – Other methods using both qualitative and quantitative approaches: case studies, consensus methods, action research and document research – Glossary – References – Index.

448pp   0 335 19885 6 (Paperback)   0 335 19886 4 (Hardback)